Y0-IWE-931

CHEMICAL INDUSTRY INSTITUTE OF TOXICOLOGY SERIES

Barrow: Toxicology of the Nasal Passages

Gibson: Formaldehyde Toxicity

Golberg: Structure-Activity Correlation as a Predictive Tool in Toxicology: Fundamentals, Methods, and Applications

Gralla: Scientific Considerations in Monitoring and Evaluating Toxicological Research

Hamm: Complications of Viral and Mycoplasmal Infections in Rodents to Toxicology Research and Testing

Popp: Mouse Liver Neoplasia: Current Perspectives

Rickert: Toxicity of Nitroaromatic Compounds

TOXICOLOGY OF THE NASAL PASSAGES

TOXICOLOGY OF THE NASAL PASSAGES

Edited by

Craig S. Barrow

Chemical Industry Institute of Toxicology

HEMISPHERE PUBLISHING CORPORATION

Washington New York London

DISTRIBUTION OUTSIDE THE UNITED STATES

McGRAW-HILL INTERNATIONAL BOOK COMPANY

Auckland Bogotá Guatemala Hamburg Johannesburg Lisbon
London Madrid Mexico Montreal New Delhi Panama Paris
San Juan São Paulo Singapore Sydney Tokyo Toronto

This book was set in Press Roman by Hemisphere Publishing Corporation. The editors were John Sealine and Allison Brown, the production supervisor was Miriam Gonzalez, and the typesetter was Shirley J. McNett.
Braun-Brumfield, Inc. was printer and binder.

TOXICOLOGY OF THE NASAL PASSAGES

Copyright © 1986 by Hemisphere Publishing Corporation. All rights reserved. Printed in the United States of America. Except as permitted under the United States Copyright Act of 1976, no part of this publication may be reproduced or distributed in any form or by any means, or stored in a data base or retrieval system, without the prior written permission of the publisher.

1 2 3 4 5 6 7 8 9 0 BRBR 8 9 8 7 6 5

Library of Congress Cataloging-in-Publication Data
Main entry under title:

Toxicology of the nasal passages.

(Chemical Industry Institute of Toxicology series)
Based on the Seventh CIIT Conference on Toxicology, held in Raleigh, N.C., Feb. 22–23, 1984.
Includes bibliographies and index.
1. Nose–Diseases–Etiology–Congresses. 2. Nose–Cancer–Etiology–Congresses. 3. Toxicology–Congresses. 4. Toxicity testing–Congresses. I. Barrow, Craig S. II. Chemical Industry Institute of Toxicology. Conference (7th : 1984 : Raleigh, N.C.) III. Series. [DNLM: 1. Nose–congresses. 2. Nose Diseases–chemically induced–congresses. WV 300 T755 1984]

RF342.T68 1986 617'.523 85-17545
ISBN 0-89116-397-2
ISSN 0278-6265

Contents

Contributors

E. D. ACHESON, D.M., F.R.C.P.
Department of Health and Social Security
London, England

M. ÅHLMAN, B.Sc.
Wallenberg Laboratory
Stockholm, Sweden

YVES ALARIE, Ph.D.
University of Pittsburgh
Pittsburgh, Pennsylvania, USA

JOHN E. AMOORE, Ph.D.
Olfacto-Labs
El Cerrito, California, USA

IB ANDERSEN, M.D.
Danish National Institute of Occupational Health
Hellerup, Denmark

CRAIG S. BARROW, Ph.D.
Chemical Industry Institute of Toxicology
Research Triangle Park, North Carolina, USA

ROBERT O. BEAUCHAMP, JR., M.A.
Chemical Industry Institute of Toxicology
Research Triangle Park, North Carolina, USA

EDILBERTO BERMÚDEZ, M.S.
Chemical Industry Institute
of Toxicology
Research Triangle Park,
North Carolina, USA

JAMES A. BOND, Ph.D.
Inhalation Toxicology Research
Institute
Albuquerque, New Mexico, USA

INGVAR BRANDT, Ph.D.
Swedish University of Agricultural
Sciences
Uppsala, Sweden

EVA B. BRITTEBO, Ph.D.
Swedish University of Agricultural
Sciences
Uppsala, Sweden

LORRENE A. BUCKLEY, M.S.
Chemical Industry Institute
of Toxicology
Research Triangle Park,
North Carolina, USA

MERCEDES CASANOVA, B.S., M.S.
Chemical Industry Institute
of Toxicology
Research Triangle Park,
North Carolina, USA

A. CASTONGUAY, Ph.D.
Naylor Dana Institute for Disease
Prevention
Valhalla, New York, USA

JANE C. F. CHANG, Ph.D.
Chemical Industry Institute
of Toxicology
Research Triangle Park,
North Carolina, USA

ALAN R. DAHL, Ph.D.
Inhalation Toxicology Research
Institute
Albuquerque, New Mexico, USA

VICTOR J. FERON, Ph.D.
Netherlands Organization for
Scientific Research
Zeist, The Netherlands

ELIZABETH A. GROSS-BERMÚDEZ,
B.A.
Chemical Industry Institute
of Toxicology
Research Triangle Park,
North Carolina, USA

HENRY d'A. HECK, Ph.D.
Chemical Industry Institute
of Toxicology
Research Triangle Park,
North Carolina, USA

RICHARD A. JAMES, B.A.
Chemical Industry Institute
of Toxicology
Research Triangle Park,
North Carolina, USA

XUE-ZHI JIANG, M.D.
Chemical Industry Institute
of Toxicology
Research Triangle Park,
North Carolina, USA

B. KOWALSKI, Ph.D.
Swedish University of Agricultural
Sciences
Uppsala, Sweden

CHIU-WING LAM, Ph.D.
Chemical Industry Institute of Toxicology
Research Triangle Park, North Carolina, USA

JI ER LUO, M.D.
University of Pittsburgh
Pittsburgh, Pennsylvania, USA

JOSEPH T. MARTIN, EMT (EMSA)
Chemical Industry Institute of Toxicology
Research Triangle Park, North Carolina, USA

MICHAEL J. McKENNA, Ph.D.
Dow Chemical U.S.A.
Midland, Michigan, USA

MICHAEL J. McNULTY, Ph.D.
Chemical Industry Institute of Toxicology
Research Triangle Park, North Carolina, USA

NANCY A. MONTEIRO-RIVIERE, Ph.D.
Chemical Industry Institute of Toxicology
Research Triangle Park, North Carolina, USA

KEVIN T. MORGAN, B.V.Sc., Ph.D.
Chemical Industry Institute of Toxicology
Research Triangle Park, North Carolina, USA

DANIEL L. PATTERSON, B.S.
Chemical Industry Institute of Toxicology
Research Triangle Park, North Carolina, USA

JAMES A. POPP, D.V.M., Ph.D.
Chemical Industry Institute of Toxicology
Research Triangle Park, North Carolina, USA

J. J. RAFTER, Ph.D.
Karolinska Institute
Huddinge, Sweden

JOHN C. RAMSEY, Ph.D.
Dow Chemical U.S.A.
Midland, Michigan, USA

HOLLY W. RANDALL, H.T., A.S.C.P.
Chemical Industry Institute of Toxicology
Research Triangle Park, North Carolina, USA

JAY P. SCHREIDER, Ph.D.
University of California, Davis
Davis, California, USA

B. J. SPIT, B.Sc.
Netherlands Organization for Applied Scientific Research
Zeist, The Netherlands

WILLIAM H. STEINHAGEN, B.S.
Chemical Industry Institute of Toxicology
Research Triangle Park, North Carolina, USA

WILLIAM T. STOTT, Ph.D.
Dow Chemical U.S.A.
Midland, Michigan, USA

JAMES A. SWENBERG, D.V.M., Ph.D.
Chemical Industry Institute of Toxicology
Research Triangle Park, North Carolina, USA

R. A. WOUTERSEN, Ph.D.
Netherlands Organization for Applied Scientific Research
Zeist, The Netherlands

JOHN T. YOUNG, D.V.M., M.S.
Dow Chemical U.S.A.
Freeport, Texas, USA

Preface

The information in this book resulted from the Seventh CIIT Conference on Toxicology entitled Toxicology of the Nasal Passages, which was held in Raleigh, North Carolina, February 22-23, 1984.

In recent years toxicologists have come to clearly recognize the nasal passages as being an important part of the respiratory system, having their own unique anatomy, physiology, and biochemistry. Widespread interest in the nasal passages has undoubtedly stemmed from the occurrence of neoplasms following chronic exposure to various substances. Along these lines, formaldehyde has perhaps received the most notoriety.

The primary motivation in organizing the conference was to review current knowledge concerning the toxicology and carcinogenicity of the nasal passages. Specific objectives were (1) to summarize present knowledge on the anatomy, physiology, and biochemistry of the nasal passages in relation to chemical injury; (2) to assess the relevance of data from experimental animals to human risk estimation; and (3) to identify areas of research that need to be expanded or initiated. Chapters 1-5 discuss comparative anatomy and function; ultra-structure; and histopathology of acute, subacute, and chronic responses of the nasal passages. Chapters 6–11 deal with sensory irritation, effects on the nasal mucociliary apparatus, epidemiology, studies in human volunteers, and effects on olfaction. Chapters 12–18 provide information on absorption of chemicals by the nasal passages, metabolism, genotoxic effects, and cell proliferation. The conference ended with a panel discussion of the research needs and state of knowledge to assess the toxicology of the nasal passages. This serves as a conclusion to the book.

Appreciation is extended to Drs. Henry d'A. Heck and Kevin Morgan for their significant contributions in assisting with the planning of the conference and serving as session chairpersons. Administratively, the conference was under the capable direction of Dr. Donald Hart and Mrs. Ann McCarthy. Final typing of the manuscripts was done by Ms. Joanne Quate and Ms. Linda Smith. Tape recording of the panel discussion was arranged by Mr. Ron Norton.

Craig S. Barrow

TOXICOLOGY OF THE NASAL PASSAGES

Chapter 1

Comparative Anatomy and Function of the Nasal Passages

Jay P. Schreider

GENERAL FUNCTIONS AND ANATOMY

The respiratory system is the portal of entry for a variety of airborne materials and life-giving oxygen. In some animals the nose is the major means of entry for air and airborne substances into the respiratory system. In others the nose is the only means of entry. In addition to the simple conveyance of air to the lungs, the nose has a variety of functions, not all related to respiration.

The nasal cavity is lined with three kinds of epithelium: squamous, ciliated secretory, and olfactory. The vestibule is lined with moderately keratinized stratified squamous epithelium and nasal hairs. The region of the nasal cavity just posterior to the vestibule contains squamous epithelium that gradually gives rise to transitional epithelium with short microvilli. The respiratory or pseudo-

The author thanks Drs. Steven Book and Otto Raabe for their helpful discussions and Charles Baty for his aid in preparing the manuscript. This work was supported by the Office of Health and Environmental Research of the U.S. Department of Energy under contract DE-AM03-76SF00472 with the University of California, Davis.

stratified column epithelium begins near the anterior portion of the turbinates (1). The respiratory region contains ciliated columnar cells and mucus-secreting goblet cells. The region also contains serous submucosal cells. The surface of the epithelium is coated with airway secretions, with a periciliary serous layer (which is necessary for ciliary action) covered by a mucous layer (which entraps and carries deposited materials). The submucosa of this region contains extensive vasculature (2). The olfactory epithelium, located generally in the more posterior portions of the nasal cavity, is less vascularized and contains neither goblet nor ciliated cells; however, it does contain serous secreting Bowman's glands. The olfactory receptor cells contain cilia, which serve to increase the surface area of the cells for the adsorption of odiferous particles to the receptor membranes (3, 4). The paranasal sinuses, depending on the species, may contain either respiratory epithelium (though with less vasculature and fewer goblet cells or secretory glands than the respiratory epithelium in the nasal cavity proper) or olfactory epithelium. In the nasopharynx there is a transition from ciliated secretory to squamous epithelium (3). The transition from one epithelial type to another is not abrupt. The extent, distribution, and specific type of epithelial cells vary with different species, depending on the activities in which they engage and the environmental conditions under which they live.

Olfaction is perhaps the main function associated with the nose, with the uses of olfaction varying somewhat from species to species. Olfaction is used for the recognition of surroundings and territory, recognition of members of the same species for both sexual and nonsexual purposes, and for warning of changes in the environment (e.g., smoke warning of fire). Some animals use smell in an indirect way, such as the skunk using it to repel enemies. The prime use of olfaction, however, is in the acquisition of food. Herbivores use smell to locate and distinguish prey. Both herbivores and carnivores utilize smell to recognize and elude other carnivores. Olfactory impulses also activate gastric activity in preparation for digestion (3).

The extent and distribution of olfactory epithelium and of accessory tissues and structures vary with the degree to which a species utilizes olfaction. In arboreal environments, odors do not remain as they do on the ground; hence, the sense of smell loses much of its usefulness and is replaced by increased visual abilities (3). As a result, arboreal and arboreal-derived species use sight to the suppression of smell, with a decrease in olfactory abilities accompanied by a decrease in olfactory structure. In microsmatic man there are approximately 10–12.5 cm^2 of olfactory epithelium, whereas in the macrosmatic rabbit and cat there are 7.4 and 20.8 cm^2 of olfactory epithelium, respectively, with the olfactory epithelium invading the sinuses in some carnivorous species. The ethmoturbinates, upon which the olfactory epithelium lies, are also more extensive in macrosmatic species. The cribriform plate, through which the nerves from the olfactory epithelium pass to the olfactory bulb of the brain, is proportional to the extent of the olfactory epithelium, again being large in macrosmatic species and relatively small in microsmatic species (3). While olfactory acuity decreases with the decrease in olfactory structures, discriminatory abilities seem to be relatively unaffected and, in fact, seem to be partially learned, as would be attested to by any wine connoisseur.

The conveyance of odiferous particles to the olfactory epithelium is accomplished by a number of means. The particles may be carried on mucus by ciliary action to the more anterior olfactory epithelium. Odiferous material may reach the more posterior or recessed olfactory epithelium by diffusion. Perhaps the most important means is by carriage in the respiratory air currents. More forceful inhalation or sniffing carries material to the more posterior epithelium. The currents may be further modified or directed by structures such as the nostrils and swell bodies.

Conditioning of the inspired air by the respiratory epithelium is another major function of the nose. Proper functioning of the olfactory tissues is dependent upon sufficient humidity of the air, with drying of the air leading to diminished olfactory abilities (3). Mammals with relatively extensive olfactory tissues also have extensive respiratory epithelium. Humidification is also necessary for efficient respiration, since moistness of the epithelial tissue lining the alveoli of the lungs enables the exchange of carbon dioxide and oxygen to take place. The relatively small turbinates of man are sufficient for the purposes of humidification for respiration (2), with humidification also occurring in the airways of the lungs. Humidification of the nasal air is essential for proper ciliary action to take place (3). As the inspired air moves through the nasal passages, it takes up moisture and heat from the mucosa, with a concomitant cooling of the mucosa. During exhalation the air passes back over the cooled mucosa and gives up heat to the mucosa with a concomitant cooling of the air. This cooling of the expired air causes a condensation of water vapor and a return of moisture to the mucosa. If the condensation is great enough, resulting from severe chilling of the nasal mucosa, a dripping nose will result (5).

In most animal species there is a close apposition between the epiglottis and the soft palate. As a result, there is normally no direct communication between the mouth and the nasal air passages. When the mouth is open, such as during fighting or feeding, the inspired air continues to pass through the nose, thus maintaining olfactory abilities. This separation is not maintained during panting or phonation (6). Negus (3) considers the maintenance of olfactory abilities during open-mouth conditions important enough that he refers to the epiglottis as an "accessory organ of olfaction." In man and the higher primates, a wide gap exists between the epiglottis and the soft palate, so that when the mouth is open there is a direct communication between the mouth and nasal airways, with oral respiration resulting. In infants, however, there is a closer apposition, with infants being obligate nose breathers (6). The tendency toward nasal breathing persists in adults, with oral or oronasal breathing taking place when the pulmonary ventilation requirements become sufficiently high that it becomes advantageous to supplement nasal breathing with oral breathing.

Another important function of the nose is its filtering action, which, while serving to protect the lungs from potentially harmful particles or gases, may as a consequence expose the tissues of the nose to the same potentially toxic materials. The role of the nose in infection and disease also seems to be somewhat paradoxical. On the one hand, the nose serves as a reservoir for various infectious agents such as staphylococcus (7), but it also serves to protect the lower respiratory airways from infectious agents. Infectious agents may be cleared from the nasal airways or may be inactivated by the immunological defenses found in the nasal airways. Immunoglobulin A (IgA), for example, forms 50 percent of the protein in the nasal secretions and is produced 80-90 percent locally (8).

ANATOMICAL METHODS

Exposures of laboratory animals such as rats, guinea pigs, dogs, and monkeys are commonly used in inhalation toxicology research as surrogates for human exposures. The toxicity of an inhaled substance depends partially on the extent and loci of deposition in the respiratory tract. Deposition, in turn, depends on particle characteristics, on physical characteristics of the airways, and on kinetics of the airflow in the airways. Differences in deposition characteristics between animals and man will influence extrapolation of toxicity results from these animals to man. An accurate knowledge of the anatomy of the nasal airways is useful for the interpretation of data from exposure studies and for the extrapolation of data found with experimental animals.

A number of methods are used for studying the anatomy of the nasal airways. Gross dissection and measurement have been used to provide a picture of the airways of man (9) and various laboratory animals (10-13). Greater detail is added through the use of transverse serial sections, which have been used in fairly complete studies of small animals: rat (14), European insectivores (15), and hamster (16). Computed tomography has been used to generate coronal tomograms of human cadavers (17). Replica casts have been an important tool for studies of the anatomy of the air passages. A number of methods have been used by investigators to produce casts of excised lungs and in some cases the nasal regions: dog (18-20), cat (21), human (22, 23).

Schreider and Hutchens (24) prepared epoxy casts of the nasal regions and excised lungs of the guinea pig. As part of this same study (25), positive casts or molds of the nasal cavities of guinea pigs and rats were prepared. A metal cast of the nasal cavity was first prepared. The casting compound was Cerrolow-117 (Christy Metals, Northfield, IL), an alloy melting at 47°C. The animals were pretreated with an aerosol of atropine sulfate to reduce the amount of mucus in the nose. Following sacrifice, the esophagus was tied off, the head removed, and the mouth and ears sealed with epoxy resin, to prevent the escape of casting material. The nasal cavity was rinsed with saline (by way of a tracheal cannula), and the head placed in a vacuum oven for 2 h at 60°C and -30 lbs/in^2, thus drying out mucus remaining in the nose and warming the head to a temperature above the melting point of the alloy. A small piece of acrylic tube was glued over the nostrils, serving as a reservoir for the molten alloy. Molten alloy was injected into the nasal cavity through the tracheal cannula. Following injection the head was replaced in the vacuum oven, and the head was allowed to cool slowly under negative pressure. Following cooling, the alloy in the reservoir was removed, excess tissue trimmed from the head, and the remaining tissue digested by placing the head in concentrated potassium hydroxide. One side of the cast was removed at the junction with the nasopharynx. The case was encased in casting acrylic and the metal melted out, leaving a mold of the nasal cavity.

Phalen et al. (26) produced in situ silicone rubber castings of the lungs of hamsters, rats, monkeys, beagles, and humans. It is useful to cast the airways as a single unit, with the casting of the nasal, tracheobronchial, and pulmonary regions from one animal at the same time, eliminating scaling problems and establishing the spatial arrangement of the regions of the respiratory airways. Schreider and Raabe (27, 28) prepared silicone rubber casts of the respiratory airways of rats (Sprague-Dawley), beagles, and monkeys (rhesus monkeys), using a method modified from Phalen et al. (26). Following sacrifice of the animal to be cast, the trachea was cannulated in two places below the larynx. The lungs were ventilated with carbon dioxide through the lower cannula. The lungs were then perfused with saline, which passed through the permeable lung tissue and out slits cut in the chest wall. A predetermined amount of silastic molding compound (Silastic E, Dow Corning, Midland, MI) was slowly pumped into the lungs. While the silastic was being introduced into the lungs, the esophagus was tied shut as close as possible to the larynx and the mouth was taped shut to prevent the casting material from exiting the mouth and bypassing the nasal cavity. The nasal region was washed with saline introduced through the upper cannula to remove blood or mucus that might interfere with casting. The region was partially dried by blowing air through the cavity. Silastic was injected through the cannula until clean material emerged from the nares. Following injection, the cannulas were clamped and the head and body positioned in a normal posture while the silastic cured overnight. Following curing, the tissues surrounding the cast airways were removed and digested in potassium hydroxide, leaving a separate cast of the lungs and nasal airways.

COMPARATIVE ANATOMY

In Fig. 1 the upper and lower airway casts have been joined by a piece of tubing, illustrating the positions of the nasal cavity in relation to the remainder of the respiratory tract. The differences in the bends of the nasopharynx are clearly

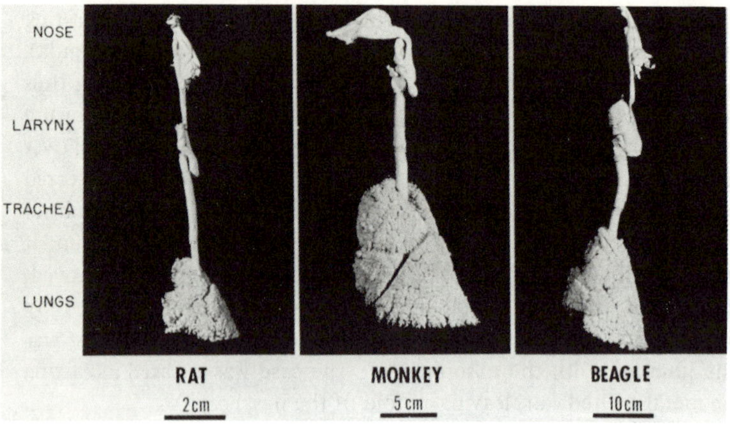

Figure 1 Silicone rubber casts of the entire respiratory airway of a rat, monkey, and beagle. [*From Chem-Orbital; Schreider and Raabe (27).*]

demonstrated and are related to the differences in the posture of the different animals. Figure 2 shows casts of the nasal regions alone. To avoid confusion when comparing these casts with diagrams of sections of the nasal cavity, it should be kept in mind that the casts delineate the airways, and the diagrams usually illustrate the tissue, one being a "negative" of the other. In general, the air inhaled by laboratory animals such as dogs and rats tends to follow a path in which the airstreams are confined to the upper one-half of the nasal passage, whereas the airstream in monkeys and man tends to be confined to the lower two-thirds of the nasal cavity (2).

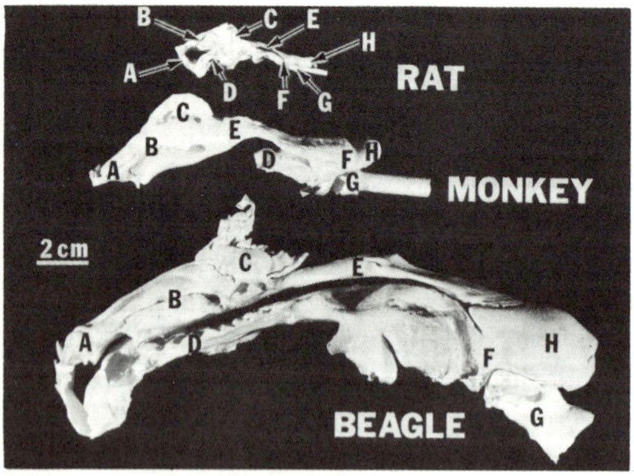

Figure 2 Silicone rubber casts of the nasal-pharyngeal airway of the rat, the rhesus monkey, and the beagle. (A) External nares; (B) maxilloturbinate region; (C) ethmoturbinate region; (D) mouth and oropharynx; (E) nasopharynx; (F) larynx; (G) trachea; (H) esophagus. [*From Schreider and Raabe (26).*]

The flexible nature of the rubber molding compound allowed the more complex parts of the casts to be unfolded and the internal portions to be examined and measured. Linear dimensions and angles were measured using a linear micrometer ocular on a dissecting microscope, an optical comparator, and, for the largest structures, a caliper. The volumes of the nasal cavities (excluding the nasopharynx) were estimated by measuring the volume of water displaced by the casts.

Following gross examination, serial cross sections were made of the most complete cast of each species (28, 29), including the previously mentioned epoxy cast of the guinea pig nasal cavity. Each of these cross sections was made in a plane perpendicular to what was estimated to be the primary local airflow direction. In all cases, cross sections were made of the right side of the cast until the two sides joined together to form a single unit, after which the cross sections were made of the entire cast. The two sides of the nose were treated as mirror images. This method of sectioning allowed each section to be seen in relation to the nasal region as a whole. In some cases, it was necessary to support the casts in an epoxy or paraffin matrix prior to sectioning, maintaining the positions of the side pockets.

Duplicate tracings were made of each of the cross sections for the dog and monkey. The small size of the rat and the guinea pig casts precluded tracing or imprinting. The cross sections were placed on finely ruled graph paper and examined under a dissecting microscope equipped with a linear micrometer ocular, and enlarged (5X) drawings were made of the sections. An image-analyzing computer was used to measure the perimeter and area of the diagram of each cross section. When a section was cut from the right half of the nasal cast, the perimeter and cross-sectional area of both the right and left sides of the nose at that point were estimated by doubling the values for the right side.

A shortcoming of studies of this type involving detailed dissection and measurement of replica airway casts is that it is practical to sufficiently evaluate only a few casts to be used as the basis for a model of the airways. While the procedure for producing replica casts is fairly straightforward, morphometric measurements can be complex and tedious. Practicality limited the number of specimens that were fully evaluated. Hence, only one representative cast for each species was chosen for detailed measurements.

While sections were made from only the right sides of the nasal casts when the two sides were separate, the left sides are drawn as mirror images for clarity in the diagrams of the cross sections (rat in Fig. 3, guinea pig in Fig. 4, beagle in Fig. 5, and rhesus monkey in Fig. 6). The diagrams of each section are numbered correspondingly for reference in both the figures and Tables 1-4 (rat, guinea pig, beagle, and monkey, respectively), which give the distance from the anterior end of the nose to the location of each section, the perimeter of the section, and the cross-sectional area of the section. The nasal-pharyngeal airway can be divided into the regions of the nares, maxilloturbinates, ethmo-

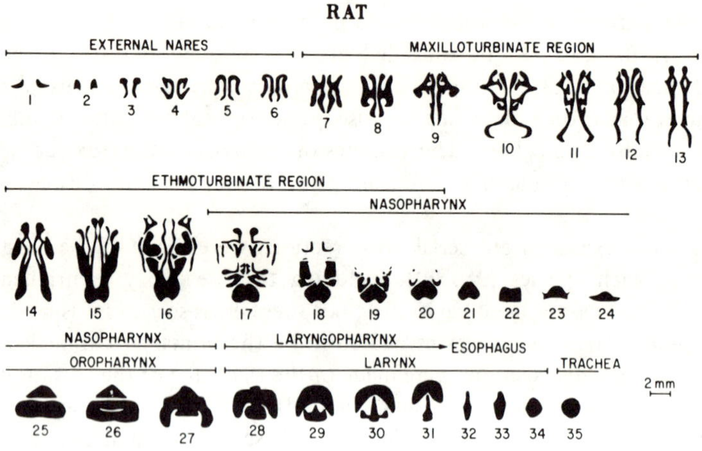

Figure 3 Cross sections of a cast of the nasal-pharyngeal airway of the rat. The numbers under each diagram correspond to the values in Table 1. [*From Schreider and Raabe (26).*]

turbinates, pharynx (including nasopharynx, oropharynx, epiglottis, and laryngopharynx), and larynx; however, the boundaries are not distinct and the regions may overlap.

The cast of the rat (Sprague-Dawley) was from a 250-g animal. The external naris is 0.5 cm long and encompasses sections 1-6 (Fig. 3). The naris makes a

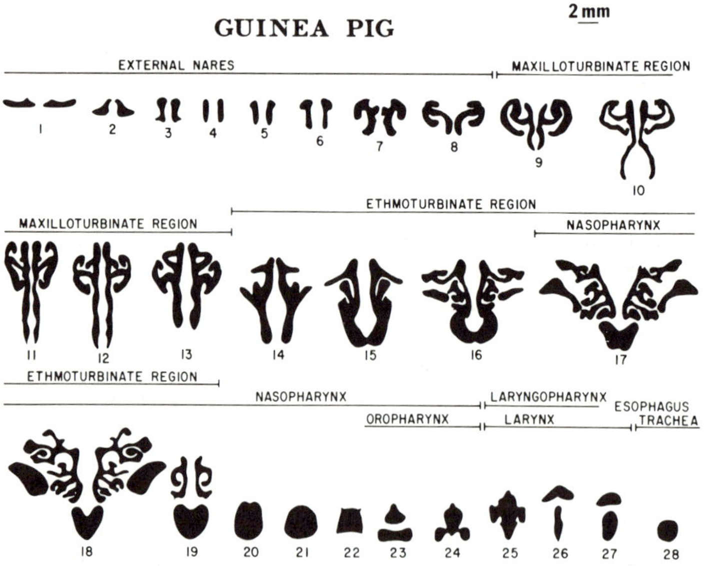

Figure 4 Cross sections of a cast of the nasal-pharyngeal airway of the guinea pig. The numbers under each diagram correspond to the values in Table 2. [*From Schreider (29).*]

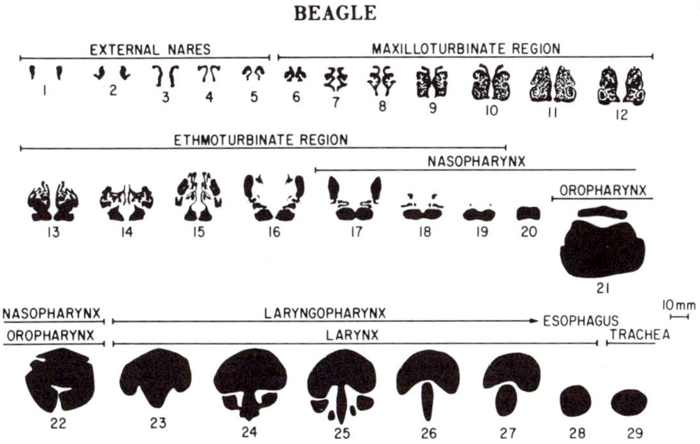

Figure 5 Cross sections of a cast of the nasal-pharyngeal airway of the beagle. The numbers under each diagram correspond to the values in Table 3. [*From Schreider and Raabe (26).*]

40° horizontal bend in sections 4 and 5. This bend brings the two sides of the nose closer together. In sections 4, 5, and 6, the nares become more platelike and folded. In the maxilloturbinates (sections 7-13) the airways become quite tortuous, forming a double scroll. This region of respiratory epithelium has a relatively large surface area, increasing the efficiency of humidification, absorption of gases, and filtration of particles. The ethmoturbinate region is made up of sections 14-20, with the olfactory epithelium in the superior portions. In

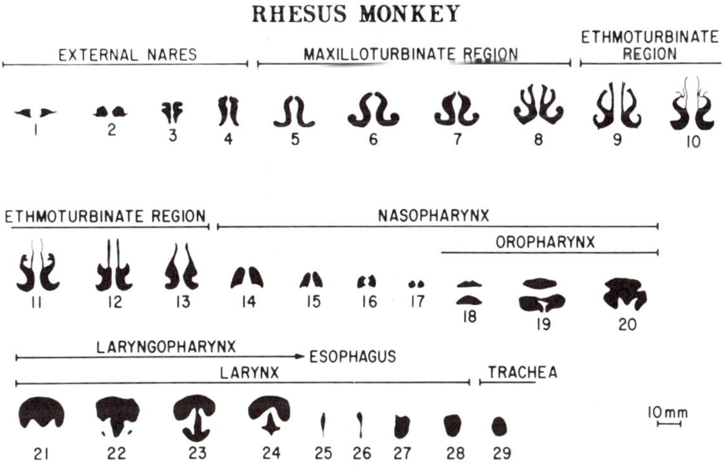

Figure 6 Cross sections of a cast of the nasal-pharyngeal airway of the rhesus monkey. The numbers under each diagram correspond to the values in Table 4. [*From Schreider and Raabe (26).*]

Table 1 Dimensions of the Cross Sections of the Nasal Cast of the Rat

Section number	Distance from anterior end of nose (mm)	Perimeter (mm)	Area (mm^2)
1	0	8.3	1.4
2	1	5.6	1.3
3	2	11.9	2.0
4	3	21.7	3.5
5	4	23.4	3.8
6	5	27.3	4.5
7	5.5	35.0	7.6
8	7	38.3	9.9
9	8	44.0	9.3
10	10	73.9	13.2
11	12	63.5	10.3
12	14	54.4	10.3
13	16	48.3	8.1
14	17	67.6	16.7
14*	17	57.8	13.0
15	18	58.4	21.7
16	19	104.1	25.8
16*	19	47.5	14.0
17	20	97.8	17.0
17*	20	9.0	5.0
18	21	44.5	12.5
18*	21	9.0	5.0
19	22	30.9	7.7
19*	22	8.5	4.2
20	23	17.4	5.9
20*	23	8.9	4.9
21	25	7.5	3.6
22	32	7.9	3.7
23	35	8.6	2.8
24	37	7.7	2.2
25	40	8.4	3.4
26	41	8.7	3.4
27	42	23.7	15.8
28	43	24.2	14.9
29	44	9.2	3.2
30	44.5	12.8	3.2
31	45	7.6	1.8
32	45.5	7.4	1.9
33	46	7.8	3.1
34	47	6.5	3.0
35	52	7.1	3.8

*Main airway alone. Does not include separate pockets. [*From Schreider and Raabe* (28).]

Table 2 Dimensions of the Cross Sections of the Nasal Cast of the Guinea Pig

Section number	Distance from anterior end of nose (mm)	Perimeter (mm)	Area (mm^2)
1	0	18.0	5.0
2	1	14.0	4.4
3	2	15.3	4.9
4	2.5	12.4	3.6
5	3	13.9	4.2
6	3.5	18.5	5.4
7	4	32.9	13.0
8	5.0	19.8	13.4
9	8	66.4	20.4
10	11	88.0	21.5
11	16	91.5	28.6
12	18	91.2	31.1
13	20	82.0	36.2
14	22	62.7	30.1
15	24	75.1	38.1
16	26	109.4	44.4
16*	26	94.3	39.2
17	28	153.5	58.1
17*	28	14.9	11.2
18	31	184.6	73.4
18*	31	14.5	10.8
19	34	14.2	13.3
19*	34	8.2	11.7
20	39	13.9	13.7
21	45	13.2	31.2
22	50	12.0	8.1
23	55	8.0	4.1
24	56	18.9	8.8
25	57	20.7	12.7
26	59	8.9	2.8
27	62	9.1	5.1
28	70	8.6	5.7

*Main airway alone. Does not include side pockets. [*From Schreider* (29).]

sections 14 and 15, the two sides of the nose make 10° inward bends and join together to form a single unit. The ethmoturbinate region is made up of both a scrolled main structure and a number of air pockets: the beginnings of the largest pocket, the maxillary recess, can be seen in section 14.

The overlapping of regions is evident in sections 17-20. The volume of the nasal cavity from nares to, but not including, the nasopharynx is 0.4 cm^3. The nasopharynx begins in section 17, but the pockets of the ethmoturbinate region

Table 3 Dimensions of the Cross Sections of the Nasal Cast of the Beagle

Section number	Distance from anterior end of nose (mm)	Perimeter (mm)	Area (mm^2)
1	0	44.0	33.3
2	5	50.3	42.3
3	10	72.5	44.8
4	15	66.5	32.0
5	20	63.8	37.6
6	25	70.1	49.6
7	30	106.3	75.9
8	35	143.4	95.5
9	40	294.8	155.0
10	43	503.0	205.8
11	50	674.3	228.4
11*	50	665.6	227.3
12	55	470.6	267.3
13	60	333.9	312.5
14	65	318.8	240.9
14*	65	64.3	91.2
15	70	424.1	277.5
15*	70	55.1	68.0
16	75	266.8	289.5
16*	75	109.1	143.8
17	80	200.9	272.5
17*	80	54.5	113.9
18	90	121.5	138.3
18*	90	52.6	105.3
19	100	44.4	95.2
19*	100	35.6	92.6
20	120	39.3	88.8
21	150	64.0	139.1
22	160	184.5	1022.5
23	170	131.0	871.3
24	180	210.0	1055.4
25	185	250.9	933.6
25*	185	53.1	89.1
26	190	50.8	112.6
27	195	50.6	175.4
28	205	57.5	251.3
29	275	57.0	237.1

*Main airway alone. Does not include separate pockets. [*From Schreider and Raabe (28).*]

Table 4 Dimensions of the Cross Sections of the Nasal Cast of the Rhesus Monkey

Section number	Distance from anterior end of nose (mm)	Perimeter (mm)	Area (mm^2)
1	0	45.8	55.6
2	3	43.3	51.0
3	8	62.3	61.0
4	13	73.8	86.2
5	18	95.6	105.6
6	23	119.3	161.1
7	25	121.0	155.0
8	28	169.1	180.8
9	33	192.9	165.6
10	38	211.8	165.3
11	40	171.8	164.1
12	43	143.4	161.7
13	48	116.1	152.6
14	53	58.5	91.5
15	58	45.0	53.2
16	63	37.9	38.0
17	68	24.0	18.8
18	73	20.0	27.3
19	78	37.9	66.0
20	80	86.5	224.9
21	83	73.6	253.1
22	88	90.5	263.0
22*	88	75.4	256.4
23	90	118.8	257.3
24	93	34.1	43.8
25	95	27.6	15.8
26	08	29.5	18.2
27	103	35.0	72.0
28	105	33.3	75.4
29	110	27.9	56.1

*Main airway alone. Does not include separate pockets. [*From Schreider and Raabe (28).*]

are still present. The nasopharynx makes a gradual downward bend of 15° in sections 22–24. The openings of the eustachian tubes can be seen in section 23. The oropharynx begins in section 25. The perimeters and cross-sectional areas of the separated sections of the oropharynx are not included in the values given in Table 1. In section 27 the nasopharynx and oropharynx join and cross in the pharyngeal isthmus. The airway makes a dorsal-ventral bend of 45° in section 27. In the upper portion of section 28, the oropharynx gives rise to the laryngopharynx. The epiglottis is found between sections 27 and 28. Since the epiglottis is in a middle position (because of casting material), the laryngopharynx forms a common chamber with the larynx. In section 29 the two passages have separated, with the larynx on the bottom and the laryngopharynx on the top (eventually giving rise on the esophagus). The side pockets on the larynx in sections 29 and 30 are the laryngeal ventricles. The larynx makes a reverse ventral-dorsal bend of 45° in sections 30 and 31. The larynx gradually assumes a rounded shape, giving rise to the trachea around section 35.

The cast of the guinea pig that was used for the generation of the cross sections was from a 600-g animal. The external naris is 0.5 cm long and encompasses sections 1-8 (Fig. 4). The naris makes an approximately 40° horizontal bend in sections 5-8. The maxilloturbinate region is made up of sections 9-13 and assumes a double scrolled structure. As with the rat, this region is also relatively extensive. The ethmoturbinate region is made up of sections 15-19 with the olfactory epithelium in the more superior areas. In section 19 the two sides of the nose join to form a single unit. As with the rat, this region is made up of both a scrolled main portion and various side pockets. Portions of the maxillary sinus or recess can be seen in sections 16-18. The volume of the nasal cavity from the nares to the beginning of the nasopharynx is 0.88 cm^3. The nasopharynx runs from section 17 to section 24. The nasopharynx makes a gradual 30° downward bend in sections 21-23. The openings of the eustachean tubes are seen in section 22. The oropharynx is seen in section 23. In section 24 the oropharynx and nasopharynx join in the pharyngeal isthmus. Between sections 23 and 24, there is a 45° downward bend in the airway. In the upper portion of section 25, the oropharynx gives rise to the laryngopharynx. The epiglottis is found between sections 24 and 25. In section 26 the two portions have separated into the laryngopharynx (top) and the larynx (bottom). The larynx is at its narrowest point in section 26. The larynx makes a reverse ventral-dorsal bend in section 27. By section 28 the airway has rounded to form the trachea.

The most complete cast of the beagle nasal passage was from a 10-kg animal. The external naris is made up of sections 1-5 (Fig. 5). The bend of the naris is 30° and takes place in sections 3 and 4. The maxilloturbinate region is made up of sections 6-12. The region is quite membranous and complex, forming a branched structure with an extensive surface area for effective humidification, gas absorption, and particle filtration. The ethmoturbinate region runs from sections 13-19. There are folded membranous portions of the airway (though less complex than the maxilloturbinates) with a large surface area available for olfaction. The maxillary sinuses begin in section 13, continue to a point between sections 13 and 14, and contain respiratory epithelium. Portions of the frontal sinuses begin in section 14, continue through section 18, and are extensively invaded by olfactory epithelium. The sphenoid sinuses begin in section 15, continue through section 20, and are also extensively invaded by respiratory epithelium. In section 17 the two sides of the nose join and form the nasopharynx. The volume of the nasal cavity from nares to nasopharynx was 20 cm^3.

The pockets end by section 19. In sections 19 and 20 there is a gradual 30° dorsal-to-ventral bend in the nasopharynx. The nasopharynx flattens in section 21. The oropharynx may also be seen in section 21. In section 22 the two passages cross in the pharyngeal isthmus. In this section the nasopharynx takes a 50° dorsal-to-ventral bend, and the oropharynx gives rise to the laryngopharynx. The epiglottis is between sections 22 and 23. The laryngeal ventricles can be seen in section 24. In section 25 the posterior portions of these ventricles are seen as distinct pockets. The larynx is at its narrowest state in this section and makes a reverse ventral-to-dorsal bend of 50°. By section 26 the larynx has separated from the laryngopharynx. The trachea, which begins at section 29, undergoes a gradual 30° dorsal-to-ventral bend over the anterior half of the trachea.

In the rhesus monkey (7 kg) the external naris is 1.3 cm long and is made up of sections 1–4 (Fig. 6). The horizonal bend of the naris in sections 2 and 3 is 30°. The maxilloturbinate region is composed of sections 5-8. This region develops from a single chamber into three connected, flattened chambers with a fairly simple scroll shape, with relatively larger, less membranous air passages and relatively less respiratory epithelium, suggesting less efficient humidification, gas absorption, and particle filtration. In the ethmoturbinate region (sections 9-13), portions of the chambers narrow to a more membranous form, with the olfactory epithelium in the superior area. The volume of the nasal cavity from nares to nasopharynx is 8 cm^3. Section 14 marks the beginning of the nasopharynx, which continues as two separate airways. The two sides of the nose join to form a single unit between sections 17 and 18 and flatten after joining. The nasopharynx makes an 80° dorsal-to-ventral bend in sections 16-18. The bottom passage in section 18 is the oropharynx. The two passages cross in the pharyngeal isthmus of section 20. The epiglottis is found between sections 20 and 21. In section 21 the nasopharynx makes a 45° dorsal-to-ventral bend, and the oropharynx gives rise to the laryngopharynx. Again, since the epiglottis is in a middle position, the larynx and the laryngopharynx form a common chamber through section 22. In section 22 the two separate pockets are the anterior portions of the laryngeal ventricles, seen more clearly in section 23. In section 23 the airway makes a reverse 45° ventral-to-dorsal bend. The larynx and laryngopharynx are separated in section 24. The larynx becomes quite narrow in sections 25 and 26, then expands to give rise to the trachea by section 29. While the rhesus monkey does not have sinuses, other monkeys do (3).

A view of a sagittal section of the human nasal cavity is shown in Fig. 7. Inside the naris is the dilated area of the vestibule. On the wall of the cavity are the superior, medial, and inferior turbinates or conchae, which divide the cavity into air passages or meatuses. The small openings to the paranasal sinuses and ethmoidal air cells are found on the lateral and rear walls of the cavity.

A number of the dimensions of the nasal cavity of an adult are given by Snyder (30) and Anson (31). In the adult male the naris is about 2.0 cm long and 0.7–0.8 cm wide. The length of the cavity is 7-8 cm from the most

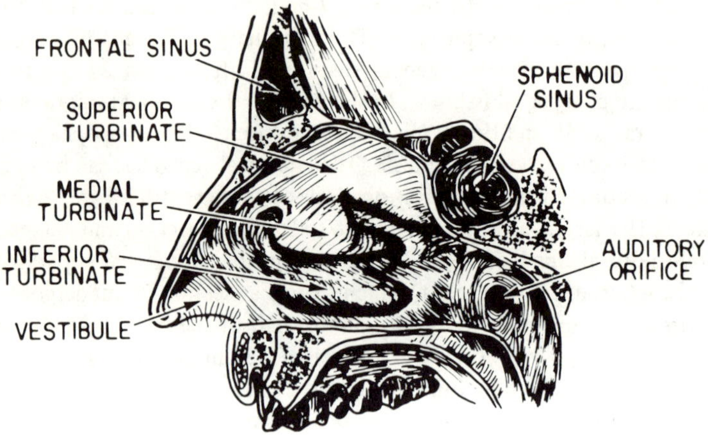

Figure 7 Sagittal section of the human nasal cavity showing the left lateral wall. [*From Schreider (29).*]

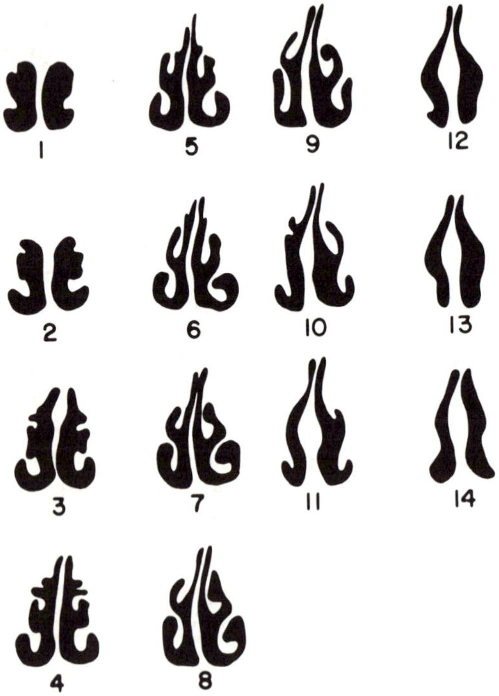

Figure 8 Tracing of tomograms of the human nasal airway. [*From Montgomery et al. (17).*]

prominent part of the naris to the posterior border of the hard palate. The greatest vertical diameter is 4.0–4.5 cm from the nasal floor to the cribriform plate. The surface area of both vestibules is 21 cm^2. The surface area of the turbinates and nasal passages (excluding the vestibules) on both sides of the nose is 160 cm^2. The volume of the nasal cavity is given as 8-9 cm^3 per side.

Using computed tomograms of the nasal airway, Montgomery et al. (17) generated a series of tracings of the nasal airway. The tracings were generated for four different human cadavers. Figure 8 shows the tracings of one of the specimens. In this specimen the inferior turbinates started in section 1 and ended in section 11, whereas the medial turbinates began in section 2 and ended in section 10. Postmortem shrinkage of the mucosa could have led to a larger than normal air passage. Table 5 gives the distance from the base of the nostrils at which each tomogram was made and the cross-sectional area of the airway at that point. These values were estimated from a graph of the cross-sectional areas of the airways. Using both casts and values from the tomograms, Montgomery et al. (17) calculated that the volumes of the right and left passages of the nose, contained in the region described above, were 11.5 and 13.5 cm^3, respectively. These volumes do not include the sinuses and are only for that region encompassed by the tomograms. The region encompassed by the human sections is approximately equivalent to sections 5-13 in the rhesus monkey. A comparison between the cross sections of the human nasal airway and that of the rhesus monkey shows a great deal of similarity, with the notable exception of the presence of paranasal sinuses in the human.

Table 5 Dimensions of the Tomograms of the Nasal Cavity of a Human Cadaver

Section	Distance from base of nostrils (mm)	Area (mm^2) Left side	Right side
1	0	2.3	2.4
2	4	2.4	2.5
3	8	2.8	2.8
4	12	2.8	2.7
5	16	2.5	2.3
6	20	2.8	2.3
7	24	2.7	2.3
8	28	3.0	2.5
9	32	3.2	2.5
10	36	2.9	2.2
11	40	2.8	2.0
12	44	2.3	1.7
13	48	2.3	1.6
14	52	2.2	2.0

[*From Schreider (29).*]

INHALATION DEPOSITION OF PARTICLES

There are five basic processes leading to particle deposition in the airways: electrostatic attraction, interception, impaction, gravitational settling, and diffusion. In all these cases, contact of the particle with the moist walls of the airways will result in the removal of the particle from the airstream. Electrostatic forces on a particle may cause that particle to be attracted to and contact the walls of an airway. Deposition by interception is caused by the noninertial incidental contact of a particle within the wall of an airway. This process depends on the physical size of the particle and will be most important for fibrous particles. As the velocity of an airstream changes direction, inertia will prevent a suspended particle from following exactly the path of the airstream. If the inertia is great enough, the particle will hit the walls of the airway. The extent of deposition by impaction depends on the velocity of the particle, the aerodynamic diameter of the particle, the dimensions of the airway, and the change of direction of the airstream. Particles settle under the influence of gravity. If the particles settle far enough, they will contact the wall of the airway. This deposition by sedimentation will depend on the residence time in the airway, the aerodynamic size of the particle, and the inclination of the airways. Small particles suspended in air are in random motion caused by the bombardment of the particles by air molecules. If the motion of the particle is great enough, the particle will contact the wall of an airway. This process is important for small particles at low air velocities.

Particles deposited in the nasal cavity may be cleared by ciliary mucous flow or may be absorbed by the blood. The extent of clearance will depend on the characteristics of the deposited particles and on the sites of deposition. Particles that are freely soluble in body fluids may be absorbed by the blood before they are cleared by mucous flow. Less soluble particles may be partially absorbed by the blood. This partial absorption, which can have important consequences, may occur in the nasal turbinates even for only moderately soluble particles. The reader is referred to Raabe (32) for an extensive review of particle deposition and clearance.

When making interspecies comparisons of particle deposition in the nasal airways, it should be remembered that there may be competing deposition factors at work in the nasal regions of various species. While the turbinates of the beagle and of rodents are more complex than those of the monkey and man, the bend in the nasopharynx of man and the monkey is much sharper, and the flow rates through the nasal cavities are higher. Since the animals all have a fairly sharp bend in the nares, and impaction is the principal means of deposition of the larger particles, it might be expected that these larger particles are deposited to a similar extent in the nares of the various animals. With the medium-size particles, where impaction in the nares decreases in importance, higher deposition would be expected in the rat, guinea pig, and the beagle because of the greater complexity, smaller airway dimensions, and greater surface areas of the turbinates. Deposition by diffusion of the very small particles might also be expected to be higher in the animals with the more complex turbinate systems and lower flow rates. In the case of very water soluble gases, under normal breathing conditions there are not expected to be major species differences in absorption (2). For less soluble gases, a situation similar to that found with particle deposition by diffusion is expected to take place, with higher absorption in those species with lower flow rates, more complex turbinates, greater relative surface areas, and smaller airway dimensions. This situation is also complicated by species differences in the response to irritants or toxicants in which the minute volume is decreased (by apnea) with a resulting decrease in absorption (33).

The previously discussed acrylic molds of the nasal cavity of guinea pigs and rats were used to study particle deposition in these animals (25, 34). Monodisperse aerosols of unit density spherical particles of methylene blue, ranging in size from 1 to 7 μm, were pulled through the mold at a rate equivalent to the normal resting minute volume of the animal in question. The amount of material depositing in the cast was measured colorimetrically and compared to the amount deposited on a filter behind the cast to give the fraction of "inhaled" material that was deposited in the cast. The results of the deposition measurements are given in Fig. 9. All the deposited material was found in the front third of the nose. The highest concentration was found just posterior to the nares, with the material fanning out in a posterior direction, in decreasing concentra-

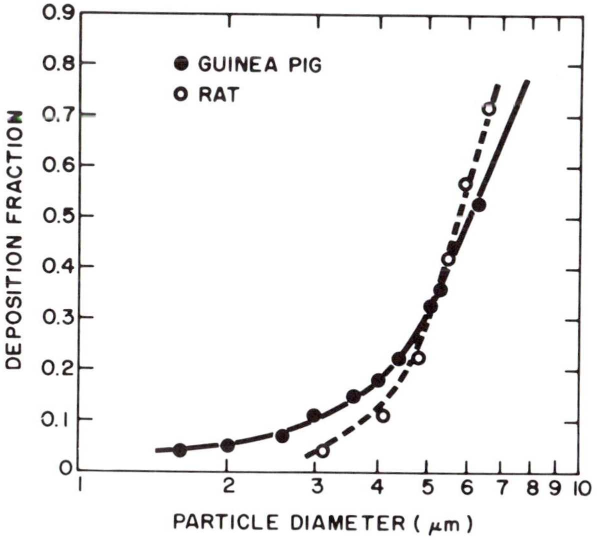

Figure 9 Particle deposition in acrylic molds of the nasal cavity of the guinea pig and rat. [*From Schreider (29).*]

tion, supporting the supposition that impaction is the main deposition process in the nasal cavity for the larger particles.

The use of acrylic nasal molds for deposition measurements has the advantages of yielding reproducible results and allowing easy visualization of the deposition sites. Like the previously discussed silicone rubber casts, the metal casts and the resulting acrylic molds were made from saline-rinsed, mucous-free noses. In addition, the walls of the mold were inflexible and devoid of nasal hairs. Because of the lack of mucus and nasal hairs, the deposition values should be treated as the lower limits of nasal deposition. It should also be noted that these deposition values do not include laryngeal deposition.

The small number of studies involving exposures to well-characterized aerosols of a series of particle sizes makes interspecies comparison of particle deposition very difficult. Raabe et al. (35) exposed hamsters and rats to a series of well-characterized, monodisperse, radiolabeled aluminosilicate aerosols. The deposition was measured for the entire nasal-pharyngeal region. Cuddihy et al. (36), again using radiolabeled, monodisperse aerosols, measured deposition in the beagle nasal-pharyngeal region. Fairchild et al. (37) used a radiolabeled polydisperse aerosol of streptococcus to measure deposition in the nose and the nasopharynx. The results of these various exposures are shown in Fig. 10. Selected data (38–41) from experimental measurements of particle deposition in the nasal-pharyngeal region of man are presented in Fig. 11. Also included are the values calculated by the ICRP Task Group on Lung Dynamics (42) for 15 breaths per minute (BPM) and a tidal volume (V_t) of 1450 ml. The deposition fraction is plotted against the characteristic term ($D_{ar}^2 Q$) that controls inertial impaction, where D_{ar} is the aerodynamic resistance diameter and Q is the

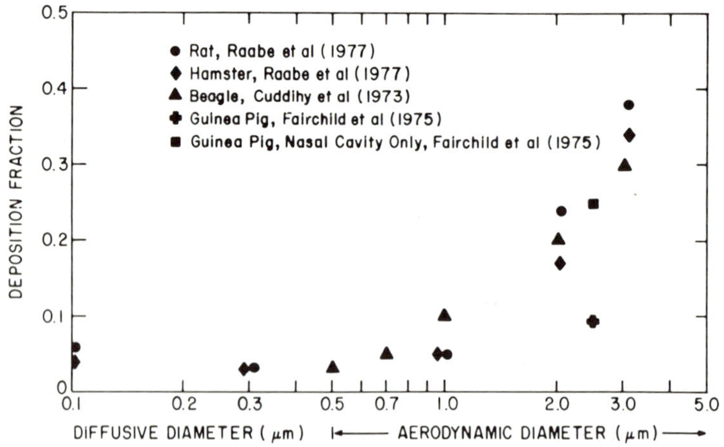

Figure 10 Selected data for the deposition of inhaled aerosols in experimental animals. [*From Schreider (29).*]

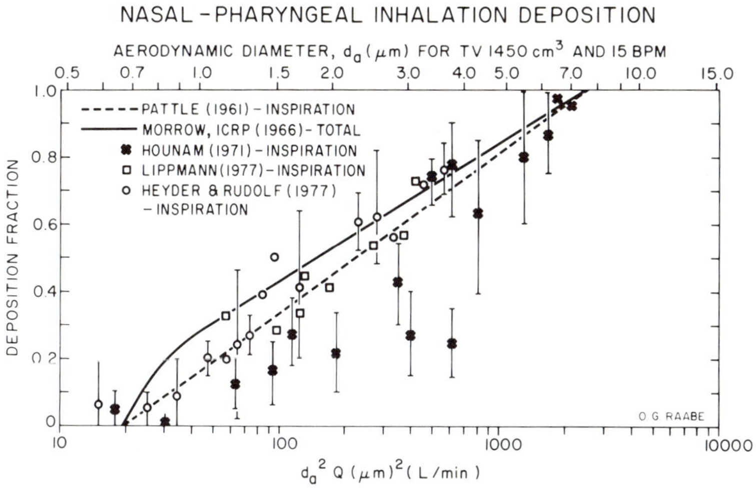

Figure 11 Selected data reported for inspiratory deposition in the nasal-pharyngeal (NP) region of monodisperse aerosols inhaled by people through the nose as reported by Hounam et al. (39), Lippmann (40), and Heyder and Rudolf (41) compared to the empirical model of Pattle (38) for inspiration alone (dashed line) as a function of the impaction parameter $d_a^2 Q$, where d_a is the aerodynamic diameter and Q is the average inspiratory flow rate. Also shown are the corresponding aerodynamic diameters for reference worker for tidal volume (V_t) of 1450 cm³ and 15 breaths per minute (BPM) and the calculated total deposition fraction for both inspiration and exhalation given by the ICRP Task Group on Lung Dynamics (42). [*Figure and caption kindly provided by O. G. Raabe.*]

minute volume. While the scarcity of animal data and the high degree of intra-experimental variation make such comparisons equivocal, a comparison of Figs. 10 and 11 suggests that the larger particle (> 1 μm) deposition values for experimental animals fall within the same range as the values for man.

CONCLUSIONS

The anatomical characteristics of the various experimental animals and man are summarized in Table 6. The surface areas of the nasal cavity of the experimental animals were estimated in a segmental calculation using the perimeter and thickness of the appropriate sections of each animal nasal cast (Tables 1-4). These surface areas do include the sinuses and air pockets, whereas the surface area of the human nasal cavity does not. The dimensions listed for the nasal cavity of man are those given by Snyder (30) and Anson (31).

There are both differences and similarities between the species. Perhaps one of the most obvious examples of anatomical differences is in the structure of the turbinate regions. Some of the differences could affect deposition of particles and gases in the nasal cavities. A degree of caution, therefore, should be

Table 6 Interspecies Comparison of Nasal Cavity Characteristics

	Rat	Guinea pig	Beagle dog	Rhesus monkey	Man
Weight	250 g	600 g	10 kg	7 kg	~ 70 kg
Naris cross section	0.7 mm^2	2.5 mm^2	16.7 mm^2	22.9 mm^2	140 mm^2
Bend in naris	40°	40°	30°	30°	n.a.
Length	2.3 cm	3.4 cm	10 cm	5.3 cm	7–8 cm
Greatest vertical diameter	9.6 mm	12.8 mm	23 mm	27 mm	40–45 mm
Surface area* (both sides of nasal cavity)	10.4 cm^2	27.4 cm^2	220.7 cm^2	61.6 cm^2	181 cm^2
Volume (both sides)*	0.4 cm^3	0.9 cm^3	20 cm^3	8 cm^3	16–19 cm^3
Bend in nasopharynx	15°	30°	30°	80°	~ 90°
Turbinate complexity	Double scroll	Double scroll	Membranous, branched	Simple scroll	Simple scroll
Sinuses	Maxillary recess, frontal sinus	Maxillary recess, frontal sinus	Maxillary, sphenoid, frontal sinuses	Maxillary recess	Frontal, sphenoid, maxillary, ethmoid sinuses

*Includes sinuses for rat, guinea pig, beagle dog, and rhesus monkey. Does not include sinuses for man.

exercised in extrapolating the nasal deposition characteristics and inhalation toxicity results from one species to another.

SUMMARY

A discussion is presented of the comparative anatomy and functions of the nasal passages for different animal species (rat, guinea pig, beagle dog, rhesus monkey, man). The functions include olfaction, air conditioning (humidification, temperature regulation), filtration, and resistance to disease. The relative importance of the different functions is reflected in the structure and distribution of the tissues necessary for these various functions. The anatomical characteristics are examined primarily through the use of casts of the airways. There are both structural differences and similarities between the species presented. Perhaps one of the most obvious examples of anatomical differences is the structure of the turbinate regions, which is relatively simple in the monkey and man, complex in the rat and guinea pig, and quite complex in the beagle. Some of the differences affect the deposition and uptake of particles and gases in the nasal passages. Therefore, caution must be exercised in extrapolating the nasal deposition characteristics and inhalation toxicity results from one species to another.

REFERENCES

1 Mygind, N, M Pederson, and M Nielsen. Morphology of the upper airway epithelium. In *The Nose: Upper Airway Physiology and the Atmospheric Environment,* edited by D Proctor and I Anderson, New York: Elsevier, pp. 71–97(1982).
2 Proctor, D, and J Chang. Comparative anatomy and physiology of the nasal cavity. In *Nasal Tumors in Animals and Man,* Vol. 1, edited by G Reznik and S Stinson. Boca Raton, FL: CRC Press, pp. 1–33 (1983).
3 Negus, V. *Comparative Anatomy and Physiology and Physiology of the Nose and Paranasal Sinuses.* Edinburgh: Livingstone (1958).
4 Berglund, B, and T Lindvall. Olfaction. In *The Nose: Upper Airway Physiology and the Atmospheric Environment,* edited by D Proctor and I Anderson, New York: Elsevier, pp. 274–305 (1982).
5 Cole, P. Modification of inspired air. In *The Nose: Upper Airway Physiology and the Atmospheric Environment,* edited by D Proctor and I Anderson, New York: Elsevier, pp. 351–375 (1982).
6 Proctor, D. The upper airway. In *The Nose: Upper Airway Physiology and the Atmospheric Environment,* edited by D Proctor and I Anderson, New York: Elsevier, pp. 12–43 (1982).
7 Gwaltney, J and F Hayden. The nose and infection. In *The Nose: Upper Airway Physiology and the Atmospheric Environment,* edited by D Proctor and I Anderson, New York: Elsevier, pp. 399–422 (1982).
8 Widdicombe J, and U Wells. Airway secretions. In *The Nose: Upper Airway Physiology and the Atmospheric Environment,* edited by D Proctor and I Anderson, New York: Elsevier, pp. 215–244 (1982).

9 Goss, C. *Anatomy of the Human Body by Henry Gray*. Philadelphia: Lea and Febiger (1973).

10 Hartman, C, and W Strauss. *The Anatomy of the Rhesus Monkey*. New York: Hafner (1933).

11 Miller, M. *Anatomy of the Dog*. Philadelphia: Saunders (1964).

12 Hebel, R, and M Stromberg. *Anatomy of the Laboratory Rat*. Baltimore: Williams and Wilkins (1976).

13 Cooper, G, and A Schiller. *Anatomy of the Guinea Pig*. Cambridge, MA: Harvard University Press (1975).

14 Leibich, H. Zum bau der oberen luftwege der weiben ratte. *Anat. Anz.* 138: 170–179 (1979).

15 Wohrmann-Repenning, A. Zur vergleichenden makro- und mikroskopischen anatomie der nasenhohle europaischer insectivoren. *Gegenbaurs Morphol. Jahrb.* 121:698–796 (1975).

16 Reznik, G, and K Jensen. Anatomy of the nasal cavity of the european hamster. *Z. Versuchstierkuade,* 21:321–340 (1979).

17 Montgomery, W, P Vig, E Stabb, and S Matteson. Computed tomography: A three-dimensional study of the nasal airway. *Am. J. Orthod.* 76:363–375 (1979).

18 Rahn, H, and B Ross. Bronchial tree casts, lobe weights and anatomical dead space measurements in the dog lung. *J. Appl. Physiol.* 10:154–157 (1957).

19 Tucker, J, and E Krementz. Anatomical corrosion specimens. II. Broncho-pulmonary anatomy in the dog. *Anat. Rec.* 127:667–676 (1957).

20 Eisman, M. Lung models, hollow flexible reproductions. *J. Appl. Physiol.* 29:531–533 (1970).

21 Frank, N, and R Yoder. A method of making a flexible cast of the lung. *J. Appl. Physiol.* 21:1925–1926 (1966).

22 Thompsett, D. *Anatomical Techniques*. London: Livingstone (1970).

23 Proctor, DF, and HN Wagner. Mucociliary clearance in the human nose. In *Inhaled Particles and Vapours II,* edited by CN Davies. Oxford: Pergamon, pp. 25–35 (1967).

24 Schreider, J, and J Hutchens. Morphology of the guinea pig respiratory tract. *Anat. Rec.* 196:313–321 (1980).

25 Schreider, J. Lung anatomy and characteristics of aerosol retention of the guinea pig. Ph.D. thesis, University of Chicago, Division of Biological Sciences, Department of Pharmacological and Physiological Sciences (1977).

26 Phalen, R, H Yeh, O Raabe, and D Velasquez. Casting of the lungs *in situ*. *Anat. Rec.* 177:255–263 (1973).

27 Schreider, J, and O Raabe. Replica casts of the entire respiratory airways of experimental animals. *J. Environ. Pathol. Toxicol.* 4:427–435 (1980).

28 Schreider, J, and O Raabe. Anatomy of the nasal pharyngeal airways of experimental animals. *Anat. Rec.* 200:195–205 (1981).

29 Schreider, J. Nasal airway anatomy and inhalation deposition in experimental animals and people. In *Nasal Tumors in Animals and Man,* Vol. III, edited by G Reznik and S Stinson. Boca Raton, FL: CRC Press, pp. 1–36 (1983).

30 Snyder WS. *International Commission on Radiological Protection (ICRP) Task Group on Reference Man.* Oxford: Pergamon, p. 151 (1975).

31 Anson, B. *Morris' Human Anatomy.* New York: McGraw-Hill, p. 1391 (1966).

32 Raabe, OG. Deposition and clearance of inhaled aerosols. In *Mechanisms in Respiratory Toxicology,* edited by H Witschi and P Nettesheim. Boca Raton, FL: CRC Press, pp. 27–76 (1982).

33 Chang, J, W Steinhagen, and C Barrow. Effect of single or repeated formaldehyde exposures on minute volume of B6C3F1 mice and F-344 rats. *Toxicol. Appl. Pharmacol.* 61:451–459 (1981).

34 Schreider, J, and J Hutchens. Particle deposition in the guinea pig respiratory tract. *J. Aerosol Sci.* 10:599–607 (1979).

35 Raabe, O, H Yeh, G Newton, R Phalen, and D Velasquez. Deposition of inhaled monodisperse aerosols in small rodents. In *Inhaled Particles IV,* edited by W Walton. New York: Pergamon, pp. 3–33 (1977).

36 Cuddihy, R, D Brownstein, O Raabe, and G Kanapilly. Respiratory tract deposition of inhaled polydisperse aerosols in beagle dogs. *J. Aerosol Sci.* 4:35–45 (1973).

37 Fairchild, G, S Stultz, and D Coffin. Sulfuric acid effect on the deposition of radioactive aerosol in the respiratory tract of guinea pigs. *Am. Ind. Hyg. Assoc. J.* 36:584–594 (1975).

38 Pattle, R. The retention of gases and particles in the human nose. In *Inhaled Particles and Vapours,* edited by CN Davies. Oxford: Pergamon, pp. 302–309 (1961).

39 Hounam, R, A Black, and M Walsh. The deposition of aerosol particles in the nasopharyngeal region of the human respiratory tract. In *Inhaled Particles,* edited by WH Walton. Surrey, England: Unwin Brothers, pp. 71–80 (1971).

40 Lippmann, M. Regional deposition of particles in the human respiratory tract. In *Handbook of Physiology, Section 9: Reactions to Environmental Agents,* edited by D Lee, H Falk, and S Murphy. Bethesda, MD: American Physiological Society, pp. 213–232 (1977).

41 Heyder, J, and G Rudolf. Deposition of aerosol particles in the human nose. In *Inhaled Particles,* edited by WH Walton. Oxford: Pergamon, pp. 107–125 (1977).

42 Morrow, P, D Bates, B Fish, T Hatch, and T Mercer. Deposition and retention models for internal dosimetry of the human respiratory tract. (Report of the International Commission on Radiological Protection, ICRP: Task Group on Lung Dynamics.) *Health Phys.* 12:173–207 (1964).

Chapter 2

Light Microscopic Examination of the Rat Nasal Passages: Preparation and Morphologic Features

John T. Young

INTRODUCTION

With the relatively recent "discovery" of the nasal passages as something more than a passageway for air to the lower respiratory tract and an organ for smell has come a need for more information about the basic functional characteristic of the nasal tissues as an organ system. It is a basic biological tenet that form and function are inseparable characteristics of an organ system, and knowledge of both is necessary for complete understanding. It is the purpose of this chapter to introduce the "form" of the nasal passage of our most useful animal model, the rat, at the light microscopic level. Subsequent chapters will deal with many aspects of "function" (and dysfunction)–absorption, metabolism, mucociliary clearance, etc.–and it is hoped that the reader will be able to integrate these anatomic and biochemical characteristics into a more complete understanding of the nasal passages as a dynamic organ system.

METHODS OF PREPARATION FOR LIGHT MICROSCOPY

A method for the preparation of the rat nasal cavity has been previously published (1). This procedure will be briefly reiterated here since the histologic descriptions in subsequent sections are based on this method. The procedure is described for rats but works equally well for mice with obvious modifications for size.

Preparations at Necropsy

Following decapitation, the eyes, skin, lower jaw, brain, and pituitary are removed from the head and the nasal cavity is gently flushed with Formalin via the pharyngeal duct. The head is then allowed to fix in Formalin for several days.

Decalcification

The formic acid-sodium citrate method of decalcification (2) is considered optimal, and 14-18 days (7-10 days for mice) with frequent changes of solution is generally adequate. Following decalcification, the tissues should be washed 8-24 h in running tap water and then trimmed or returned to Formalin.

Trimming

The objective of trimming the heads is to produce four tissue slices which, after embedding and sectioning, will permit histopathologic examination of the nasal cavity at the following levels: (1) immediately posterior to the upper incisor teeth, (2) at the incisive papilla, (3) at the second palatal ridge, and (4) at the middle of the first upper molar teeth. The decalcified head should be placed on a cutting board so that the roof of the mouth (hard palate) is facing upward. With a sharp razor blade or scalpel, the cuts outlined in Fig. 1 are made perpendicular to the plane of the hard palate and perpendicular to the nasal septum. The four slices are examined for discrete lesions and placed anterior side down in a cassette for processing.

Processing, Embedding, Sectioning, and Staining

The nasal tissues are processed in a conventional manner, embedded anterior face downward, sectioned at 5-6 μm, and stained with hematoxylin and eosin in the usual manner.

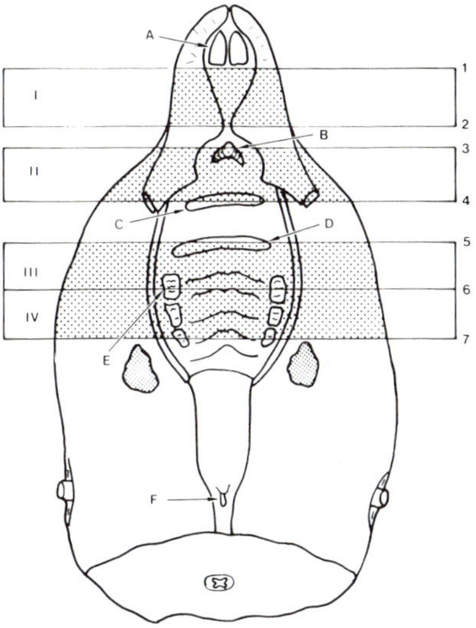

Figure 1 Ventral view of the rat hard palate region, with the lower jaw removed, indicating the four tissue slices, I–IV (stippled areas), which will be embedded anterior face down. The numbers on the right-hand side indicate the levels of the seven cuts necessary to produce the four slices. (A) Upper incisor teeth; (B) incisive papilla; (C) first palatal ridge; (D) second palatal ridge; (E) first upper molar tooth; (F) posterior opening of the pharyngeal duct (nasopharynx). [*Reprinted with permission (1).*]

GENERAL HISTOLOGIC FEATURES OF THE RAT NASAL CAVITY

The paired, slitlike nostrils of the rat open into a short vestibule which is supported almost entirely by cartilage. The nasal cavity is divided longitudinally into two approximately equal halves by the cartilaginous nasal septum. Each half contains a dorsal, middle, and ventral meatus. At the posterior end of the nasal cavity lies a blind-ended cavity known as the ethmoid recess. The ventral meatus extends along the floor of the nasal cavity proper and terminates at the nasopharyngeal duct, which is the functional air passage to the respiratory pharynx. The dorsal meatus extends into the dorsal part of the ethmoid recess, and the middle meatus ends at the ostium of the maxillary sinus, a pocketlike recess outside the nasal cavity lateral to the ethmoid recess (3).

The nasal septum does not completely divide the right and left sides of the cavity. At the base of the septum just anterior to the nasopharyngeal duct is a septal "window" that permits luminal continuity between the right and left halves of the nasal cavity (4). Each half also has an independent connection to the oral cavity by way of the paired incisive ducts. These stratified squamous epithelial lined ducts exit the ventral meatus near its midpoint and emerge from slitlike openings on the incisive papilla in the roof of the mouth. Lying in the lower part of the nasal septum and parallel to the plane of the septum is a paired tubular structure known as the vomeronasal organ of Jacobson. The tubes are lined medially by a specialized type of olfactory epithelium, extend from the vestibule to the incisive duct, and are blind on both ends but communicate with the vestibule laterally by a short tube (3).

In the nasal cavity proper there are two pairs of turbinates or concha: the nasoturbinates and the maxilloturbinates. The former originate in the roof of the nasal cavity, project ventrally, and extend from the vestibule to a point posterior to the incisive ducts. The maxilloturbinates arise from the maxillary bone medial to the root of the upper incisor, project dorsally, and are roughly in the same plane as the nasoturbinates but somewhat smaller. Although the terminology for the turbinates of the ethmoid recess is confusing in the literature, there appear to be six pairs in the rat nose: two ectoturbinates and four endoturbinates (5). These are usually designated by Roman numerals, and several of them have more than one lamella greatly expanding the potential surface area.

Three basic epithelial types line the mucosa of the nasal cavity: stratified squamous epithelium, respiratory epithelium, and olfactory epithelium. Stratified squamous epithelium lines only the vestibule, the most anterior end of the nasal cavity, and the floor of the ventral meatus as far as the incisive ducts. The nasal cavity proper is lined almost entirely by respiratory epithelium with the exception of the upper part of the dorsal meatus near the posterior end. This area is lined by olfactory epithelium which also lines most of the ethmoid recess and its turbinates. A small patch of specialized olfactory epithelium, known as the septal organ of Rodolfo-Masera, is also located on the nasal septum posterior to the vomeronasal organ (6). The stratified squamous epithelium lines only about 3–4 percent of the total nasal surface area, and respiratory and olfactory epithelia each line approximately half of the remainder (7).

The volume of the nasal cavity in adult rats has been determined to be approximately 257 mm^3 (7); however, the volume is dynamic. Because of the presence of "swell bodies," focal collections of distensible vascular channels along the lateral wall and tip of maxilloturbinates, a cyclic alteration in conductivity between the two halves of the nasal cavity has been demonstrated in rats (8).

SPECIFIC HISTOLOGIC CHARACTERISTICS AT FOUR LEVELS

Level 1 (Fig. 2)

The first level of examination is immediately posterior to the upper incisor teeth, and the roots of the teeth are present laterally in the sections. At this level the entire cavity, with the exception of the lower ventral meatus, is lined by respiratory epithelium. The nasoturbinates, and to a lesser degree the maxilloturbinates, have a hooklike appearance with the curve directed laterally. At the base of the cartilaginous septum, the paired tubes of the vomeronasal organ bulge into the ventral meatus, and the paired nasolacrimal ducts are present ventrolateral to the maxilloturbinates nearing their anterior termination in the vestibule.

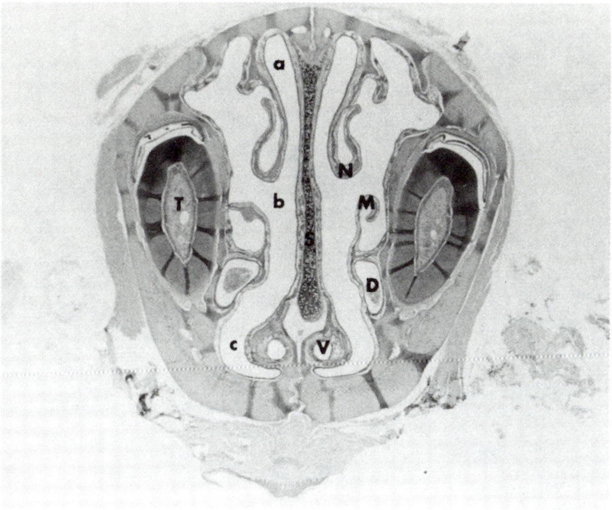

Figure 2 Level 1 of the rat nasal cavity. This section is just posterior to the upper incisor teeth and consists primarily of respiratory epithelium except for the ventral meatus. Dorsal meatus (a), middle meatus (b), ventral meatus (c), nasoturbinate (N), maxilloturbinate (M), nasolacrimal duct (D), vomeronasal organ (V), nasal septum (S), root of upper incisor tooth (T). H&E stain (X1.5). [*Reprinted with permission (1).*]

Level 2 (Fig. 3)

Level 2 is a transverse section at the incisive papilla, and the continuity of the nasal and oral cavities by way of the incisive ducts can be seen. The upper incisor roots are still prominent and the nasolacrimal ducts are now lateral to the teeth, having passed ventrally under the teeth between levels 1 and 2. The maxilloturbinates are near their posterior end and are reduced to a small projection from the lateral wall. The nasoturbinates have lost their characteristic hooklike profile, and the lumina of the vomeronasal organ are no longer visible. At this level the dorsal meatus is lined by olfactory epithelium, but the remainder of the nasal cavity and septum with the exception of the incisive ducts is lined by respiratory epithelium.

Level 3 (Fig. 4)

The third level of examination is at or near the anterior end of the nasopharyngeal duct, where the two halves of the nasal cavity communicate. The two ectoturbinates occupy the dorsal part of the section, and three endoturbinates project inward from the lateral walls on either side. Most of the mucosa in the section is olfactory with the exception of the pharyngeal duct area, lower septum, and the inner portion of some lamellae, which are relatively inaccessible

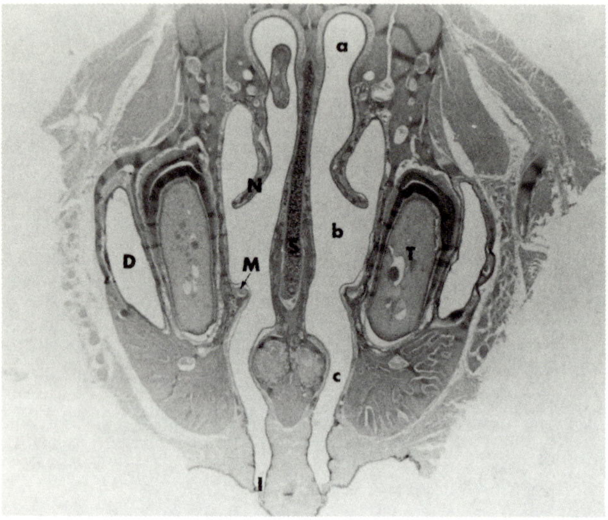

Figure 3 Level 2 of the rat nasal cavity. This section is at the incisive papilla and contains all three epithelial types—respiratory, olfactory, and stratified squamous. Dorsal meatus (a), middle meatus (b), ventral meatus (c), nasoturbinate (N), maxilloturbinate (M), incisive duct (I), nasolacrimal duct (D), root of upper incisor tooth (T), nasal septum (S). H&E stain (X1.5). [*Reprinted with permission (1).*]

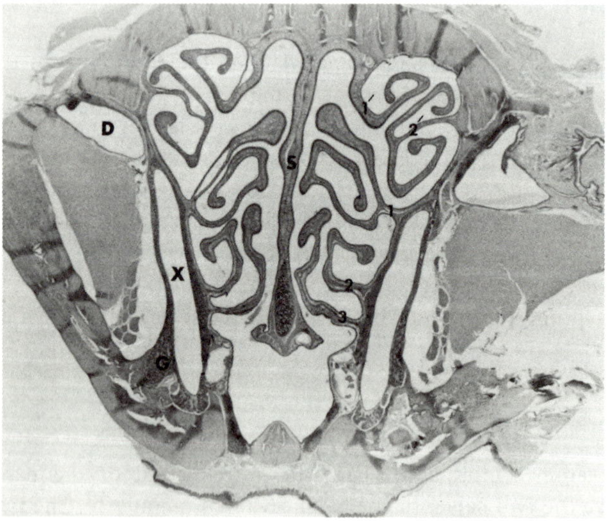

Figure 4 Level 3 of the rat nasal cavity. This section of the ethmoid recess, taken at the level of the second palatal ridge, is lined primarily by olfactory epithelium. Ectoturbinates (1', 2'), endoturbinates (1, 2, 3), nasolacrimal duct (D), maxillary sinus (X), lateral nasal glands (G), nasal septum (S). H&E stain (X1.5). [*Reprinted with permission (1).*]

to inspired air. The maxillary sinus, which opens by a wide ostium anterior to the plane of section, is situated lateral to the ethmoid recess and is surrounded by the lateral nasal glands of Steno and the maxillary glands. Respiratory epithelium lines the maxillary sinus. The nasolacrimal ducts at this level are adjacent to the dorsal part of the recess nearing their origin at the medial canthus of the eyes.

Level 4 (Fig. 5)

The fourth level is deep in the blind end of the ethmoid recess and is lined almost entirely by olfactory mucosa. The pharyngeal duct is fully formed in the ventral part of the section and does not again communicate with the nasal cavity on its course to the respiratory pharynx. In the dorsal part of the section, the olfactory lobes of the brain can be seen and the Harderian glands are present laterally in the orbits.

SPECIFIC EPITHELIAL TYPES

Stratified Squamous Epithelium

The lining epithelium of the vestibule and ventral meatus is similar to nonkeratinizing stratified squamous epithelium found elsewhere. The lamina propria is a

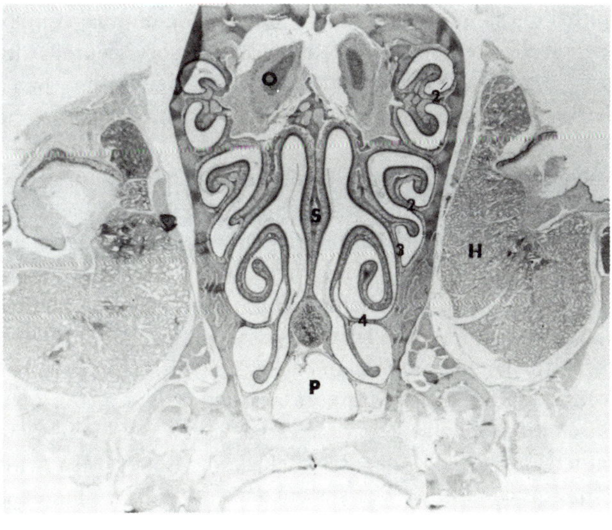

Figure 5 Level 4, which occurs at the level of the first upper molar teeth, is deep in the ethmoid recess and is lined primarily by olfactory epithelium. Ectoturbinate (2′), endoturbinates (2, 3, 4), pharyngeal duct (P), olfactory lobe of brain (O), Harderian gland (H), nasal septum (S). H&E stain (X1.5). [*Reprinted with permission (1).*]

simple collagenous stroma poor in glands, and the epithelium in general has no features particularly distinct to the region.

Respiratory Epithelium

The respiratory epithelium is generally considered to be a ciliated simple cuboidal or tall columnar epithelium with abundant goblet cells, and this description applies to much of the surface area. However, the character of the epithelium varies considerably with location. A functional mucociliary apparatus requires cilia and mucus, so the epithelium of the septum and medial aspects of the nasoturbinates and maxilloturbinates is heavily ciliated and has numerous goblet cells and mucus producing glands in the lamina propria. In the dorsal meatus the epithelium is pseudo-stratified in appearance. In contrast, the lining of the lateral portion of the nasoturbinates and dorsal portions of the lateral wall are sparsely ciliated and the epithelial cells are low cuboidal and almost squamous in appearance, and few goblet cells are present. In general, the epithelium appears taller and more ciliated more posteriorly near the termination of the naso- and maxilloturbinates.

The lamina propria is collagenous and contains nerves, glands for serous and mucous secretions, and numerous distensible vascular channels, particularly in the region of the "swell bodies."

Olfactory Epithelium

The olfactory neuroepithelium is by far the most complex and unusual component of the nasal mucosa. In vertebrates the olfactory sensory neurons are the only neurons whose perikarya are located in a neuroepithelium rather than a sensory ganglion, and they are unique in their capacity to turn over and to be replaced after injury (9).

The olfactory epithelium is a pseudo-stratified neuroepithelium consisting of three cell types: sustentacular or support cells, neurons, and basal cells—all supported by a basal lamina (Fig. 6). The basal cells are usually seen as a single layer adjacent to the basal lamina, and above them are numerous strata of mature neurons with hyperchromatic nuclei and scant cytoplasm. Each neuron has a single axon that passes down through the basal lamina and into the olfactory nerve bundles in the lamina propria, and a single dendritic process that extends upward between the single layer of support cells and ends as a vesicle on the luminal surface. Each of the olfactory vesicles has a few cilia extending radially; however, neither the vesicles nor their cilia are usually seen with standard light microscopic preparations. The sustentacular cells have abundant columnar cytoplasm with a microvillous border and round to oval, less hyperchromatic nuclei that appear as a single row. The subnuclear part of the sustentacular cytoplasm extends all the way to the basal layer but is not very apparent between the neuronal layers.

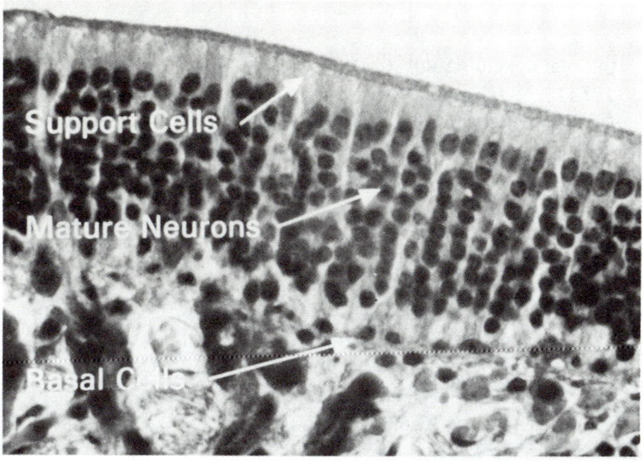

Figure 6 Olfactory epithelium from the region of the dorsal meatus. A single row of basal cells lies above the basal lamina, and 8–10 layers of mature neurons occupy the midportion of the epithelium. The sustenacular or support cells with their prominent cytoplasm and microvillous border form the luminal boundary. H&E stain (X20).

Since the basal cells are the stem cells for the neurons, and the rat neuroepithelium turnover time is approximately 30 days (10), some areas will have multiple layers of basal cells associated with a decrease in the numbers of mature neurons. These multiple basal layers are differentiating into mature neurons in a mosaic pattern throughout the entire olfactory neuroepithelium at any given time (10).

The lamina propria of the olfactory epithelium contains numerous nerve bundles of the olfactory nerve, blood vessels, and "Bowman's glands." These glands have small ducts with a very flattened epithelial lining that can be seen passing through the neuroepithelium to the luminal surface.

SUMMARY

The general structure and histologic features of the nasal passages of the rat are presented. A method for the histologic preparation of rat noses is briefly described that permits evaluation of transverse sections at four levels: (1) immediately posterior to the upper incisor teeth, (2) at the incisive papilla, (3) at the second palatal ridge, and (4) at the middle of the first upper molar teeth. A detailed description of the anatomic features present in each of these sections is discussed, as well as the specific light microscopic characteristics of the three types of epithelium that line the nasal mucosa: stratified squamous epithelium, respiratory epithelium, and the olfactory neuroepithelium.

REFERENCES

1 Young, JT. Histopathologic examination of the rat nasal cavity. *Fundam. Appl. Toxicol.* 1:309-312 (1981).

2 Luna, LG. *Manual of Histologic Staining Methods of the Armed Forces Institute of Pathology*, 3d ed. New York: McGraw-Hill, pp. 8-9 (1968).

3 Hebel, R, and MW Stromberg. *Anatomy of the Laboratory Rat.* Baltimore: Williams and Wilkins (1976).

4 Kelemen, G. The junction of the nasal cavity and the pharyngeal tube in the rat. *Arch. Otolaryngol.* 45:159-168 (1947).

5 Kelemen, G, and F Sargent. Nonexperimental pathologic nasal findings in laboratory rats. *Arch. Otolaryngol.* 44:24-42 (1946).

6 Rodolfo-Masera, DT. Su l'esistenza di un particolare organo olfaltivo nel setto nasale della civia e di altri roditori. *Arch. Ital. Anat. Embriol.* 48:157-212 (1943).

7 Gross, EA, JA Swenberg, S Field, and JA Popp. Comparative morphometry of the nasal cavity in rats and mice. *J. Anat.* 135:83-88 (1982).

8 Bojsen-Moller, F, and J Fahrenkrug. Nasal swell bodies and cyclic changes in the air passages of the rat and rabbit nose. *J. Anat.* 110:25-37 (1971).

9 Graziadei, PPC, and GA Monti Graziadei. Neurogenesis and neuron regeneration in the olfactory system of mammals. I. Morphological aspects of differentiation and structural organization of the olfactory sensory neurons. *J. Neurocytol.* 8:1-18 (1979).

10 Monti Graziadei, GA, and PPC Graziadei. Neurogenesis and neuron regeneration in the olfactory system of mammals. II. Degeneration and reconstitution of the olfactory sensory neurons after axotomy. *J. Neurocytol.* 8:197-213 (1979).

Chapter 3

Ultrastructure of the Rat Nasal Mucosa

James A. Popp, Nancy A. Monteiro-Riviere,
and Joseph T. Martin

INTRODUCTION

The nasal cavity has an important physiologic function in warming, humidifying, and cleansing the inspired air prior to reaching the lung. Extensive literature characterizes these physiologic functions in multiple species. Likewise, the general structure of the lining epithelium and the glands of the nasal cavity have been described by light microscopy. More specifically, use of the light microscope has demonstrated that the nasal passages are lined by three types of epithelium: squamous, respiratory, and olfactory. Despite its characterization as pseudo-stratified ciliated epithelium, it is obvious by light microscopy that the respiratory epithelium varies from area to area and is composed of more than one cell type. Unfortunately, the complexity of the cell types in the nasal cavity epithelium has not been completely evaluated by ultrastructural studies until very recently.

The authors thank Linda K. Garvey for preparing the photographs and aiding in the preparation of the manuscript.

In the past few years we have studied the ultrastructure of the normal nasal mucosa of the rat. Although our primary interest was in the morphologic response of the nasal cavity epithelium to inhaled toxicants, it was clear that inadequate information was available concerning the normal ultrastructure of the rat nasal mucosa. The baseline information of the normal structure was necessary before one could adequately evaluate any toxin-induced changes in this tissue. The rat was chosen for study since it is one of the primary animals used in chronic inhalation toxicology research and testing programs. The information obtained has already provided a useful background for toxicological studies underway at the Chemical Industry Institute of Toxicology.

METHODS

CDF (F344) rats (150–200 g) of both sexes were obtained from Charles River Breeding Laboratories (Kingston, NY). They were quarantined for 2 weeks in a mass air displacement room (Bioclean, Hazleton Systems, Inc., Vienna, VA). During this preconditioning period, animals were found to be free of common pathogenic viruses using a standard virus antibody screening battery of tests (Microbiological Associates, Bethesda, MD). Lights were automatically controlled to provide 12 h of light per day. The temperature and humidity were maintained at 22 ± 2°C and 50 ± 5%, respectively. Animals were given NIH-07 diet (Ziegler Bros., Gardner, PA) that was analyzed for nutrients and contaminants (Lancaster Labs, Lancaster, PA) and purified tap water ad libitum (1).

The preparative procedure, previously described in detail by Popp and Martin (2), will be briefly described here. The rats were anesthetized with sodium pentobarbital (50 mg/kg). The nasal cavity was flushed with 10 ml of bacteriostatic sodium chloride (Cutter Lab., Berkeley, CA) to remove excess mucus. The vascular system was first flushed with 10% Dextran 40 in 0.9% sodium chloride for 1 min (Cutter Lab., Berkeley, CA) by cannulating the left side of the heart. For fixation the animal was then perfused for approximately 30 min with Karnovsky's fixative in cacodylate buffer (pH 7.4) which contained glutaraldehyde and paraformaldehyde. Excess skin, muscle, and fascia were removed from the head which was then placed in fixative for an additional 2 h. The skulls were subsequently decalcified in 10% EDTA in 0.1 M cacodylate buffer (pH 7.4) at 4°C for approximately 2 weeks.

After decalcification, samples were selected for ultrastructural observation. For transmission electron microscopy (TEM), a system for block selection has been described by Monteiro-Riviere and Popp (3). This procedure allowed for the comparison of any area of the nasal mucosa to adjacent areas. For scanning electron microscopy (SEM), the skull was opened in various ways to allow visualization of all nasal surfaces as previously described by Popp and Martin (4).

Morphometric evaluation of nasal surfaces utilized a Zeiss Videoplan to measure areas on scanning electron micrographs which were enlarged to a final magnification of 12,000X.

RESULTS

The nasal cavity is lined by three types of epithelium: squamous, respiratory, and olfactory. The squamous epithelium of the anterior and ventral surfaces has ultrastructural characteristics similar to this type of epithelium on other mucosal surfaces. Using SEM, the individual flattened cells were easily identified by distinct borders and an irregular surface. On higher magnification, the surface was composed of numerous microridges. Occasionally cells were observed sloughing off the surface and were characterized by having nonadherent edges. There was a sharp border between squamous epithelium and the adjacent respiratory epithelium.

SEM and TEM demonstrated distinct cell types that were unevenly distributed in the respiratory epithelium of the rat nasal mucosa. The ciliated cell had the largest apical appendages, making this cell obvious when observed by TEM, SEM (Figs. 1, 2), or light microscopy. Each ciliated cell had between 50 and 100 cilia, which usually obliterated other apical surface structures when viewed by SEM. However, TEM demonstrated numerous slender, long, and sometimes branching microvilli between the cilia (Fig. 2). The ciliated cell extended from the lumen of the nasal cavity to the basal lamina but, with the exception of cilia, contained no uniquely identifying structure. The cytoplasm was frequently stained lighter than the cytoplasm of other cell types. Mitochondria were numerous, but very little rough endoplasmic reticulum (ER) was found.

Typical of an active secretory cell, the goblet cell had variable ultrastructural characteristics depending on its stage in the secretory cycle. The apical surface frequently formed a bleb that protruded into the lumen of the nasal

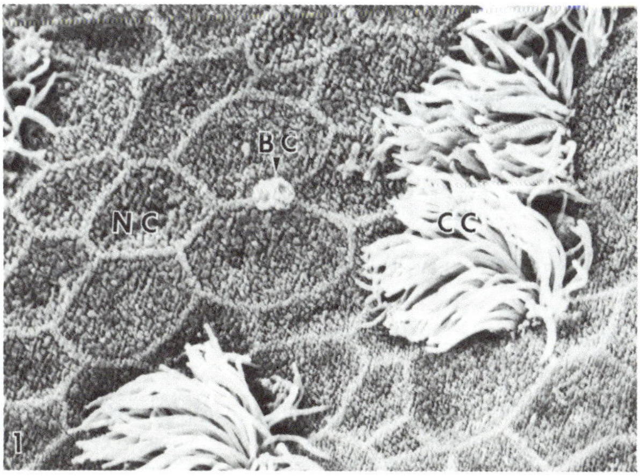

Figure 1 Ciliated cells (CC), nonciliated columnar cells (NC), and a single brush cell (BC) are demonstrated in this scanning electron micrograph of the nasal respiratory epithelium. Original magnification X900.

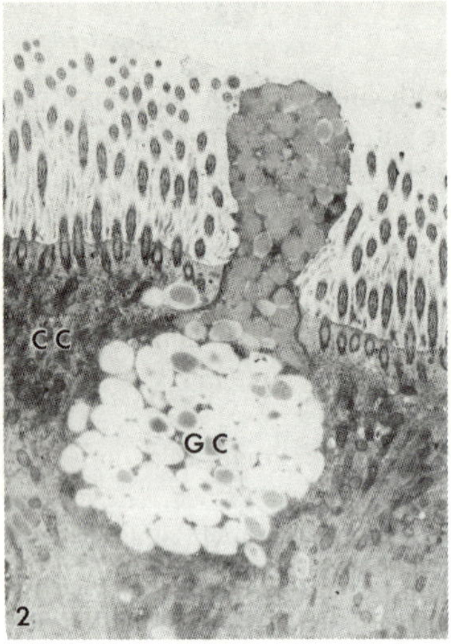

Figure 2 This transmission electron micrograph shows a goblet cell (GC) containing numerous secretory granules in an apical bleb and the underlying cytoplasm. The ciliated cells (CC) have numerous cilia and long branching microvilli. Original magnification X2280.

cavity (Figs. 2, 3). When present, this bleb was multilobulated as viewed from the surface and was sometimes covered by short microvilli. Very few cells were actively discharging the secretory granules. Some cells contained few secretory granules and were presumed to have recently completed the secretory phase. In the latter instance the surface of the cell was flat, or in some cases indented, with a disrupted plasma membrane. By TEM the secretory granules varied in

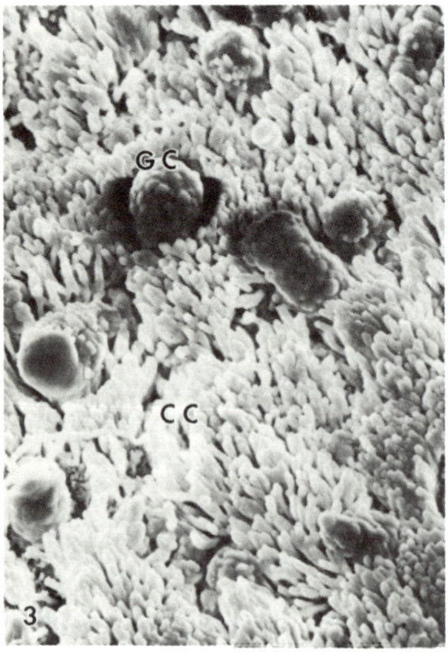

Figure 3 By scanning electron microscopy, the apical blebs of goblet cells (GC) are observed to be protruding between the ciliated cells (CC). Original magnification X780.

electron density but were the most striking morphologic feature of this cell type. The goblet cell was also characterized by a columnar shape and extensive smooth and rough ER. As the secretory granules filled the apical end of the cell, other organelles were concentrated below the nucleus.

The nonciliated columnar cell had a flat apical surface covered with numerous short (0.3 μm in length), nonbranching microvilli (Figs. 1, 4). As viewed by SEM, the borders of the cells were distinct since they formed ridges covered with microvilli (Fig. 1). The apical surface of the cells was variable in size and irregular in shape, usually consisting of 4-7 relatively straight sides. TEM demonstrated irregular lateral walls on the cells, which formed extensive interdigitations between the lower half of adjacent nonciliated cells. The most striking feature of this cell type was the extensive smooth ER, which typically filled much of the apical end of the cell, excluding other organelles (Fig. 4). Single or multiple well-developed Golgi complexes were usually found within the extensive smooth ER. Mitochondria were moderate in number and equally distributed throughout the cytoplasm.

The cuboidal cell was identified as either a simple cuboidal cell or a stratified cuboidal cell. The simple cuboidal cell extended from the nasal lumen to the basement membrane (Fig. 5). The apical surface had short microvilli (0.3 μm in length), which were much less numerous than the microvilli of the nonciliated columnar cell. On the apical surface the nonbranching microvilli were more numerous on the borders of the cell. The lateral plasmalemma formed extensive interdigitations with adjacent cells. Mitochondria and rough ER were sparse but evenly distributed throughout the cytoplasm. A small amount of smooth ER was identified in the apical end of the cell. The surface of the

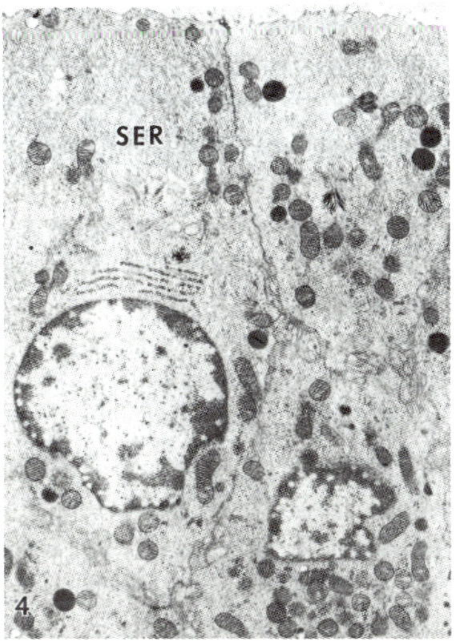

Figure 4 The extensive smooth endoplasmic reticulum (SER) in the apical end of the cell is the most striking feature of the nonciliated columnar cell as viewed by transmission electron microscopy. Original magnification X1824.

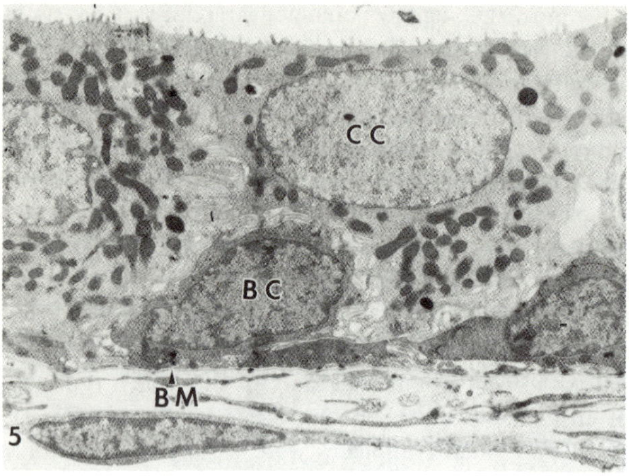

Figure 5 The basal cell (BC) is a flattened or cuboidal cell adjacent to the basement membrane (BM) as seen in this transmission electron micrograph. The simple cuboidal cell (CC) has no unique intracellular characteristic but does have extensive interdigitation of the plasma membrane with adjacent cells. Original magnification X1665.

stratified cuboidal epithelium was distinct when viewed by SEM. The cells were dome-shaped with moderate numbers of microvilli.

The basal cells were observed only by TEM since they were covered by other cell types and therefore not visible by SEM observation of the lumenal surface. The basal cells had a cuboidal or flattened shape but were always adjacent to the basement membrane (Fig. 5). They had a large nucleus and little cytoplasm. A few mitochondria and limited rough ER were found in the cytoplasm. The basal cells were variable in staining density, with some cells stained either lighter or darker than adjacent cells. They were characterized by dispersed or bundled microfilaments although extensive variation existed in the numbers of these filaments from cell to cell. Desmosomes connected the irregular lateral plasmalemmae of adjacent cells; hemidesmosomes connected the basal cell to the basement membrane.

The brush cell had distinct ultrastructural characteristics when viewed by both TEM and SEM. The cell typically had a pear shape with a wide base containing the nucleus and a narrow apical tip (1.5 μm in diameter) that projected into the lumen of the nasal meatus (Figs. 1, 6). The apical tip had dense nonbranching microvilli (0.7 μm in length), which made them easily distinguishable from any other cell type when viewed by both SEM and TEM. When viewed by SEM, this cell was always found at the junction of three or more cells. Typically, brush cells were found between nonciliated columnar cells. When observed by TEM, the brush cell had numerous bundles of microfilaments and microtubules in the apical end of the cell including the internal space of the microvilli. Small clear vesicles (0.09 μm in diameter) were usually found between the microfilaments and microtubules. Mitochondria were moderate in number and frequently irregular in shape. Long mitochondria invariably had the long axis perpendicular to the apical surface. Rough and smooth ER were poorly developed although a well-developed Golgi complex was frequently observed in the supranuclear region. Paired cisternae, composed of parallel rows of membrane without ribosomes on the external surface, were observed. This structure was typically adjacent to the nuclear membrane and usually found in a supranuclear location. The lateral plasmalemmae of adjacent cells were moderately interdigitated.

Intraepithelial axons were also noted between cells in the respiratory epithelium. They were characterized by pale-staining cytoplasm and contained a small number of neurotubules and small mitochondria. Small clear vesicles were sometimes observed. Rarely, membrane-bound vesicles contained dense core granules. Intraepithelial axons were usually found adjacent to the basement membrane, although they were occasionally found between the lateral plasmalemmae of epithelial cells. In the latter location they were always found in the lower half of the epithelium and were never observed extending into the apical half of the epithelium or into the lumen of the nasal cavity. Intraepithelial axons were found adjacent to all cell types and did not have a preferential location adjacent to any single cell type. Synapses between axons and epithelial cells were never observed.

Inflammatory cells were rarely encountered in the respiratory epithelium. An occasional neutrophil could be found between the various cell types.

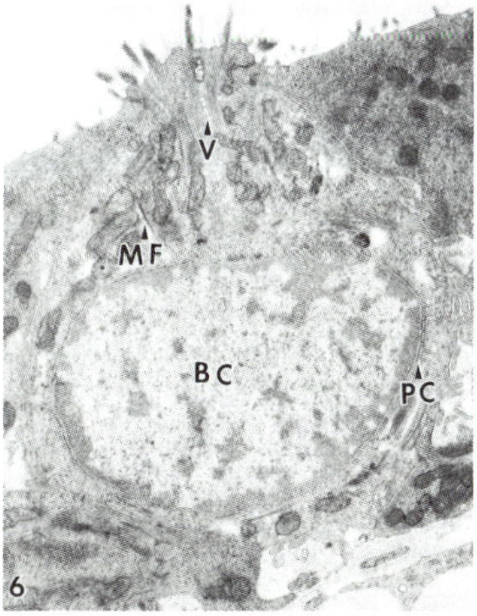

Figure 6 On the cross section, the brush cell (BC) frequently has a pear shape when viewed by transmission electron microscopy. Characteristic features include numerous clear vesicles (V) in the apical cytoplasm, bundles of microfilaments (MF), and paired cisternae (PC) adjacent to the nucleus. Original magnification X2280.

As previously shown by SEM, the cells of the respiratory epithelium were not uniformly distributed in the nasal mucosa. Starting just posterior to the squamous epithelium, a thin zone of stratified cuboidal cells was observed. Posterior to this zone, the anterior one-third of the maxilloturbinate, the nasoturbinate, and the lateral wall were generally composed of nonciliated cells. A few brush cells were observed between the nonciliated cells. Ciliated cells were few but, when observed, were individual cells surrounded by nonciliated cells. Goblet cells were randomly scattered in this area.

The middle third of the respiratory epithelium had more ciliated cells than the anterior third of the nasal mucosa. Ciliated cells were found individually, in short rows or in small clusters, until increased density obscured any pattern. Although generally more numerous in the middle third than the anterior third of the nasal mucosa, the distribution of ciliated cells varied on the different surfaces at the same level of the nasal cavity (Table 1). The medial side of the nasoturbinate had the highest density of ciliated cells when compared to other surfaces. The density of ciliated cells differed greatly on the two sides of a nasoturbinate, with ciliated cells covering 71% of the medial surface but only 4% of the lateral surface. Goblet cells were relatively uncommon at this level of the nasal cavity. Brush cells covered less than 1% of any nasal surface in the middle third of the respiratory epithelium.

In the distal third of the respiratory epithelium, all surfaces were covered primarily with ciliated cells. When compared to the middle third of the respiratory epithelium, goblet cells were more common and nonciliated cells were less common at this location. Brush cells were never observed, although they may have been obscured by the cilia or adjacent cells when SEM was used to map the various cell types.

Simple cuboidal cells were found primarily in the anterior respiratory epithelium and on the lateral wall. However, small areas of simple cuboidal cells

Table 1 Distribution of Various Cell Types in the Middle Third of the Respiratory Epithelium

	Percent of surface area			
Surface	Ciliated cells	Nonciliated cells	Brush cells	No. of brush cells (45600 μm^2)
Lateral wall	9.07	90.39	0.54	25
Lateral maxilloturbinate	20.25	79.12	0.63	32
Medial maxilloturbinate	15.30	84.66	0.04	4
Lateral nasoturbinate	4.46	95.35	0.19	14
Medial nasoturbinate	70.81	29.19	0.00	<1

[*Reproduced by permission (4).*]

were also found on the turbinates, particularly on the lateral surface of the nasoturbinate.

Although the respiratory epithelium is composed of extremely different proportions of the six cell types described depending on the location in the nose, a gradual transition exists in the proportions of these cell types. An abrupt change from one cell type to another was never seen.

The nasal septum had a relatively constant mixture of cell types from anterior to posterior. The septum was essentially covered with ciliated cells with numerous interspersed goblet cells. When viewed by TEM, the ciliated cells and goblet cells appeared to be longer and more slender than the same cells at other locations. Areas of nonciliated columnar cells or individual brush cells were not identified on the nasal septum. A focal area of olfactory epithelium was identified on the ventral posterior surface of the nasal septum anterior to the septal window.

The transition between respiratory epithelium and olfactory epithelium was generally abrupt at every location; however, the line of demarcation was irregular. Occasionally a single or few olfactory cells could be identified near the edge of the respiratory tissue but were separated from the olfactory tissue by a few respiratory epithelial cells.

The ultrastructure of the normal olfactory epithelium, as described previously by Graziadei (5), Jourdan (6), and Ohno et al. (7), was less complex than the ultrastructure of the normal respiratory epithelium for two reasons. First, only three or four cell types had been identified; second, they were uniformly distributed throughout the olfactory epithelium. The basal cell found in the olfactory epithelium was similar to the basal cell found at other locations, such as in the respiratory epithelium. However, the supporting cell (sustentacular cell) and the olfactory bipolar neuron had distinguishing ultrastructural characteristics.

The supporting cells were tall columnar cells with long, branched microvilli on the apical surface, which were intermingled with the cilia of the adjacent neuronal cells. The supporting cells also contained a large amount of smooth ER in the apical end, a well-developed Golgi apparatus, and numerous mitochondria. Other organelles were relatively modest in number, but electron-dense pigment granules were present. The nucleus of the supporting cell was located in the upper third of the epithelial layer.

The neuronal cells were tall and columnar with a centrally located nucleus and a narrow dendritic process leading to the apical surface. At the mucosal surface the dendritic process had an apical enlargement (2 μm in diameter), which is referred to as an olfactory vesicle. This structure contained numerous mitochondria, neurotubules, and neurofilaments. The olfactory vesicle protruded above the general level of the apical surface of the adjacent cells and was between the long microvilli of the supporting cells. It contained numerous basal bodies that gave rise to long cilia that protruded in all directions from the bulbous olfactory vesicle. These long cilia often covered the microvilli of the adjacent supporting cells and thus obstructed them from view when the apical surface was examined by SEM. By SEM the apical surface of the olfactory epithelium therefore consisted of a tangled web of cilia derived from the olfactory cell. Beneath the centrally placed nucleus, the cytoplasm of the olfactory cell formed a narrow axon which penetrated the basement membrane. In the submucosa the axons of numerous olfactory cells formed nerve bundles that became the olfactory nerve.

DISCUSSION

Recent ultrastructural studies by Monteiro-Riviere and Popp (3) and Popp and Martin (4) have provided an increased understanding of the complexity of the normal respiratory epithelium of the rat nasal cavity. The comparison of the cell types previously described in other areas of the respiratory tract and in other experimental species has been adequately discussed in these two papers. Clearly, the respiratory epithelium is composed of several different cell types which are unevenly distributed. This fact mandates that ultrastructural studies of either normal or pathologic nasal tissue include a clear definition of the area examined and a standardized procedure to assure that precisely the same area was examined in all animals. Orientation of tissue blocks from the turbinates also becomes critical since the ratio of the various cell types was normally very different on the two sides of a single turbinate even at a single cross-sectional level.

The normal olfactory epithelium of the rat has been described by electron microscopy by Ohno et al. (7) but appears to be less well defined than the olfactory epithelium of other species as reviewed by Graziadei (5). In addition to the three cell types described in the results, Jourdan (6) has described an additional cell type referred to as a type C cell. However, the brief description of this cell and the photograph presented both suggest that the type C cell is morphologically similar to the brush cell described in the respiratory epithelium by Monteiro-Riviere and Popp (3).

From information available at present, the selection and documentation of sample sites would appear to be less critical in studies of olfactory epithelium versus respiratory epithelium. Although the rat olfactory epithelium appears to be composed of only a few cell types, which are apparently uniformly mixed and distributed, caution in documenting the site of sample selection is still recommended until additional information is available.

It had become clear to us over the past several years that ultrastructural studies of toxin-induced nasal lesions could proceed only after a better understanding of the normal nasal mucosa was obtained. The definition of the multiple cell types in the rat respiratory epithelium now allows future ultrastructural studies to focus on possible cell specificity of toxin-induced damage to the nasal respiratory epithelium. It is possible, although not shown to date, that some toxins may affect only one cell type based on the biochemical or morphologic characteristics of the cell and not on the location of the cell in the nasal mucosa. For example, it is possible that toxins requiring metabolic activation may result in toxicity of only one cell type if that cell type is the only one capable of the metabolic process required. In addition, a basic understanding of the cell distribution in the normal rat nasal mucosa is essential before studies can clarify whether alterations in the cell distribution have resulted from a nasal toxicant. It is certainly possible that a subchronic or chronic toxic response of the nasal cavity could result in normal-appearing cells but with an abnormal distribution. SEM has proved to be a useful tool in determining cell distribution in the normal nasal mucosa and will certainly continue to be useful in documenting abnormal distributions of cell types. Abnormal distribution of cell types in response to a nasal toxicant could be due to the loss of ciliated cells or other specific cells within the nasal cavity with the abnormality restricted to a small portion of the nasal mucosa.

Since most rodent toxicity studies are performed to assess potential toxicity in man, the similarities or dissimilarities of the nasal mucosa in rat and man are of primary importance. Jafek (8) recently provided a review of the literature as well as additional observations on the ultrastructural characteristics of human nasal mucosa. This work, however, clearly demonstrated that the descriptive information for man is very limited compared to the information available for rats. Obvious technical and ethical problems in obtaining well-fixed tissue from well-defined areas of the human nasal cavity account for this difference in available information. Nevertheless, some comparisons can be made between the ultrastructural characteristics and cell types in the nasal cavity of man and rat.

Jafek (8) reiterates the long-held impression that the human respiratory epithelium is a pseudo-stratified, ciliated, columnar epithelium in at least some areas of the nasal cavity. In contrast, no truly pseudo-stratified columnar epithelium was noted in our rodent studies, where the tallest epithelium was simple columnar. TEM and SEM studies led Jafek (8) to conclude that the human nasal respiratory epithelium was composed of four cell types: ciliated, goblet, intermediate, and basal. Whereas the ciliated, basal, and actively secreting goblet cells are very similar in man and rat, no cell type was described in man that would be the counterpart to the nonciliated columnar cells described in the rat. Nonciliated cells were certainly observed between ciliated cells in the human respiratory epithelium but were interpreted to be resting goblet cells. While the distinction between a resting goblet cell and a nonciliated columnar cell may be difficult when viewing an individual cell, the observation of numerous nonciliated columnar cells in areas where few to no goblet cells existed clearly demonstrated that the nonciliated columnar cells were distinct from goblet cells in the rat. Whether a counterpart to the nonciliated columnar cell of the rat exists in human nasal mucosa is uncertain at this time. The brush cell found in other areas of the respiratory tract in man and in the nasal mucosa (respiratory epithelium) in the rat was not identified in human nasal mucosa even though the cell was specifically sought by Jafek (8). In addition to the questions arising on the existence of comparable cell types in the nasal mucosa of rat and man, a greater question exists as to the distribution of the various cell types in the nasal mucosa of man. Although mapping studies are incomplete in the rat, available information obtained by Popp and Martin (4) showed that great differences in cell distribution do occur. In contrast, essentially no information was available on the distribution of various cell types in the human nasal respiratory epithelium.

The ultrastructural features of human olfactory epithelium have been well described in a recent report by Moran et al. (9). The basal cell, supporting cell, and olfactory cell were morphologically similar to the same cell types in a variety of other species as reviewed by Graziadei (5). However, Moran et al. (9) clearly described a "microvillar cell" similar to the brush cell Monteiro-Riviere and Popp (3) described in the respiratory epithelium of the rat. The comparable cell is apparently also found in the olfactory mucosa of rats since the type C cell described by Jourdan (6) in rats is morphologically similar to the microvillar cell described by Moran et al. (9). It should be noted that sex differences were described by Saini and Breipohl (10) in the ultrastructural characteristics of olfactory mucosa in rhesus monkeys. While the morphology of the olfactory epithelium was constant in males, the length of the olfactory vesicles and apical projections of the supporting cell varied with the ovulatory cycle in females. Although sex differences and differences in relation to the ovulatory cycle have apparently not been described in rat or man, these differences should be kept in mind if comparisons of olfactory epithelium ultrastructure are made between rats and humans.

In summary, available ultrastructural studies on the normal epithelium lining the rat nasal cavity have provided information on the complexity of the normal structure and a baseline of information for subsequent toxicity studies. This information will be useful in characterizing and understanding the mechanisms of future nasal toxicity studies. However, additional information is needed on the ultrastructural characteristics of the normal human nasal mucosa, particularly the distribution of various cell types, before one can ascertain the relevance of ultrastructural studies of the rodent nasal mucosa to potential injury of the human nasal mucosa.

SUMMARY

The ultrastructure of the rat nasal mucosa has recently been investigated. TEM and SEM demonstrated that six morphologically distinct cell types were found in the respiratory epithelium of the rat nasal mucosa. These included ciliated, goblet, nonciliated columnar, cuboidal, basal, and brush cells. SEM clearly demonstrated that these cell types were not distributed uniformly in the respiratory epithelium. In general, the density of ciliated cells increased from the anterior to the posterior areas of the respiratory epithelium; however, the degree of ciliation was variable when the different surfaces were compared at a single cross-sectional level of the nasal cavity. The olfactory epithelium was composed of three cell types: basal, supporting, and neuronal. These cell types appeared to be evenly distributed in the olfactory epithelium.

REFERENCES

1 Raynor, TH, EL White, JM Cheplen, JM Sherrill, and TE Hamm, Jr. An evaluation of a water purification system for use in animal facilities. *Lab. Anim.* 18:45–51 (1984).
2 Popp, JA, and JT Martin. Method for the ultrastructural evaluation of rodent nasal mucosa. In *39th Annual Proceedings, Electron Microscopy Society of America,* edited by GW Bailey. Baton Rouge, LA: Claitors Publishing, pp. 594–595 (1981).
3 Monteiro-Riviere, N, and JA Popp. Ultrastructural characterization of the nasal respiratory epithelium in the rat. *Am. J. Anat.* 169:31–43 (1984).
4 Popp, JA, and JT Martin. Surface topography and distribution of cell types in the rat nasal respiratory epithelium: Scanning electron microscopic observations. *Am. J. Anat.* 169:425–436 (1984).
5 Graziadei, PPC. The ultrastructure of vertebrate olfactory mucosa. In *The Ultrastructure of Sensory Organs,* edited by I Friedman. Amsterdam: Elsevier North Holland, pp. 269–305 (1973).
6 Jourdan, MF. Ultrastructure de l'epithelium olfactif du rat: Polymorphisme des recepteurs. *C. R. Acad. Sci. Paris* 280:443–446 (1975).
7 Ohno, I, M Okyama, Y Hanamure, and K Ogawa. Comparative anatomy of olfactory epithelium. *Biomed. Res. Suppl.* 2:455–458 (1981).
8 Jafek, BW. Ultrastructure of human nasal mucosa. *Laryngoscope* 93:1576–1599 (1983).
9 Moran, DT, JC Rowley, BW Jafek, and MA Lovell. The fine structure of the olfactory mucosa in man. *J. Neurocytol.* 11:721–746 (1982).
10 Saini, KD, and W Breipohl. Surface morphology in the olfactory epithelium of normal male and female rhesus monkeys. *Am. J. Anat.* 147:433–445 (1976).

Chapter 4

Histopathology of Acute and Subacute Nasal Toxicity

Xue-Zhi Jiang, Kevin T. Morgan, and Robert O. Beauchamp, Jr.

INTRODUCTION

Laboratory animals, especially rats and mice, have been widely used for inhalation toxicology studies, but the majority of these investigations were confined to the lower respiratory tract, while the nasal passages received much less attention (1). A review of the literature on inhalation studies of gaseous irritants and other airborne contaminants revealed detailed descriptions of neoplastic findings in the nasal passages with little or no mention of nonneoplastic effects, except for the more recent studies (2-7). The purpose of this chapter is to present a general description and classification of acute and subacute nonneoplastic responses observed in the nasal passages of rodents, with most of the material being derived from studies at the Chemical Industry Institute of Toxicology (CIIT). The nasal passages of rodents are complex, and the precise localization of lesions often presents a problem, especially if various treatments are to be compared. Procedures developed at CIIT to address this problem will also be discussed.

DETECTION OF NASAL LESIONS

Nasal lesions may be suspected on the basis of clinical signs, such as nose rubbing and nasal or ocular discharge. Gross observations during necropsy are generally not very helpful unless a large space-occupying lesion is present, resulting in protrusions beyond the normal limits of the nasal passages. However, during preparation of tissue blocks for embedding, following the procedures described by Young (1), careful examination of the cut surface will often reveal lesions. After fixation and decalcification, multiple transverse blocks are needed so that the major regions of the nose are represented in sections. Generally, lesions induced by highly water soluble gaseous irritants are localized in the anterior portion of the nose. It is important to prepare appropriate blocks to include the nasal vestibule, in addition to the sections recommended by other workers (1, 5) and not to discard residual tissue, as localized lesions may be lost. Tissues may be embedded in paraffin, but the use of glycol methacrylate (GMA) is recommended, as this medium provides superior resolution of toxic effects.

Familiarity with the complex arrangement of the three types of epithelium in the nose and their morphologic characteristics in the species under study is essential. For instance, the anterior limit of the olfactory epithelium in the dorsal meatus has a transitional zone, which is sparsely populated with sensory cells and which may be readily confused with toxin-induced olfactory epithelial degeneration. The morphologic features of the olfactory epithelium vary considerably between species (8). In the respiratory epithelium, goblet cells have a clear distribution pattern in rodents, and knowledge of this distribution pattern assists the diagnosis of goblet cell hyperplasia. The shape of the nasoturbinates and other structures changes with age (unpublished observations), as do the distribution and morphologic characteristics of the nasal epithelia. Furthermore, infectious agents may induce lesions in the nasal mucosa. A detailed description of aging lesions and effects of a range of infectious agents on the nasal passages of laboratory animals is not available, and careful examination of control animals is probably the best way to avoid confusion of aging lesions with treatment-related effects.

MAPPING OF NASAL LESIONS

The nasal passages of rodents are very complex, and lesions may occur in small but distinct regions. Mapping procedures may be useful when recording toxic responses to gaseous irritants. The precise determination of lesion distribution in the nose may be of value as it can lead to (1) the identification of sensitive or susceptible sites, (2) correlations with factors that influence the delivery of inhaled irritants to specific regions of the nose, such as mucus flow and air flow patterns, (3) comparison of acute with chronic effects, and (4) comparisons between different irritants for effects on each of the epithelial types.

The type and distribution of lesions may be recorded on complex or simple maps that portray the nose in either the transverse or longitudinal axis. Each of the major regions of the nose has distinct functions, and thus it is important that the maps indicate the location of each of the three principal epithelial types. Different lesions, such as epithelial erosions, ulceration, or squamous metaplasia, may be recorded with different-colored markers or cross-hatching (Fig. 1). A simple map, such as that shown in Fig. 2, combined with a table summarizing the nature and severity of lesions, was found to facilitate comparison of the effects of 10 different gaseous irritants in a recent study (9).

RESPONSES TO TOXIC AGENTS

Nasal epithelial lesions, following exposure to noxious air contaminants, can generally be placed in one or more of the following categories: degeneration,

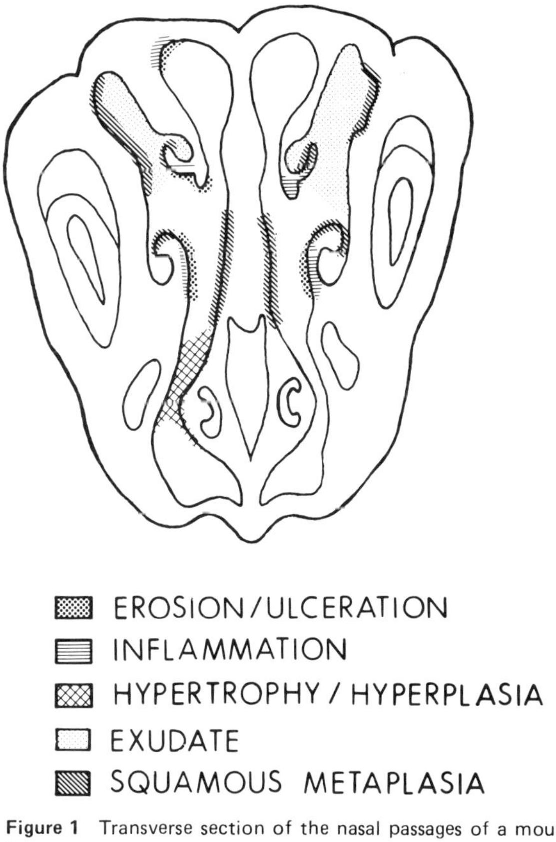

Figure 1 Transverse section of the nasal passages of a mouse to show the major structures for mapping of lesions. The locations of lesions in a mouse exposed to acrolein gas for 5 days are shown.

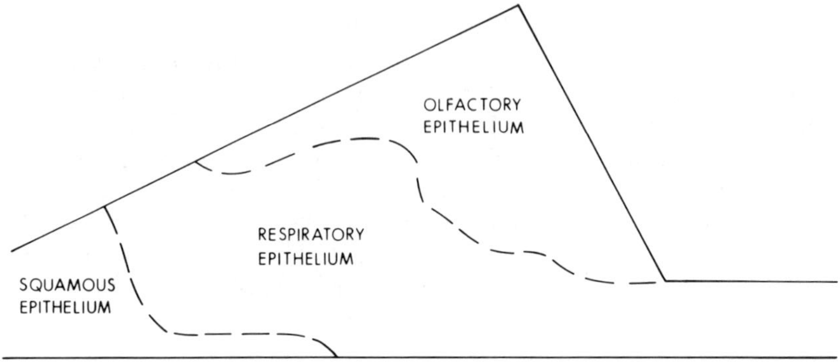

Figure 2 Simple diagram of rodent nasal passages in the longitudinal axis. The broken lines indicate the boundaries of the three major epithelial types. This diagram is suitable for recording lesion location in the long axis of the nose.

inflammation, repair, defense or adaptation, and proliferation. If airway defenses are overcome, degenerative changes will be induced in the nasal epithelial cells, which will lead to inflammation and subsequent repair. Continued exposure to the agent may result in adaptive or defensive responses such as squamous metaplasia or goblet cell hyperplasia. Repair of damaged epithelium requires cell proliferation to cover erosions or ulcerations of the nasal epithelium, and excessive proliferation will result in hyperplasia or even neoplasia. Several stages of these responses are often present in the same animal, with varying severity from one region of the nose to another, presumably as a result of local differences in exposure or tissue susceptibility. A valuable indication of nasal toxicity, which is readily detected by low-power light microscopy, is exudate in the nasal lumen (Fig. 3). If the nasal passages are flushed with fixative, exudate may be lost in the major airway while being retained in the complex ethmoid region (Fig. 4). The morphologic features of toxic effects on the three main regions of the nose—i.e., those lined by squamous, respiratory, or olfactory epithelium—will be described, with examples from studies carried out at CIIT.

Region of Squamous Epithelium

Generally, the squamous epithelium is unresponsive and it may exhibit little or no change while very severe lesions are present in other regions of the nose. However, with a sufficiently high concentration of a gaseous irritant, this epithelium may be damaged. Erosions or ulceration are usually focal, being most frequently present on the margins of the naso- and maxilloturbinates in the vestibule (Fig. 5) and the lateral wall adjacent to these free margins. Generally, these lesions are bilateral and often symmetric, but in some cases they are present in only one of the nasal passages. When the squamous epithelium is breached there are generally lesions in the underlying tissues such as cartilage

(Fig. 5) or bone (Fig. 6). The thin strip of squamous epithelium in the ventral meatus is sometimes affected, giving rise to small lesions (Fig. 7) that may be overlooked. Less severe changes in the squamous epithelium include increased numbers of surface squames, which are best revealed by scanning electron microscopy (SEM).

Region of Respiratory Epithelium

Lesions in the respiratory epithelium may be superficial or extend to the subepithelial tissues (Fig. 8). The mildest effects generally involve the cilia, which may be lost over extensive areas, with only minimal changes in the underlying epithelial cells. This effect was frequently seen in mice and rats exposed to chlorine gas (7). Persistence of a deciliated epithelium with apparently little effect on the underlying epithelial cells may depend on continued mucus flow over the surface, which has been reported in rats exposed to chlorine (Morgan et al., Chapter 8).

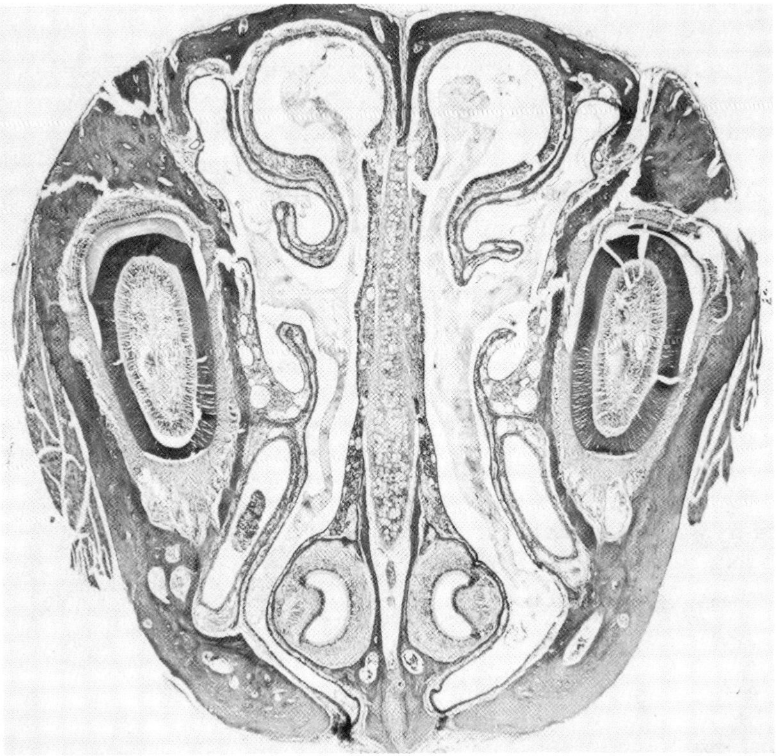

Figure 3 Paraffin section of the nose of a mouse (male, Swiss Webster) exposed to 9 ppm chlorine gas for 5 days (6 h/day). The nasal cavity contains serocellular exudate, and lesions in the nasal epithelium are not so distinct at this magnification. H&E X26.

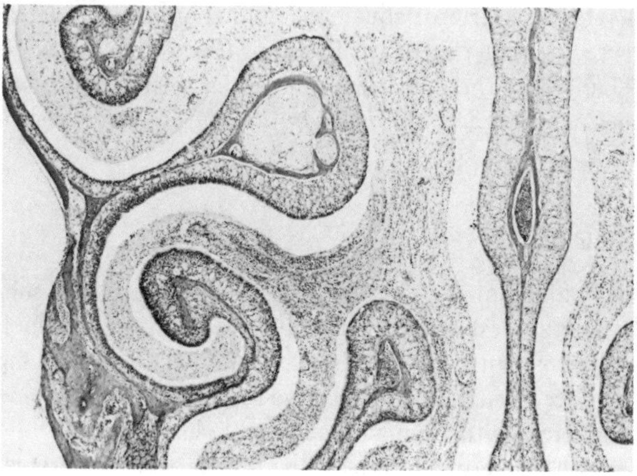

Figure 4 Paraffin section of a mouse exposed to chlorine (as in Fig. 3) to show highly cellular exudate enmeshed in the complex ethmoid turbinates in the posterior region of the nose. H&E X29.

In chlorine toxicity, cilia were replaced by numerous microvilli, whereas remaining ciliated cells had only very short cilia (7). The fate of the cilia has yet to be established; however, recent work on nasal toxicity of formaldehyde revealed that loss of cilia from the surface may be due to their internalization by the epithelial cells (Monteiro-Riviere and Popp, unpublished observations). Loss of cilia is best demonstrated in scanning electron micrographs, but it is readily identified by light microscopy.

Rodents exposed to highly water soluble, gaseous irritants most often have

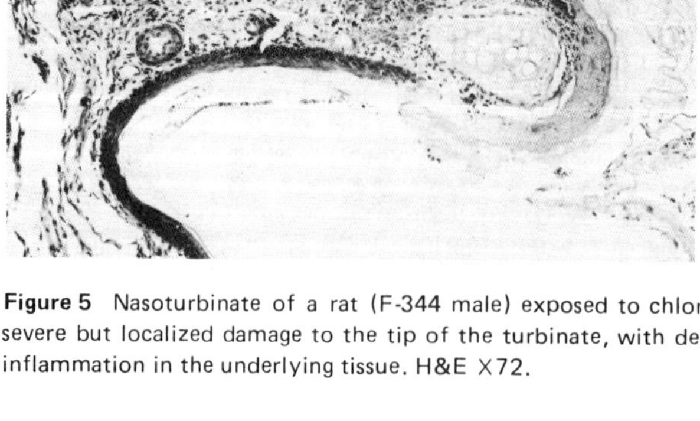

Figure 5 Nasoturbinate of a rat (F-344 male) exposed to chlorine (as in Fig. 3), to show severe but localized damage to the tip of the turbinate, with degeneration of cartilage and inflammation in the underlying tissue. H&E X72.

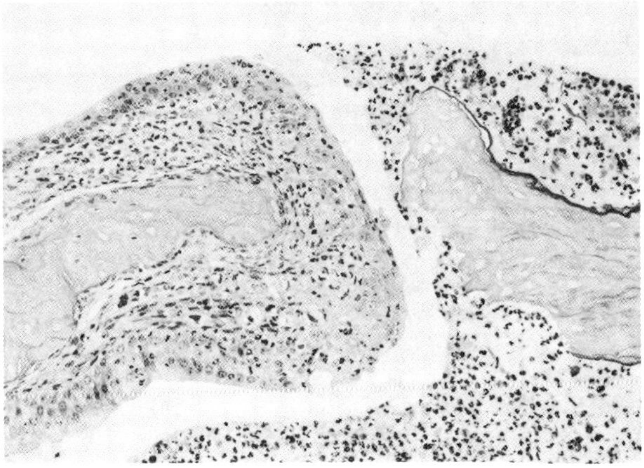

Figure 6 Glycol methacrylate (GMA) section of a mouse exposed to 175 ppm dimethylamine (6 months, 6 h/day, 5 days/week) to show the tip of the nasoturbinate in the vestibule. The squamous epithelium is thickened and infiltrated by inflammatory cells; much of the bone is necrotic, as very few lacunae contain osteocytes. Lees methylene blue basic fuchsin (LMB) X72.

lesions on the free margins of the naso- and maxilloturbinates (Fig. 9) and the adjacent lateral wall. There is generally a distinct anteroposterior gradient of lesion severity, with the greatest effect in the anterior nose. Early degeneration of epithelial cells is characterized by bleb formation, cell separation, and

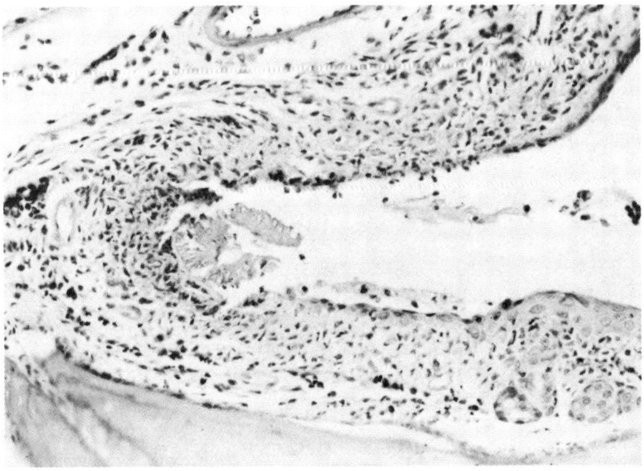

Figure 7 Ventral meatus of a mouse (B6C3F1) exposed to approximately 50 ppm hydrogen chloride (unpublished observations; 6 h/day, 5 days/week). There is severe degeneration, and almost complete loss of the squamous epithelium of the floor of the ventral meatus, with inflammation in the underlying tissue. This lesion extended posteriorly to the incisive canal. H&E X142.

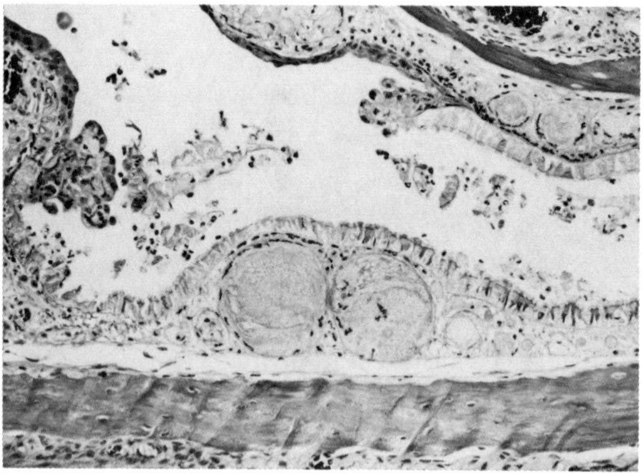

Figure 8 Paraffin section of the ventral meatus of a mouse (Swiss Webster) exposed to 300 ppm hydrogen chloride (1 day, 6 h/day, found moribund). The respiratory epithelium of the ventral meatus is necrotic, having lost much of the normal staining affinity, and several small blood vessels are plugged by fibrin thrombi or erythrocyte ghosts. H&E X142.

exfoliation, which are readily observed by both light (Fig. 10) and scanning electron microscopy (7). Fairly extensive loss of epithelial cells is often associated with an apparently intact basement membrane, and more severe lesions lead to frank ulceration. Once the epithelium is disrupted, the affected areas

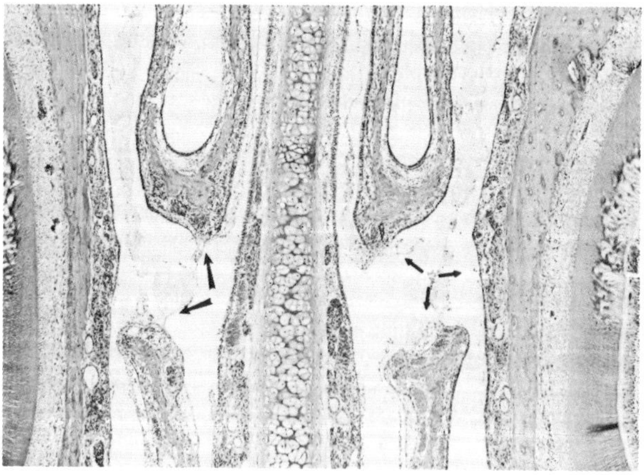

Figure 9 Paraffin section of the nasal passages of a mouse (Swiss Webster) exposed to 9 ppm chlorine (3 days, 6 h/day) to show regions where lesions were most frequently encountered with gaseous irritants—i.e., margins of turbinates and adjacent lateral wall (small arrows). This mouse had focal ulceration on the naso- and maxilloturbinates (large arrows), and exudate adhering to some of the ulcerated areas. H&E X28.

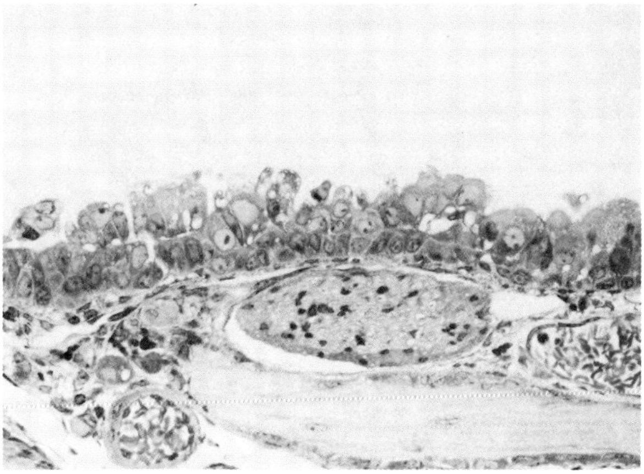

Figure 10 GMA section of the ventral nasal septum bordering the nasal window of a mouse (Swiss Webster) exposed to 1.7 ppm acrolein (5 days, 6 h/day). Respiratory epithelial cells are in various stages of degeneration, some being shed into the lumen. LMB X284.

become covered by a crust or "scab" of fibrinocellular material, which is variably infiltrated by inflammatory cells. If the exposure is not repeated, the affected areas are repaired, being covered finally by normal respiratory epithelium.

Repeated exposure most frequently leads to foci or zones of squamous metaplasia in which the normal respiratory epithelium is replaced by squamous epithelium. This squamous epithelium is presumably more resistant to the toxic effects of the gas and represents a very common adaptive response by the nose. A characteristic feature of early squamous metaplasia, which assists in its identification, is altered orientation of epithelial cell nuclei, which become more parallel to the epithelial basement membrane (Fig. 11*a*). Thin, fusiform, or squamous cells then become more numerous (Fig. 11*b*), and in extreme instances there may be extensive keratinization of the epithelium (5). In our experience, irritants differ considerably in their ability to induce squamous metaplasia (9).

A response that is frequently observed following repeated exposure to gaseous irritants is goblet cell hyperplasia, as has been reported following exposure to formaldehyde gas (5). This response may be associated with increased amounts of mucus with altered staining properties due to increased quantities of acidic mucous glycoproteins (10). The significance of the altered staining characteristics is unknown, but it may reflect changes in the viscoelastic properties of the mucus and indicate possible effects on airway clearance mechanisms.

Other incidental lesions that occur in respiratory epithelium with some frequency include small foci of mineralization that are often found adjacent to the basement membrane, and folding of the respiratory epithelium (Fig. 12) with

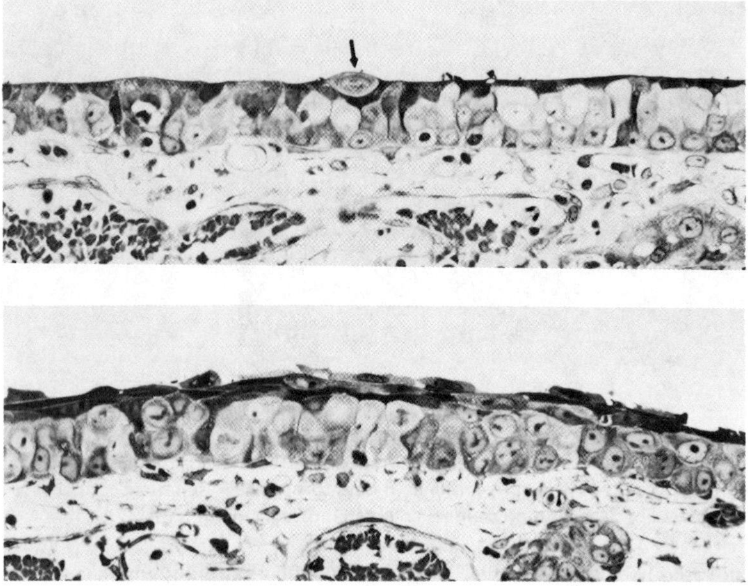

Figure 11 (*a*) GMA section of the lateral wall of a mouse (Swiss Webster) exposed to 9 ppm chlorine (5 days, 6 h/day) in a region normally lined by ciliated respiratory epithelium. The cilia are gone, and a superficial cell exhibits a 90° rotation of its axis to lie parallel to the basement membrane (arrow), indicating an early stage of squamous metaplasia. LMB X365. (*b*) Area adjacent to that in Fig. 11*a* exhibiting numerous superficial squames, a more advanced stage of squamous metaplasia. LMB X365.

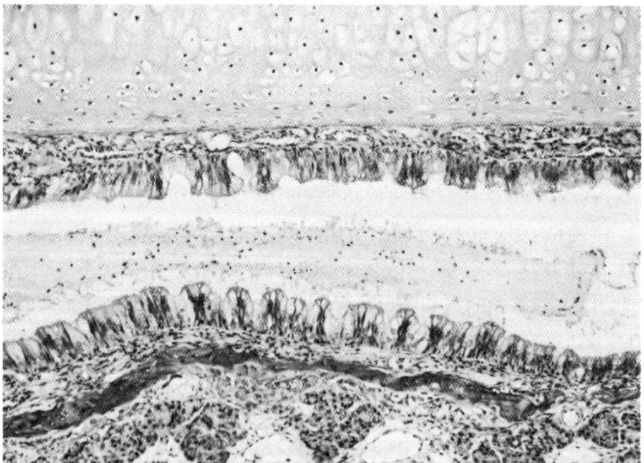

Figure 12 Paraffin section of the nasal septum (top) and medial nasoturbinate (bottom) of a mouse (Swiss Webster) exposed to 9 ppm chlorine gas (see Fig. 11*a*) to show folding and thickening of the respiratory epithelium. H&E X142.

or without goblet cell accumulation in the folds. The folds that are lined by goblet cells sometimes resemble small glands. Certain areas of the nose, such as the posterior ventral margin of the nasoturbinate, are normally folded and this could lead to confusion.

Another change observed in rats and mice exposed to gaseous irritants, and less frequently in untreated controls, is the intraepithelial, eosinophilic, or hyaline globule (11). These globules are distinctly eosinophilic in H&E-stained sections observed by light microscopy, and they vary in size (generally 2-10 μm diameter) and number. The globules are round and generally lie intracellularly between the nucleus and the base of cells of the respiratory epithelium (Fig. 13). The nature of this material and the reason for its increase in association with exposure to inhaled irritants are unknown, but in some cases it is present extensively throughout the respiratory epithelium, especially on the nasoturbinate and the nasal septum. Morphologically similar material is seen in the olfactory epithelium (see below).

Region of Olfactory Epithelium

It is important to also be familiar with the normal structure of the olfactory mucosa, and changes associated with aging in the species under study. The height of the olfactory epithelium, the number of sensory cells, and the number and size of olfactory nerves and features of Bowman's glands vary considerably. If sections from controls do not include the same regions (almost exactly),

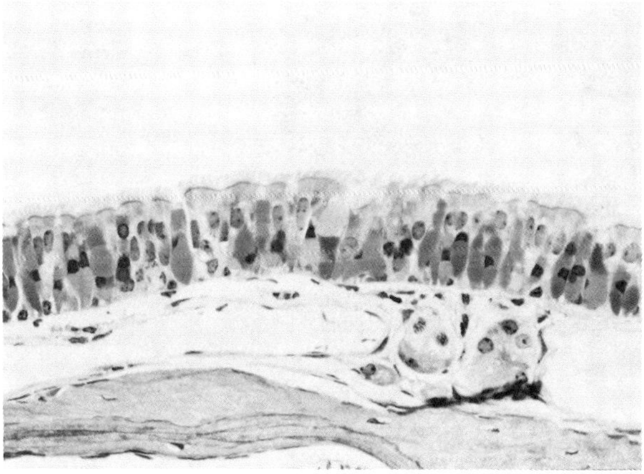

Figure 13 GMA section of respiratory epithelium on the nasoturbinate of a mouse exposed to dimethylamine for 6 months (see Fig. 6) to show numerous hyaline globules or droplets in the columnar epithelial cells. These globules are strongly eosinophilic. LMB X284.

inexperience with nasal morphology of the species under study could lead to misinterpretation.

Many of the gaseous irritants studied recently at CIIT have been found to induce lesions in the olfactory epithelium of rats and mice (7, 9, 11). These lesions ranged from slight disruption or loss of olfactory cilia to complete destruction of the olfactory epithelium in certain regions of the nose. The most frequently affected site in rats and mice is the anteriodorsal extension of the olfactory mucosa into the middle third of the dorsal meatus (Fig. 14). This region of the nose should be examined routinely in inhalation studies of gaseous irritants, as lesions may be very severe in this small region of the nose while being slight or absent more posteriorly. Because of hardness of the nasal bones and the delicate nature of the olfactory mucosa, this region of the rodent nose is prone to artifacts such as folding of the section, which will obscure lesions. Rotation of the block in the microtome prior to sectioning will sometimes alleviate this problem.

Loss of sensory cells may be fairly severe without apparent disruption of the general structure of the olfactory epithelium and may thus be overlooked. Acute exposure of mice to chlorine resulted in stripping of the olfactory epithelium in some regions of the nose (cf. Fig. 15 and 16), with fragments of degenerating epithelium lying in serofibrinous exudate in the nasal lumen (7). The denuded areas were subsequently covered by fusiform cells, which appeared to spread in from the side of the lesion, or from the ducts of Bowman's glands in the damaged region. The progression of repair of the olfactory region subse-

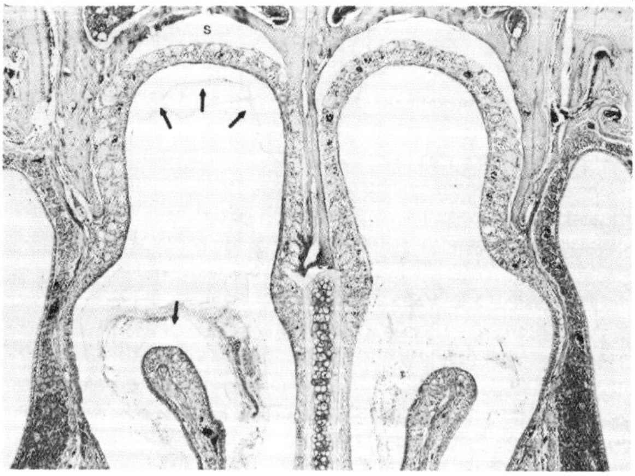

Figure 14 Paraffin section of a mouse (Swiss Webster) exposed to 9 ppm chlorine (see Fig. 12) to show the regions in which olfactory lesions frequently occur (arrows). The olfactory epithelium is almost completely destroyed in this case, leaving just a thin layer of fusiform cells covering the basement membrane. The separation (S) or space between the nasal bones and the olfactory mucosa in the dorsal meatus is a common artifact. H&E X28.

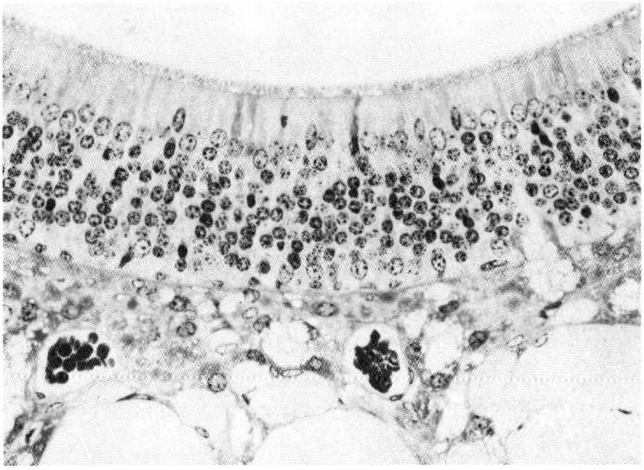

Figure 15 GMA section of olfactory epithelium in the dorsal meatus of a normal control mouse. LMB X284.

quently followed a number of distinctly different paths, which have yet to be reported in detail for gaseous irritants. The alternatives based on our observations include (1) recovery of the olfactory epithelium, (2) formation of a squamous epithelium which superficially resembles squamous metaplasia, or (3) replacement of the olfactory epithelium with well-differentiated, ciliated respiratory epithelium (Fig. 17). The factors that control the type of differentiation during the recovery or adaptive stages of responses to irritant gases, which presumably include the

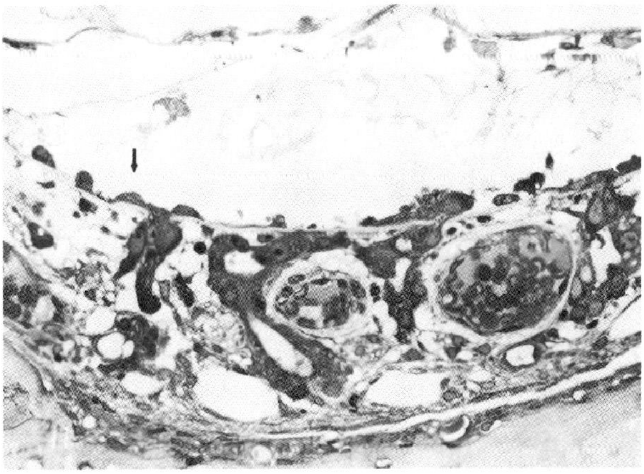

Figure 16 GMA section of olfactory mucosa of a mouse (B6C3F1) exposed to 9 ppm chlorine gas (5 day, 6 h/day). The olfactory epithelium has been completely destroyed, leaving a naked basement membrane in some areas. Note fusiform cells, contiguous with epithelium of hypertrophic ducts of Bowman's glands (arrow). LMB X284.

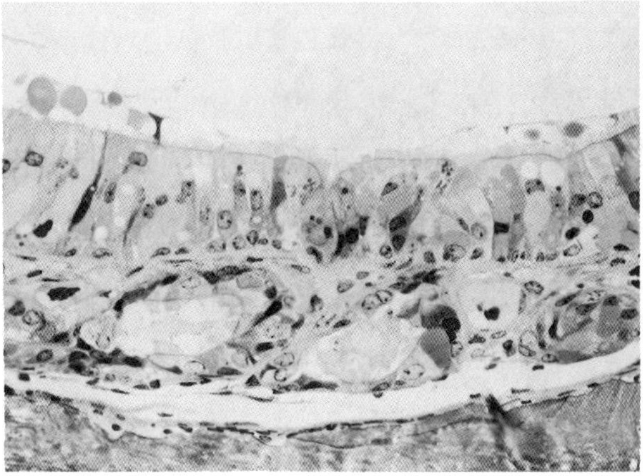

Figure 17 An area adjacent to that shown in Fig. 17. The olfactory epithelium in the center of the field has been replaced by an epithelium resembling tall, ciliated respiratory type. LMB X284.

degree and extent of damage inflicted, have yet to be determined. The metaplastic ciliated respiratory epithelium was seen in some cases to be continuous with ciliated epithelium lining ducts of hypertrophic Bowman's glands (11), which lends support to the proposal of Schultz (12) that these glands may play an important role in response of the olfactory mucosa to chemical damage.

A change that is seen in aging control animals, and that is augmented by exposure to at least one gaseous irritant, dimethylamine (11), is the accumu-

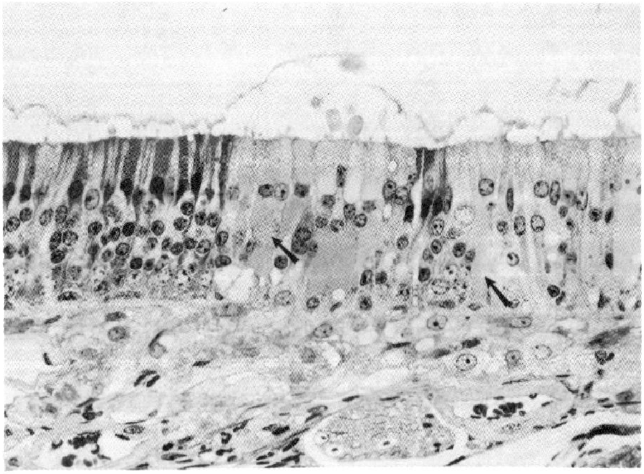

Figure 18 GMA section of olfactory epithelium in the dorsal meatus of a mouse (B6C3F1) exposed to dimethylamine (see Fig. 6). Note loss of sensory cells and accumulations of hyaline material in hypertrophied sustentacular cells (arrows). LMB X284.

lation of eosinophilic material as globules or lakes in olfactory epithelial sustentacular cells. This material resembles that found in respiratory epithelium, except for its location in the affected cells (Fig. 18). The nature of this material, which is presumed to be secretory in nature (11), has yet to be characterized.

SUMMARY

Selected examples of toxic responses by the nasal passages of rodents are described. It is evident that much remains to be learned about the nature and significance of lesions induced by inhaled gaseous irritants in the nasal passages of laboratory animals. Because nasal lesions associated with aging have yet to be adequately described, appropriate material from untreated control animals of the same age and sex is essential when attempting to interpret treatment-related changes in inhalation studies. Mapping of lesion type and distribution provides a valuable tool for histopathology studies and should lead to the identification of more sensitive or susceptible sites in nasal passages for toxic effects. One site that is readily damaged by gaseous irritants is the olfactory epithelium of the dorsal meatus in rats and mice. Further work is needed to assess the value of the rodent for human risk assessment with respect to damage of the complex mucosa of the nasal airway.

REFERENCES

1 Young JT. Histopathologic examination of the rat nasal cavity. *Fund. Appl. Toxicol.* 1:309–312 (1981).
2 Feron VJ, and A Kruysse. Effects of exposure to furfural vapour in hamsters simultaneously treated with benzo[*a*]pyrene or diethylnitrosamine. *Toxicology* 11:127–144 (1978).
3 Miller RR, JF Quast, JA Ayres, and MJ McKenna. Inhalation toxicity of butylene oxide. *Fund. Appl. Toxicol.* 1:319–324 (1981).
4 Haschek WM, CC Morse, MR Boyd, PJ Hakkinen, and HP Witschi. Pathology of acute inhalation exposure to 3-methylfuran in the rat and hamster. *Exp. Mol. Pathol.* 39:342–354 (1983).
5 Kerns WD, KL Pavkov, DJ Donofrio, EJ Gralla, and JA Swenberg. Carcinogenicity of formaldehyde in rats and mice after long-term inhalation exposure. *Cancer Res.* 43:4382–4392 (1983).
6 Chang JCF, EA Gross, JA Swenberg, and CS Barrow. Nasal cavity deposition, histopathology, and cell proliferation after single or repeated formaldehyde exposures in B6C3F1 mice and F-344 rats. *Toxicol. Appl. Pharmacol.* 68:161–176 (1983).
7 Jiang, XZ, LA Buckley, KT Morgan. Pathology of toxic responses to the RD50 concentration of chlorine gas in the nasal passages of rats and mice. *Toxicol. Appl. Pharmacol.* 71:225–236 (1983).

8 Negus V. *The Comparative Anatomy and Physiology of the Nose and Paranasal Sinuses.* Edinburgh and London: Livingstone (1958).
9 Buckley LA, XZ Jiang, RA James, KT Morgan, and CS Barrow. Respiratory tract lesions induced by sensory irritants at the RD50 concentration. *Toxicol. Appl. Pharmacol.* 74:417–429 (1984).
10 Jones R, P Bolduc, and L Reid. Goblet cell glycoprotein and tracheal gland hypertrophy in rat airways: The effect of tobacco smoke with or without the anti-inflammatory agent phenylmethyloxadiazole. *Br. J. Exp. Pathol.* 54:229–239 (1973).
11 Buckley LA, KT Morgan, JA Swenberg, RA James, TE Hamm Jr, and CS Barrow. The toxicity of dimethylamine in F-344 rats and B6C3F1 mice following a 1 year inhalation exposure. *Fund. Appl. Toxicol.* 5:341–352 (1985).
12 Schultz EW. Repair of the olfactory mucosa. *Am. J. Pathol.* 37:1–19 (1960).

Chapter 5

Pathology of Chronic Nasal Toxic Responses Including Cancer

V. J. Feron, R. A. Woutersen, and B. J. Spit

INTRODUCTION

Nasal cancer is comparatively rare in the general population but relatively common in nickel refinery workers and in workers engaged in the manufacture of wooden furniture or leather boots and shoes. In these industries there is clear evidence that the causative factor is in or associated with dust particles (1, 2).

It is well known that a series of nitrosamines is capable of inducing nasal tumors in rats and hamsters (3). In addition, in the past 5 years, tumors of the nose have been reported to occur in experimental animals after inhalation exposure to a variety of important industrial chemicals such as formaldehyde (4), bis(chloromethyl) ether (5), hexamethylphosphoramide (6), phenylglycidyl ether (7), epichlorohydrin (8), and vinyl chloride (9). Although workers have

The authors thank Dr. A. P. de Groot and Professor Dr. Ir. R. J. J. Hermus for critically reviewing the manuscript, Mr. F. van Welie for the photographic work, and Mrs. Nora Polter for typing the manuscript. The long-term inhalation study with 2,3,4-trichlorobutene-1 in rats was sponsored by the Joint Industry Committee on Chloroprene.

been exposed to some of these chemicals for many years, epidemiological studies do not indicate an increased risk for nasal cancer in the groups of workers concerned. However, rodents are obligatory nose breathers in contrast to humans, and, as a result, changes found in the noses of rodents after inhalation exposure may be predictive of effects on more distal parts of the respiratory tract in humans (4, 10).

A number of studies have been reported on the ultrastructure, histogenesis, and pathogenesis of experimentally induced nasal cavity tumors (7, 11-13), and an impressive amount of information on nasal tumors in animals and man has recently been collected by Reznik and Stinson (14). However, when tumors of the nose are seen in carcinogenicity studies, relatively little detail is given on any observed nonneoplastic nasal changes. This is even true for many reports on experiments concerning the induction of nasal tumors.

In our chronic inhalation studies with aldehydes and some other compounds, a wide array of nonneoplastic and/or neoplastic changes of the nasal respiratory and olfactory mucosa have been observed. In the present paper these pathological changes are described and compared with similar lesions observed by other investigators.

CLINICAL SIGNS AND GROSS PATHOLOGY

An early clinical sign of tumor formation in the nose is unilateral or bilateral ocular discharge (4, 12). Focal swelling on the back of the nose in the orbital region (Fig. 1) has frequently been reported as an indication of a nasal tumor (9, 15-17). Other signs reported to accompany nasal tumors are exophthalmus, spinning and loss of balance (16), bloody nasal discharge (12, 18), and a tissue mass bulging out of the nasal orifices (15). Dyspnea, stridor, and mouth breathing often accompanied by rapid weight loss are common in animals of which the nose is partially or completely occluded by a tumor or a plug of inflammatory exudate (12, 15). In our chronic inhalation study with acetaldehyde in rats many top-concentration animals (initially exposed to 3000 ppm and then decreased to 1000 ppm after 52 weeks) that died during the first 15 months of the study were emaciated, had dirty coats, and showed a bloody, greenish mucoid nasal discharge (19). Microscopic examination revealed that the nose of nearly all these rats was partially or completely occluded by a tumor or a plug of keratin with or without inflammatory exudate, and that most of the animals suffered from severe acute bronchopneumonia. An interesting finding was the presence of feed particles in the tracheobronchial tree and lungs of all rats with bronchopneumonia. One might speculate that rats, being obligatory nose breathers, easily inhale feed particles while eating and inhaling through the mouth.

Noses deformed owing to nasal swellings varying from small thickenings just

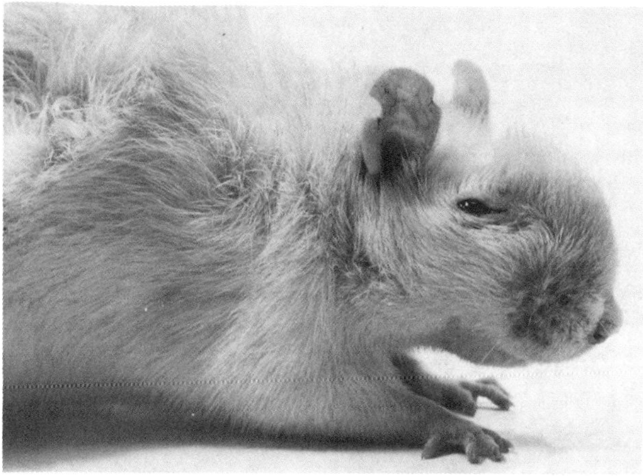

Figure 1 Deformed nose due to nasal carcinoma (an adenocarcinoma of the olfactory epithelium) extending into the subcutis over the premaxilla. Female rat exposed for 83 weeks to 2 ppm trichlorobutene (decreased to 1.5 ppm after 12 weeks).

visible with the naked eye to large protrusions measuring 3 X 2 cm have been reported by many investigators (14). The neoplastic tissue was yellowish, grayish-white or grayish-pink, varied from soft to relatively firm, partially or completely filled the nasal cavity, occasionally was heavily necrotic, often destroyed and perforated the nasal bones, infiltrated the subcutis over the premaxilla, and extended into the brain (Fig. 2). The impression is that squamous cell carcinomas prefer invasion of the subcutis to extension into the forebrain, whereas adenocarcinomas and neuroepitheliomas extend in both directions. Main clinical signs and gross pathology of nasal tumors are summarized in Table 1.

NONNEOPLASTIC CHANGES OF THE RESPIRATORY MUCOSA

Effects on the Respiratory Epithelium

Hyperplasia and (keratinized) stratified squamous metaplasia of the nasal respiratory epithelium are common findings in experimental animals exposed by inhalation to effective concentrations of irritants. Examples of irritants inducing this type of effect are acetaldehyde (20, 21), peroxyacetyl nitrate (22), butenolide (23), formaldehyde (4, 17, 24), 1,2-dibromo-3-chloropropane (25), α-ethylacrolein (26), hexamethylphosphoramide (6), mixture of radon, uranium or dust, and cigarette smoke (27), and phenylglycidyl ether (7). Heavy keratinization has been observed in hamsters and rats exposed to acetaldehyde at levels

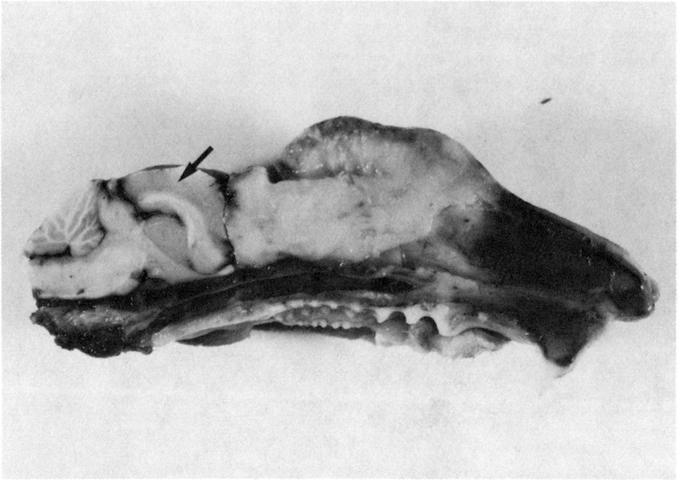

Figure 2 Nasal carcinoma (an adenocarcinoma of the olfactory epithelium) destroying the nasal bones and extending into the brain (arrow). Male rat exposed to 2 ppm trichlorobutene for 83 weeks (decreased to 1.5 ppm after 12 weeks).

of 2000 ppm and above (19, 21). In hamsters the keratinization was mainly found on the nasomaxillary turbinates and the anterior half of the nasal septum, the inner side of the ventral endoturbinates, and in the nasopharyngeal region (Fig. 3). In several rats, plugs of keratin, with or without inflammatory exudate, occluded the nose, which caused dyspnea and death. In these severely affected areas, papillomatous hyperplasia and focal proliferation of atypical basal cells were occasionally seen. Rarefaction of turbinate bones was also a conspicuous finding. In both rats and hamsters these alterations were often accompanied by rhinitis, seen as inflammatory exudate in the nasal cavity or inflammatory cell infiltration in the mucosa and submucosa.

Table 1 Main Clinical Signs and Gross Appearance of Nasal Tumors in Experimental Animals

Clinical signs	Gross pathology
Ocular discharge	Grayish-white, grayish-pink, yellowish
Swelling on the back of the nose	Soft to relatively firm
Exophthalmus	Necrotic areas
Spinning	Destruction of bones
Loss of balance	Infiltration of subcutis
Bloody nasal discharge	Extension into the brain
Tissue mass bulging out of nasal orifices	
Dyspnea, stridor, and mouth breathing	

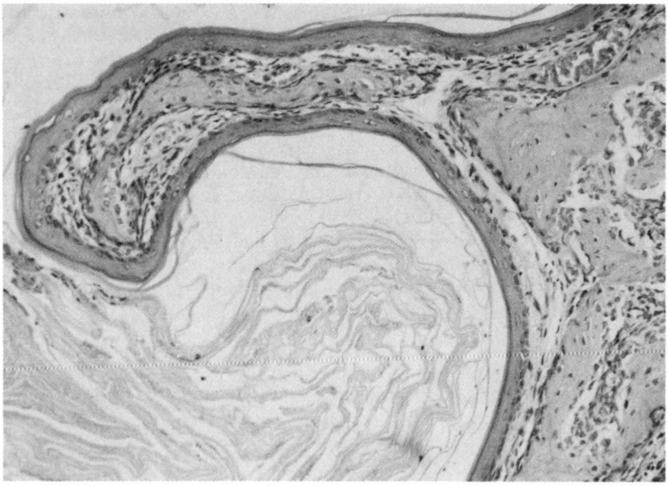

Figure 3 Maxillary turbinate covered by metaplastic heavily keratinized stratified squamous epithelium. Male Syrian hamster exposed to 4560 ppm acetaldehyde for 13 weeks. H&E, X263.

These acetaldehyde effects in rats closely resembled the lesions of the respiratory epithelium found in rats after chronic exposure to formaldehyde (28). In many rats of the high-concentration group (15 ppm formaldehyde), excessive keratosis and inflammatory exudate in the lumen of the nasal cavity caused severe dyspnea and death. In addition, squamous metaplasia with zones of epithelial hyperplasia and keratin production appeared to precede areas of papillary hyperplasia with foci of cellular atypia (24). An interesting difference with the response to acetaldehyde was that initially the formaldehyde effects were restricted to the anterior part of the nasal septum and the nasomaxillary turbinates and, as the study progressed, extended to the posterior segments of the nose.

Antecedent to tumors of the respiratory epithelium, different types of hyperplasia (simple, papillary, nodular, or pseudo-epitheliomatous) and stratified squamous metaplasia with keratinization have been found in experimental animals following oral or subcutaneous administration of various nitrosamines or other compounds (11, 29-32).

Takano et al. (12) studied the sequential changes in the development of preneoplastic and neoplastic lesions in the nasal respiratory epithelium of rats given 1, 4-dinitrosopiperazine in their drinking water. With respect to the non-neoplastic lesions they distinguished simple hyperplasia, papillary hyperplasia, and nodular hyperplasia. Simple hyperplasia was defined as focal thickening of the mucosa with slightly irregular cells; papillary hyperplasia consisted of exophytic protrusions with a thin fibrovascular stalk; and nodular hyperplasia was seen as downward growth into the submucosa which occasionally showed glandular structures containing periodic acid-Schiff-positive material. There was evidence that the papillary hyperplasia progressed to papillomas and the nodular hyperplasia to adenocarcinomas.

Rats exposed to phenylglycidyl ether developed hyperplastic and metaplastic respiratory epithelium occasionally showing invaginations, cystic infoldings, and dysplastic glandular acini with hyperplastic goblet cells (7). This type of hyperplasia and metaplasia seems to resemble closely the nodular hyperplasia described by Takano et al. (12).

Effects on Submucosal Glands

In a few experiments glandular hyperplasia or squamous metaplasia with hyperkeratosis of submucosal glands has been observed. Reznik et al. (11) described squamous metaplasia and hyperkeratosis of both respiratory epithelium and submucosal glands in rats fed diets containing p-cresidine. They also observed glandular hyperplasia of submucosal glands resembling adenomatosis. These nonneoplastic changes were often seen in combination with nasal squamous cell carcinomas or adenocarcinomas. Hyperplasia, squamous metaplasia, and dysplasia of submucosal glands have also been seen in rats after inhalation exposure to 1,2-dibromo-3-chloropropane (25).

Reversible versus Irreversible "Metaplasia"

Extensive hyperplasia and metaplasia with severe keratinization of the respiratory epithelium were found in Syrian hamsters exposed to 1500 ppm acetaldehyde for 52 weeks (7 h/day, 5 days/week) (33). These lesions had disappeared or were markedly reduced in severity and extent after a recovery period of 26 weeks. In this study no nasal (or laryngeal) tumors were observed. In a subsequent study very similar nasal lesions were found in hamsters exposed to 2500 ppm acetaldehyde which was gradually decreased to 1650 ppm after 45 weeks and under comparable experimental conditions (21). However, in this study the nasal lesions were not visibly reduced in severity after a withdrawal period of 26 weeks. On the contrary, some of the hamsters had developed a nasal tumor (and several had a laryngeal carcinoma). It is obvious that the higher exposure level of acetaldehyde in the latter study was responsible for the induction of irreversible metaplastic and neoplastic changes in the nose (and larynx).

Squamous metaplasia with often severe keratinization of the respiratory epithelium occurred in nearly all rats exposed to 3000 ppm acetaldehyde (decreased to 1500 ppm after 45 weeks) for 12 months (19). Animals that died or that were killed in extremis after a recovery period of 6-12 months still showed hyper- and metaplasia of the respiratory epithelium to about the same degree and extent, indicating that no appreciable regression of the acetaldehyde effects had occurred.

A comparable response has been found in mice and rats exposed to formaldehyde gas (24, 28). Mice exposed to 6 or 15 ppm and rats exposed to 2, 6, or 15 ppm developed hyperplasia and keratinized stratified squamous metaplasia of the nasal respiratory epithelium. At 27 months, after a 3-month postexposure period, regression of the metaplastic alterations was found at the 2- and 6-ppm level, but not at the 15-ppm level. Nasal tumors occurred only at the 15-ppm level in mice, and almost exclusively at the 15-ppm level in rats.

A summary of the main chronic nonneoplastic changes of the respiratory mucosa is given in Table 2.

TUMORS OF RESPIRATORY MUCOSA

Many compounds have been reported to induce tumors of the nasal respiratory epithelium in experimental animals. The tumors vary from small exophytic or endophytic papillomas, adenomas, and polypoid adenomas to large squamous cell carcinomas, adenocarcinomas, adenosquamous carcinomas, and anaplastic carcinomas partially or completely occluding the nose, destroying nasal bones, infiltrating the subcutis over the premaxilla, and extending into the brain; metastases have occasionally been reported. Detailed descriptions of the morphology of the tumors have been given by several authors (7, 11, 12, 25, 29, 30, 32, 34). Moreover, the recent book edited by Reznik and Stinson (14) is a storehouse of information on the pathology, pathogenesis, histogenesis, and ultrastructure of nasal tumors in experimental animals.

In our chronic inhalation study with acetaldehyde in rats, squamous cell carcinomas were mainly found in the top-concentration group (3000 ppm decreased to 1000 ppm after 52 weeks), in which a nearly 100% incidence of keratinized stratified squamous metaplasia of large areas of the nasal respiratory epithelium occurred (19). A similar response of the nasal respiratory epithelium has been reported in rats exposed to 15 ppm formaldehyde for life (17, 24).

Table 2 Main Chronic Nonneoplastic Lesions of the Nasal Respiratory Mucosa in Experimental Animals

Simple, papillary, and nodular epithelial hyperplasia with or without atypia
Stratified squamous metaplasia with or without keratinization of the epithelium (reversible/irreversible)
Excessive hyperkeratosis (with or without inflammatory exudate) leading to obstruction of the nose
Glandular hyperplasia of submucosal glands (adenomatosis)
Rhinitis/infiltration of the mucosa and submucosa with inflammatory cells
Rarefaction of turbinate bones

However, chronic exposure of hamsters to a high concentration of acetaldehyde (2500 ppm decreased to 1650 ppm after 45 weeks) resulted in only a few nasal tumors (1 adenoma, 1 adenocarcinoma, and 1 anaplastic carcinoma in a total of 53 animals), despite severe and extensive keratinized squamous metaplasia of the respiratory epithelium (21). Also, hamsters exposed to 10 ppm formaldehyde gas for life showed hyper- and metaplasia of the respiratory tract, but had no nasal tumors (35). Apparently, the nasal respiratory epithelium of hamsters is less susceptible to the carcinogenic activity of these aldehydes than that of rats. The main types of tumors of the nasal respiratory mucosa in experimental animals are summarized in Table 3.

NONNEOPLASTIC CHANGES OF THE OLFACTORY MUCOSA

Effects of Acrolein

Syrian hamsters exposed to 4.0 ppm acrolein vapor for 52 weeks (7 h/day, 5 days/week) showed slight to moderate inflammatory changes and metaplastic epithelium in the dorsomedial part of the nose, which is normally lined by olfactory epithelium (36). The lesions consisted of infiltration of neutrophilic and mononuclear inflammatory cells in the mucosa and submucosa, thickening of the submucosa due to an increased amount of loosely arranged fibrous tissue, a reduced number of Bowman's glands, and metaplastic stratified epithelium that occasionally showed keratinization. Other areas of the nose lined by olfactory epithelium or the respiratory mucosa were not clearly affected by acrolein. After a withdrawal period of 6 months the affected mucosa had partially recovered in most animals. Generally the regenerated "olfactory" epithelium at the site of damage still looked disarranged and was relatively thin and occasionally edematous. The presence of sensory cells was not clear and, if present, they most probably represented preexisting ones. In some animals severe

Table 3 Main Types of Tumors of the Nasal Respiratory Mucosa in Experimental Animals

Papilloma
Exophytic
Endophytic (inverted)
Adenoma (of submucosal glands)
Polypoid adenoma (exophytic)
Squamous cell carcinoma
Adenocarcinoma
Adenosquamous carcinoma
Anaplastic carcinoma

thickening of the submucosa and neutrophilic exudation in the lumen were still visible. Atypical hyperplasia or neoplasia of nasal epithelium was not seen at all after acrolein exposure.

Very similar nasal lesions at the same site have been found in rats and mice after inhalation exposure to acrylic acid (37), a compound very similar in structure to acrolein. In mice, degeneration of the olfactory epithelium was seen along with partial replacement by an epithelium resembling respiratory epithelium. Unlike what Miller et al. (37) stated, such a type of response had already been reported before in hamsters after prolonged exposure to furfural vapor (38). These authors pointed out that the respiratorylike epithelium possibly represents olfactory epithelium having lost its sensory cells and, therefore, being composed of basal and sustentacular cells, the latter of which may easily be mistaken for ciliated cells (Fig. 4). Ultrastructural studies are indicated to establish the true nature of such respiratorylike epithelium.

Effects of Furfural

Highly characteristic alterations of the olfactory mucosa have been found in Syrian hamsters exposed to furfural vapor (115-552 ppm) for 13 or 52 weeks (6 or 7 h/day, 5 days/week) (38, 39). Regressive changes were seen as focal thinning of the olfactory epithelium, which was mainly due to a nearly complete atrophy of the sensory cells. This atrophy was paralleled by irregular groups of sensory cells with their typical "owl eye" nuclei in the lamina propria (Figs. 5, 6). These sensory cells seemed to be part of the lining of cystlike structures which most probably represent endophytically moved surface epithelium. Another explanation may be that these glandular structures represent altered Bowman's glands partly lined by (proliferated) sensory cells, the neural origin of which still has to be confirmed by electron microscopy. In some animals hyperplasia of olfactory epithelium was visible as small papillary formations or intraepithelial, cystlike structures.

Another remarkable finding in furfural-exposed hamsters was the occurrence in the glands of Bowman of very large epithelial cells with abundant cytoplasm and huge nuclei (Fig. 7). To the best of our knowledge karyo- and cytomegaly of Bowman's glands as well as the occurrence of accumulations of sensory cells in the lamina propria have never been reported after treatment with other compounds.

Another striking but less unique observation in furfural-exposed hamsters was the presence of great numbers of large cystlike structures in the lamina propria beneath the affected olfactory epithelium (Fig. 8). Their lumen was often filled with homogeneous, eosinophilic, periodic acid-Schiff-positive material often containing cellular debris and polymorphonuclear leukocytes. The structures were lined by flat or cuboidal epithelium, or often by tall columnar cells with cilia or ciliumlike projections. Occasionally, the epithelium of the

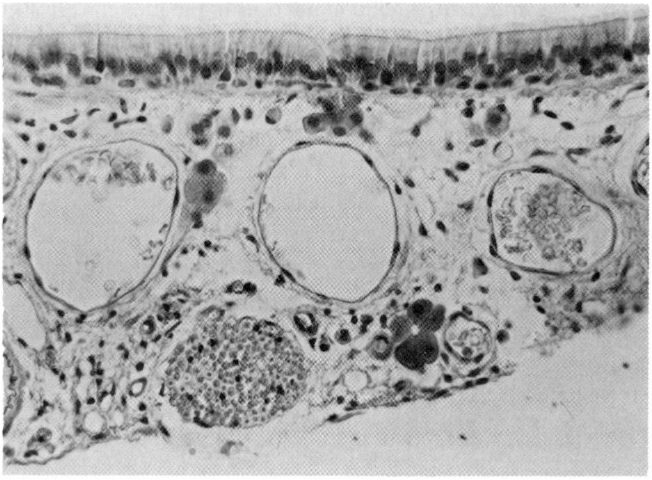

Figure 4 Respiratory(like) epithelium in the dorsomedial area of the nose normally lined by olfactory epithelium. Syrian hamster exposed to 4 ppm acrolein for 52 weeks followed by a recovery period of 26 weeks. H&E, X263.

cystlike formations, in which goblet cells were never found, was seen to be continuous with the altered surface epithelium. This finding suggests that infolding and downward growth of surface epithelium are main factors in the genesis of these cystlike structures. However, genesis from Bowman's glands is an obvious alternative.

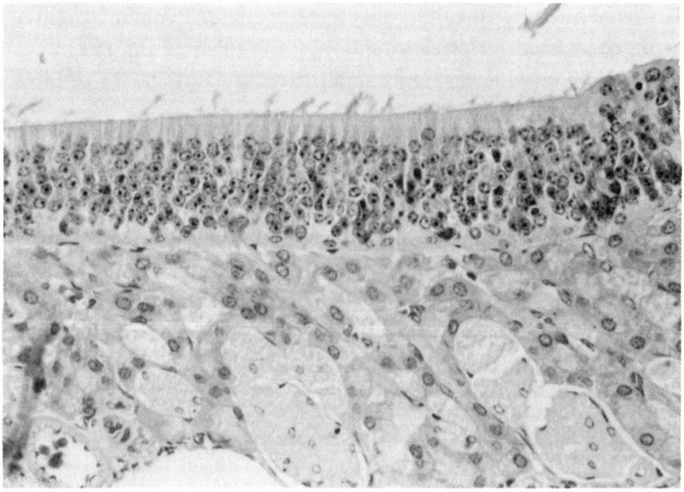

Figure 5 Normal olfactory epithelium of an untreated Syrian hamster. H&E, X280.

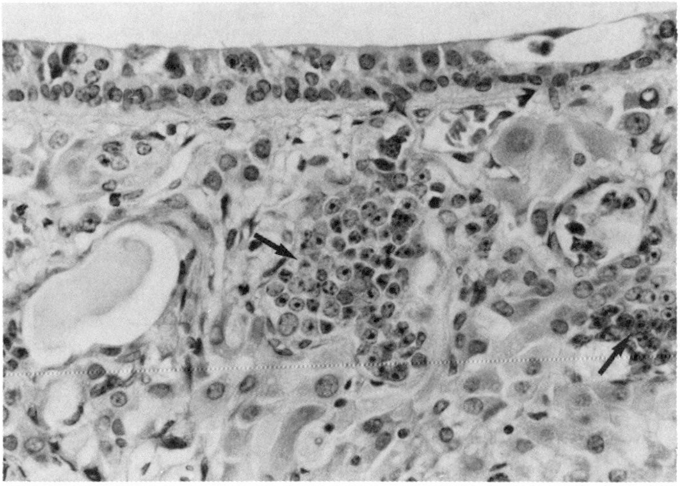

Figure 6 Thinned layer of olfactory epithelium without sensory cells. Accumulations of sensory cells (arrows) in the lamina propria. Syrian hamster exposed to 400 ppm furfural for 22 weeks (decreased to 330 ppm after 9 weeks). H&E, X280.

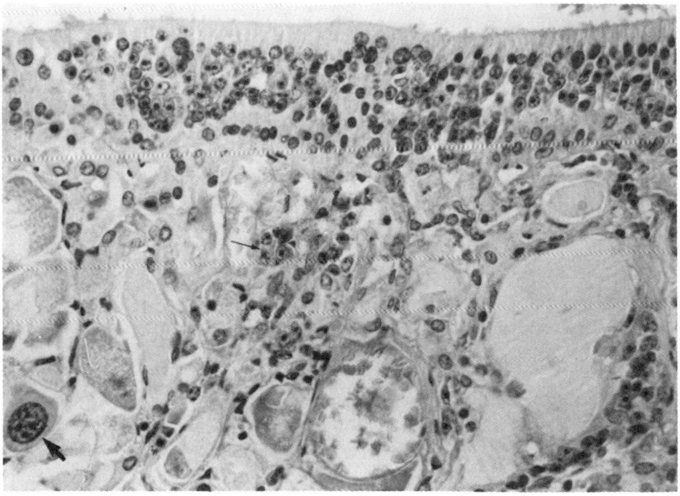

Figure 7 Irregular olfactory epithelium. Sensory cells (thin arrow) in the lamina propria. Greatly enlarged epithelial cells of the glands of Bowman. Note the huge nucleus (thick arrow) in one of the enlarged cells. Male Syrian hamster exposed for 52 weeks to 400 ppm furfural (decreased to 250 ppm after 45 weeks) followed by a recovery period of 29 weeks. H&E, X123.

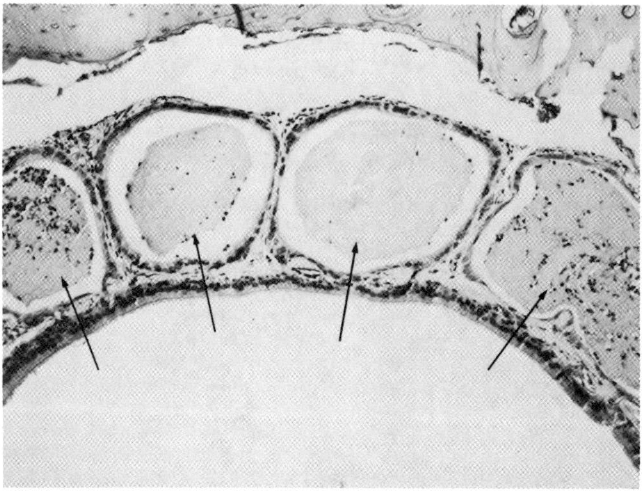

Figure 8 Cystlike structures (arrows) in the lamina propria of the olfactory mucosa. Male Syrian hamster exposed to 400 ppm furfural for 52 weeks (decreased to 250 ppm after 45 weeks) followed by a recovery period of 29 weeks. H&E, X123.

It is of interest to note that after a withdrawal period of 6 months there was no evidence of recovery of the furfural-induced lesions in the olfactory mucosa; neither was there any indication of progression of the lesions, and nasal tumors were not seen at all.

Effects of Trichlorobutene

Cystlike structures along with severe atrophy of the olfactory epithelium such as seen in furfural-exposed hamsters have also been found in rats following chronic exposure (6 h/day, 5 days/week for at most 25 months) to 2,3,4-trichlorobutene-1 (TCB) (40). However, in contrast to furfural exposure, TCB exposure did not lead to groups of sensory cells in the lamina propria and cytomegaly of Bowman's glands. On the other hand, the submucosa of TCB-treated rats appeared to be markedly thickened owing to edema, infiltration of inflammatory cells, and an increased amount of loose connective tissue. In addition, in severely affected areas, nerve bundles were absent and glands of Bowman were either absent or reduced in number. Such submucosal changes were not seen at all in furfural-exposed hamsters.

Effects of Formaldehyde and Acetaldehyde

Focal atrophy with or without hyperplasia of olfactory epithelium and Bowman's glands has been found to accompany the development of tumors of the olfactory epithelium in rats exposed to quinoxaline 1,4-dioxide (18), to 1,2-dibromo-3-chloropropane (25), or to vinyl chloride (9). Atrophy of the olfactory epithelium accompanied by loss of nerve bundles and a thickened submucosa have been observed in mice and rats after prolonged exposure to high concentrations of formaldehyde (6 or 15 ppm) (28) and in Syrian hamsters and rats exposed to acetaldehyde (Fig. 9) at concentrations of 1500 ppm and above (19, 21, 33). Proliferation of (most probably) basal cells was occasionally seen in rats exposed to lower concentrations of acetaldehyde (750 or 1500 ppm). Cystlike structures beneath the olfactory epithelium as seen with furfural or TCB were never encountered after exposure to formaldehyde or acetaldehyde. On the other hand, replacement of the atrophic olfactory epithelium by metaplastic keratinized stratified squamous epithelium, or zones of goblet or ciliated cells, was occasionally noted (19, 28). One might speculate that such a replacement occurs in case of very severe damage to the olfactory mucosa due to prolonged exposure to the causative agent.

The severely damaged olfactory mucosa of rats exposed to 3000 ppm acetaldehyde (decreased to 1500 ppm after 45 weeks) for a period of 12 months hardly showed signs of restoration after withdrawal periods of 6 to 12 months. A few female rats killed after a 6-month recovery period showed minimal proliferation of putative olfactory basal cells. In addition, some rats exhibited glandlike formations in the thickened submucosa, possibly representing regenerative hyperplasia of Bowman's glands. In the lower-dose rats (750 or 1500 ppm acetaldehyde) killed at the end of a 12-month exposure period, the olfactory

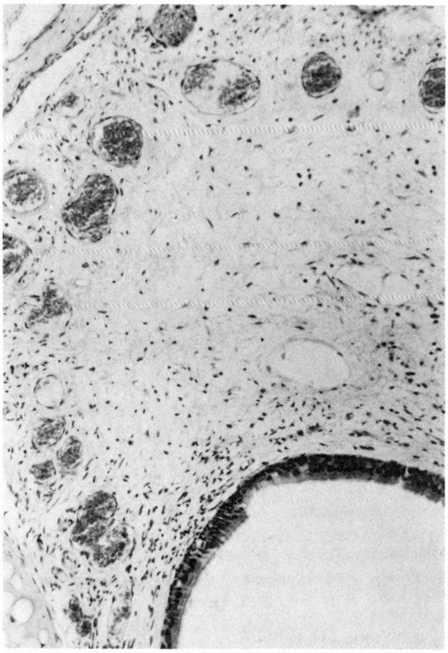

Figure 9 Thickened submucosa beneath the olfactory epithelium due to abundant, loosely arranged fibrous tissue. Note loss of nerve bundles and glands of Bowman. Female rat exposed to 3000 ppm acetaldehyde for 52 weeks (decreased to 1500 ppm after 45 weeks). H&E, X104.

epithelium in the dorsomedial region was seen to be replaced by one or a few layers of cuboidal cells, of which the superficial cells occasionally were provided with cilia or ciliumlike projections. In several of these rats there was a slight to moderate focal hyperplasia of basal cells. After a recovery period of 6-12 months, extensive proliferation of these basal cell-like cells were found in many animals. The proliferations consisted of 5-10 layers of cells and occurred along a large portion of the dorsomedial region. These cells rested on a thickened basal membrane and were covered by a more or less separate layer of cuboidal or columnar epithelial cells. A most remarkable finding was the presence of smaller or larger nerve bundles within this layer of proliferated epithelial cells (Fig. 10).

Summary of Effects

A summary of the main chronic, nonneoplastic lesions of the olfactory mucosa in experimental animals occurring either separately or in certain combinations is given in Table 4. As far as the localization of the effects is concerned, it seems justified to designate the dorsomedial region of the nasal cavity as the vulnerable site.

TUMORS OF THE OLFACTORY MUCOSA

Adenocarcinomas

Adenocarcinomas of the olfactory epithelium or of Bowman's glands were found in rats exposed to acetaldehyde vapor at levels of 750, 1500, or 3000 ppm

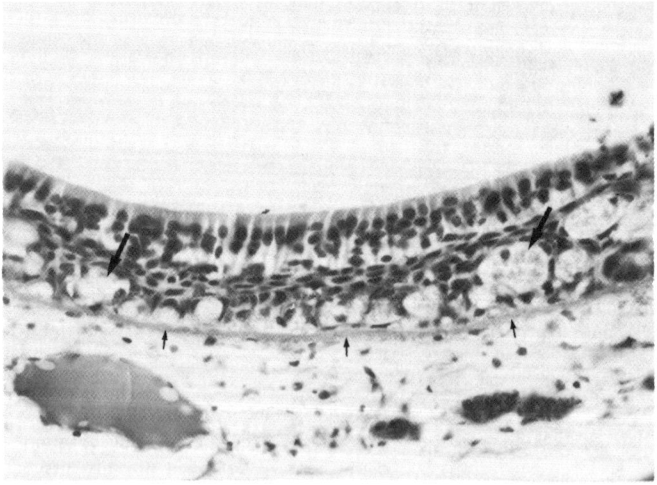

Figure 10 Regeneration of olfactory epithelium. Two more-or-less separated layers of epithelium are visible. The lowest layer seems to contain small nerve bundles (thick arrows). Note the thick basal membrane (thin arrows). Male rat exposed to 1500 ppm acetaldehyde for 52 weeks followed by a recovery period of 26 weeks. H&E, X245.

Table 4 Main Chronic Nonneoplastic Lesions of the Nasal Olfactory Mucosa in Experimental Animals

Atrophy of sensory cells
Atrophy of olfactory epithelium
Replacement of olfactory epithelium by respiratorylike epithelium
Replacement of olfactory epithelium by goblet or ciliated cells
Replacement of olfactory epithelium by keratinized squamous epithelium
Accumulations of sensory cells in the submucosa
Karyo- and cytomegaly of epithelial cells of Bowman's glands
Reduced number or loss of Bowman's glands
Cystlike structures in the submucosa
Rhinitis or necrotizing rhinitis
Infiltration of the mucosa and submucosa with inflammatory cells
Thickened submucosa due to edema and increased amount of loosely arranged fibrous tissue
Loss of nerve bundles in the submucosa

(decreased to 1000 ppm after 52 weeks) for a period of at most 27 months (19). The tumors varied in size from small carcinomas located in the mucosa and submucosa to large, osteolytic tumors growing outside the nose and often invading the brain. They consisted of sheets or cords of densely packed cells with little cytoplasm, and round to oval large nuclei with often one or two big nucleoli (Fig. 11). Mitotic figures were very common. Rosettes and glandular formations were occasionally encountered in the larger tumors. Many of the small tumors were seen to originate from olfactory epithelium or remnants of Bowman's glands. From preliminary electron microscopical studies it appeared

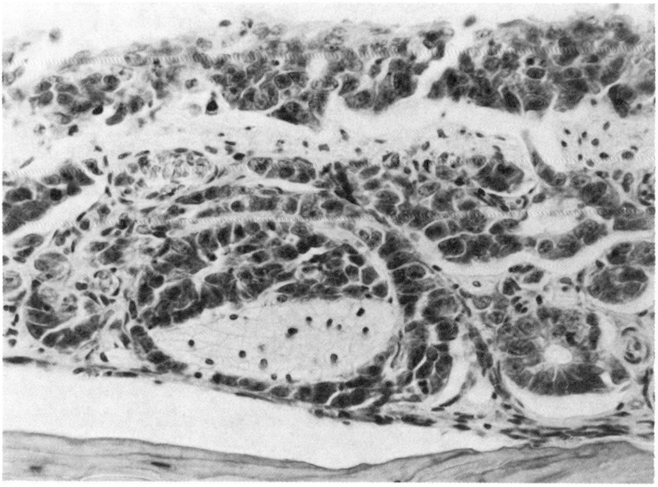

Figure 11 Adenocarcinoma of the olfactory epithelium. Male rat exposed to 3000 ppm acetaldehyde (decreased to 1000 ppm after 52 weeks) for 56 weeks. H&E, X280.

that the cytoplasm of the tumor cells did not contain very characteristic structures: small mitochondria, a few strands of rough endoplasmic reticulum, and many free polyribosomes. The nuclei were big and indentated, and had large compact nucleoli. Desmosomelike structures occurred between the cells (Fig. 12). The lack of differentiation may point to the olfactory basal cells as the cells from which the acetaldehyde-induced adenocarcinomas are derived.

In our institute we have seen this type of carcinoma of the olfactory epithelium in two other inhalation studies using the same strain of rats—viz., a 1-year study with a high concentration (5000 ppm) of vinyl chloride (9) and a 25-month study with TCB (40). Behavior and gross appearance, growth pattern, and cytology of these tumors indeed were very similar in each of the three studies (Figs. 13, 14).

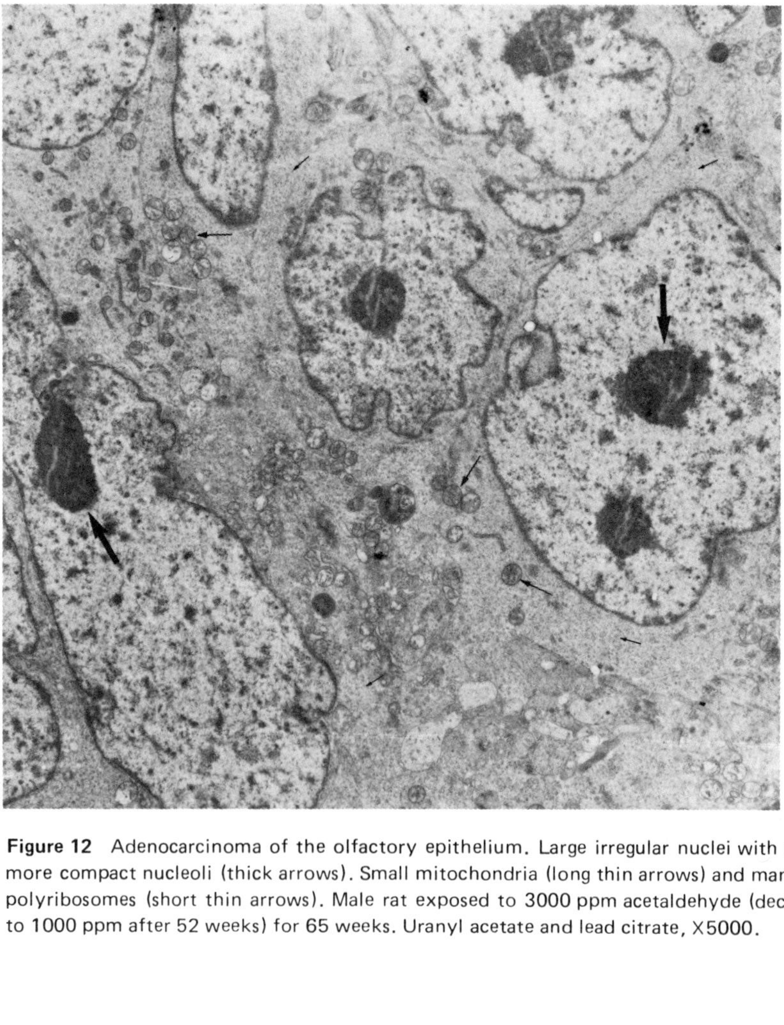

Figure 12 Adenocarcinoma of the olfactory epithelium. Large irregular nuclei with one or more compact nucleoli (thick arrows). Small mitochondria (long thin arrows) and many free polyribosomes (short thin arrows). Male rat exposed to 3000 ppm acetaldehyde (decreased to 1000 ppm after 52 weeks) for 65 weeks. Uranyl acetate and lead citrate, X5000.

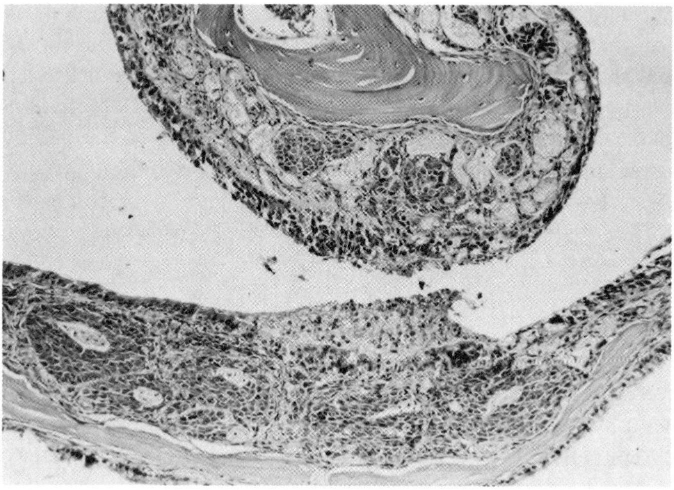

Figure 13 Adenocarcinoma of the olfactory epithelium. Male rat exposed to 5000 ppm vinyl chloride for 52 weeks. H&E, X112.

From the literature it also appears that this type of nasal carcinoma is not uncommon in experimental animals exposed to respiratory tract carcinogens. Examples of compounds capable of inducing such neoplasms are di-n-propyl-nitrosamine in Syrian golden hamsters (30), 1,2-dibromo-3-chloropropane in rats and mice (25, 41), N-nitrosomethyl(2-oxopropyl)amine in Syrian hamsters (31), p-cresidine in rats (11), nitroso-2,6-dimethylmorpholine in Syrian hamsters

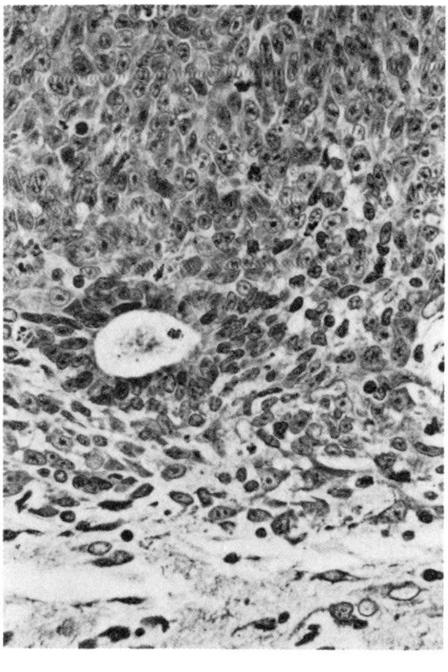

Figure 14 Metastasis of an adenocarcinoma of the olfactory epithelium in the brain. Female rat exposed to 5000 ppm vinyl chloride for 46 weeks. Reticulin stain, X228.

(42), and N-nitrosomethylpiperazine in rats (13). From electron microscopical studies it appeared that adenocarcinomas induced in rats by 1,2-dibromo-3-chloropropane were most probably derived from the olfactory basal cells and consisted of neoplastic basal cells displaying different stages of differentiation into mature sustentacular cells (25). Reznik-Schüller (13) examined the pathogenesis of N-nitrosomethylpiperazine-induced adenocarcinomas using light and electron microscopy. Basal cells of the olfactory epithelium were found to proliferate and differentiate into neuroendocrinelike cells giving rise to the adenocarcinomas.

Neuroepitheliomas

A number of investigators reported neuroepitheliomas, esthesioneuroepitheliomas, (esthesio)neuroblastomas, esthesioneuromas, or esthesioneurocytomas of the nasal olfactory epithelium in experimental animals treated with carcinogens (5, 16, 34, 43–48). The diagnosis is often mainly, if not exclusively, based on the formation of rosettes or pseudo rosettes, but the definitive neurogenic origin of such tumors should appear from the unequivocal presence of neurotubules, neurosecretory granules, or neuritic processes in the tumor cells (3, 11, 25, 49). Indeed, demonstration of features of sensory cells in tumor cells by electron microscopy seems to be a prerequisite for the diagnosis (esthesio)neuroepitheliomas. However, according to Rivenson et al. (50), all tumors from the olfactory epithelium should be classified as neuroepitheliomas. They elucidated their view by making the following interesting statement: "Calling the sustentacular and basal cells nonneurogenic would implicitly remove all gliomas (including Schwannomas) from the group of neurogenic tumors." The main types of tumors of the nasal olfactory mucosa in experimental animals are summarized in Table 5.

Table 5 Main Types of Tumors of the Nasal Olfactory Mucosa in Experimental Animals

Adenocarcinoma
From basal cells
From glands of Bowman
With sustentacular cell differentiation
With neuroendocrine cell differentiation
Esthesioneuroepithelioma
From sensory cells
Neuroepithelioma
See text for explanation

CONCLUSIONS

A wide variety of pathological changes has been reported to occur in the nasal passages of experimental animals after chronic exposure by inhalation to a variety of irritant vapors or carcinogenic compounds. Chronic exposure to toxicants by other routes has also been found to result in neoplastic and non-neoplastic changes of the nasal mucosa. We therefore support the view of Reznik et al. (25) that in experimental animals "the nasal cavity has a high sensitivity to a wide range of environmental carcinogens, and should hence be routinely examined, grossly and histologically, in all standard rodent carcinogenesis bioassays." Research on the nasal pathology in rodents should be extended and intensified. Priorities are investigations into the histogenesis of experimentally induced tumors of the olfactory mucosa and studies aimed at elucidating the significance of chronic irritation of the nasal mucosa for the development of nasal cancer.

SUMMARY

A survey is given of clinical signs and gross and microscopic pathology of chronic nasal toxic effects in experimental animals with emphasis on the nasal lesions found in rats or Syrian hamsters after chronic inhalation exposure to acrolein, furfural, or acetaldehyde.

Nasal tumors may lead to dyspnea, stridor and mouth breathing, nasal and ocular discharge, swellings on the back of the nose, exophthalmus, and loss of balance. The tumors are often osteolytic, invade the subcutis over the premaxilla, and extend into the brain.

Main chronic nonneoplastic changes of the respiratory mucosa include simple, papillary, and nodular hyperplasia with or without atypia, stratified squamous metaplasia, hyperkeratosis, rhinitis, and rarefaction of turbinal bones. Common types of tumors of the respiratory epithelium are exophytic and endophytic papilloma, adenomas of submucosal glands, polypoid adenomas, squamous cell carcinomas, adenocarcinomas, adenosquamous carcinomas, and anaplastic carcinomas.

Chronic nonneoplastic changes of the olfactory mucosa of frequent occurrence are atrophy of sensory cells, replacement of olfactory epithelium by goblet or ciliated cells or by respiratory(like) epithelium, loss of nerve bundles and glands of Bowman, rhinitis, and a thickened submucosa due to abundant loosely arranged fibrous tissue. Atrophy of olfactory epithelium accompanied by accumulations of sensory cells in the submucosa and karyo- and cytomegaly in the glands of Bowman are highly characteristic lesions in hamsters exposed to furfural. Main types of neoplasms of the olfactory mucosa are adenocarcinomas of different cell types and esthesioneuroepitheliomas.

REFERENCES

1 Pedersen, E, AC Hgetviet, and A Andersen. Cancer of respiratory organs among workers at a nickel refinery in Norway. *Int. J. Cancer* 12:32–41 (1973).

2 Acheson ED. Nasal cancer in the furniture and boot and shoe manufacturing industries. *Prev. Med.* 5:295–315 (1976).

3 Reznik-Schüller, HM. Nitrosamine-induced nasal cavity carcinogenesis. In *Nasal Tumors in Animals and Man,* edited by G Reznik, SF Stinson. Vol. III, *Experimental Nasal Carcinogenesis.* Boca Raton, FL: CRC Press, pp. 47–78 (1983).

4 Swenberg, JA, WD Kerns, RI Mitchell, EJ Gralla, and KL Pavkov. Induction of squamous cell carcinomas of the rat nasal cavity by inhalation exposure to formaldehyde vapor. *Cancer Res.* 40:3398–3402 (1980).

5 Leong, BKJ, RJ Kociba, and GC Jersey. A lifetime study of rats and mice exposed to vapors of bis(chloromethyl)ether. *Toxicol. Appl. Pharmacol.* 58:269–281 (1981).

6 Lee, KP, and HJ Trochimowicz. Metaplastic changes of nasal respiratory epithelium in rats exposed to hexamethylphosphoramide (HMPA) by inhalation. *Am. J. Pathol.* 106:8–19 (1982).

7 Lee, KP, PW Schneider, and HJ Trochimowicz. Morphological expression of glandular differentiation in the epidermoid nasal carcinomas induced by phenylglycidyl ether inhalation. *Am. J. Pathol.* 111:140–148 (1983).

8 Laskin, S, AR Sellakumar, M Kuschner, N Nelson, S La Mendola, GM Rusch, GV Katz, NC Dulak, and RE Albert. Inhalation carcinogenicity of epichlorohydrin in noninbred Sprague-Dawley rats. *JNCI* 65:751–757 (1980).

9 Feron VJ, and R Kroes. One year time-sequence inhalation toxicity study of vinyl chloride in rats. II. Morphological changes in the respiratory tract, ceruminous glands, brain, kidneys, heart and spleen. *Toxicology* 13: 131–141 (1979).

10 Page NP. Concepts of a bioassay program in environmental carcinogenesis. In *Environmental Carcinogenesis,* edited by H Kraybill, H Mehlman. Washington, DC: Hemisphere, pp. 87–171 (1977).

11 Reznik, G, HM Reznik-Schüller, DW Hayden, A Russfield, and AS Krishna Murthy. Morphology of nasal cavity neoplasms in F-344 rats after chronic feeding of p-cresidine, and intermediate of dyes and pigments. *Anticancer Res.* 1:279–286 (1981).

12 Takano, T, T Shirai, T Ogiso, H Tsuda, S Baba, and N Ito. Sequential changes in tumor development induced by 1,4-dinitrosopiperazine in the nasal cavity of F-344 rats. *Cancer Res.* 42:4236–4240 (1982).

13 Reznik-Schüller, HM. Pathogenesis of tumors induced with N-nitrosomethylpiperazine in the olfactory region of the rat nasal cavity. *JNCI* 71: 165–172 (1983).

14 Reznik, G, and SF Stinson. *Nasal Tumors in Animals and Man.* Boca Raton, FL: CRC Press (1983).

15 Hoch-Ligeti, C, MF Argus, and JC Arcos. Induction of carcinomas in the nasal cavity of rats by dioxane. *Br. J. Cancer* 24:164–170 (1970).

16 Pelfrene, A, and H Garcia. Chemically induced esthesioneuroblastomas in rats. *Z. Krebsforsch.* 86:113–119 (1976).
17 Albert RE, AR Sellakumar, S Laskin, M Kuschner, N Nelson, and CA Snyder. Gaseous formaldehyde and hydrogen chloride induction of nasal cancer in the rat. *JNCI* 68:597–603 (1982).
18 Tucker, MJ. Carcinogenic action of quinoxaline 1,4-dioxide in rats. *JNCI* 55:137–146 (1975).
19 Woutersen, RA, LM Appelman, VJ Feron, and CA Van der Heijden. Inhalation toxicity of acetaldehyde in rats. II. Carcinogenicity study: Interim results after 15 months. *Toxicology* 31:123–133 (1984).
20 Kruysse, A, VJ Feron, and HP Til. Repeated exposure to acetaldehyde vapor. Studies in Syrian golden hamsters. *Arch. Environ. Health* 31: 449–452 (1975).
21 Feron, VJ, A Kruysse, and RA Woutersen. Respiratory tract tumours in hamsters exposed to acetaldehyde vapour alone or simultaneously to benzo(a)pyrene or diethylnitrosamine. *Eur. J. Cancer Clin. Oncol.* 18: 13–31 (1982).
22 Kruysse, A, VJ Feron, HR Immel, BJ Spit, and GJ Van Esch. Short-term inhalation toxicity studies with peroxyacetyl nitrate in rats. *Toxicology* 8:231–249 (1977).
23 Feron, VJ, A Kruysse, HR Immel, and HP Til. Repeated exposure to butenolide vapour: Sub-acute study in Syrian golden hamsters. *Toxicology* 9:65–68 (1979).
24 Kerns, WD, KL Pavkov, DJ Donofrio, EJ Gralla, and JA Swenberg. Carcinogenicity of formaldehyde in rats and mice after long-term inhalation exposure. *Cancer Res.* 43:4382–4392 (1983).
25 Reznik, G, HM Reznik-Schüller, JM Ward, and SF Stinson. Morphology of nasal-cavity tumours in rats after chronic inhalation of 1,2-dibromo-3-chloropropane. *Br. J. Cancer* 42:772–781 (1980).
26 Appelman LM, CFM Hendriksen, and VJ Feron. Repeated exposure to α-ethylacrolein vapour: Subacute toxicity study in rats. *Toxicology* 22:79–87 (1981).
27 Cross, FT, RF Palmer, RE Filipy, GE Dagle, and BO Stuart. Carcinogenic effects of radon daughters, uranium ore dust and cigarette smoke in beagle dogs. *Health Phys.* 42:33–52 (1982).
28 Battelle. A chronic inhalation toxicology study in rats and mice exposed to formaldehyde. Final report, CIIT, December 31, 1981. Batelle Columbus Laboratories, p. 173 (1981).
29 Herrold, K. Epithelial papillomas of the nasal cavity. Experimental induction in Syrian hamsters. *Arch. Pathol.* 78:189–195 (1964).
30 Pour, P, FW Krüger, A Cardesa, J Althoff, and U Mohr. Carcinogenic effect of di-n-propylnitrosamine in Syrian golden hamsters. *JNCI* 51:1019–1027 (1973).
31 Pour, P, R Gingell, R Langenbach, D Nagal, C Grandjean, T Lawson, and S Salmasi. Carcinogenicity of N-nitrosomethyl(2-oxopropyl)amine in Syrian hamsters. *Cancer Res.* 40:3585–3590 (1980).

32 Reznik-Schüller, HM, and U Mohr. Ultrastructure of N-nitrosodibutylamine-induced tumours of the nasal cavity in the European hamster. *JNCI* 57:401–407 (1976).
33 Feron, VJ. Effects of exposure to acetaldehyde in Syrian hamsters simultaneously treated with benzo(a)pyrene or diethylnitrosamine. *Prog. Exp. Tumor Res.* 24:162–176 (1979).
34 Althoff J, A Cardesa, P Pour, and U Mohr. Carcinogenic effect of N-nitrosohexamethylenimine in Syrian golden hamsters. *JNCI* 50:323–329 (1973).
35 Dalbey, WE. Formaldehyde and tumors in hamster respiratory tract. *Toxicology* 24:9–14 (1982).
36 Feron, VJ, and A Kruysse. Effects of exposure to acrolein vapor in hamsters simultaneously treated with benzo(a)pyrene or diethylnitrosamine. *J. Toxicol. Environ. Health* 3:379–394 (1977).
37 Miller, RR, JA Ayres, GC Jersey, and MJ McKenna. Inhalation toxicity of acrylic acid. *Fund. Appl. Toxicol.* 1:271–277 (1981).
38 Feron, VJ, and A Kruysse. Effects of exposure to furfural vapour in hamsters simultaneously treated with benzo(a)pyrene or diethylnitrosamine. *Toxicology* 11:127–144 (1978).
39 Feron, VJ, A Kruysse, and HC Dreef-Van der Meulen. Repeated exposure to furfural vapour: 13-week study in Syrian golden hamsters. *Zentralbl. Bakteriol. Parasitenk. Infektionskr. Hyg. Abt. 1 Orig. Reihe B* 168:442–451 (1979).
40 Reuzel, PGJ, VJ Feron, HR Immel, and HC Dreef-Van der Meulen. Chronic (25-month) inhalation toxicity/carcinogenicity study with 2,3,4-trichlorobutene-1 in rats. Report No. V81.133/267399. CIVO Institutes TNO, Zeist, The Netherlands (1980).
41 Reznik, G, B Ulland, SF Stinson, and JM Ward. Morphology and sex-dependent manifestation of nasal tumors in B6C3F1 mice after chronic inhalation of 1,2-dibromo-3-chloropropane. *J. Cancer Res. Clin. Oncol.* 98:75–83 (1980).
42 Lijinsky, W, MD Reuber, and HM Reznik-Schüller. Contrasting carcinogenic effects of nitroso-2,6-dimethylmorpholine given by gavage to F-344 rats and Syrian golden hamsters. *Cancer Lett.* 16:281–286 (1982).
43 Herrold, K. Induction of olfactory neuroepithelial tumors in Syrian hamsters by diethylnitrosamine. *Cancer* 17:114–121 (1964).
44 Thomas, C. Zur Morphologie der Nasenhöhlentumoren bei der Ratte. *Z. Krebsforsch.* 67:1–10 (1965).
45 Garcia, H, L Keefer, W Lijinsky, and CEM Wenyon. Carcinogenicity of nitrosomorpholine and 1-nitrosopiperazine in rats. *Z. Krebsforsch.* 74:179–184 (1970).
46 Rivenson, A, T Ohmori, SS Hecht, and D Hoffmann. Organotropic carcinogenicity of tobacco specific N-nitrosamines. In *Biology of the Cancer Cell,* edited by K Letnansky. Amsterdam: Kugler, pp. 51–62 (1980).
47 Preussmann, R, M Habs, H Habs, and D Schmähl. Carcinogenicity of N-nitrosodiethanolamine in rats at five different dose levels. *Cancer Res.* 42:5167–5171 (1982).
48 Hecht, SS, JD Adams, S Numoto, and D Hoffmann. Induction of respira-

tory tract tumors in Syrian golden hamsters by a single dose of 4-(methyl-nitrosamino)-1-(3-pyridyl)-1-butanone (NNK) and the effect of smoke inhalation. *Carcinogenesis* 4:1287–1290 (1983).

49 Cardesa, A, P Pour, H Haas, J Althoff, and U Mohr. Histogenesis of tumors from the nasal cavities induced by diethylnitrosamine. *Cancer* 37:346–358 (1976).

50 Rivenson, A, K Furuya, SS Hecht, and D Hoffmann. Experimental nasal cavity tumors induced by tobacco-specific nitrosamines (TSNA). In *Nasal Tumors in Animals and Man,* edited by G Reznik, SF Stinson. Vol. III, *Experimental Nasal Carcinogenesis.* Boca Raton, FL: CRC Press, pp. 79–114 (1983).

Chapter 6

Sensory Irritation by Airborne Chemicals: A Basis to Establish Acceptable Levels of Exposure

Yves Alarie and Ji Er Luo

INTRODUCTION

Kratschmer (1), in 1870, was the first to report on the effects of a variety of airborne chemicals on the nasal mucosa. He introduced the concept of reflex reactions from stimulation of trigeminal nerve endings located in the respiratory epithelium of the nasal mucosa. He also correctly demonstrated the variety of reflex reactions that follow stimulation of the nasal mucosa. More organ systems are affected from trigeminal stimulation than from any other peripheral nervous receptors (2). These reactions included inhibition of respiration with a lengthening of the expiratory phase, bradycardia, and a rise in systemic blood pressure, as shown in Fig. 1. Closure of the glottis and constriction of the nares also occurred in expiration, and thus impeded airflow movement out of the lungs. Indeed, Kratschmer described the entire process as an expiratory tetanus. This occurs with very high concentrations of airborne irritants, which he was using. His results were fully confirmed by Magne et al. in 1925 (3, 4). Allen (5) confirmed that the trigeminal reflex is present in man, as was demonstrated in rabbits by Kratschmer (1) and in dogs by Magne et al. (3, 4). Since then, many other

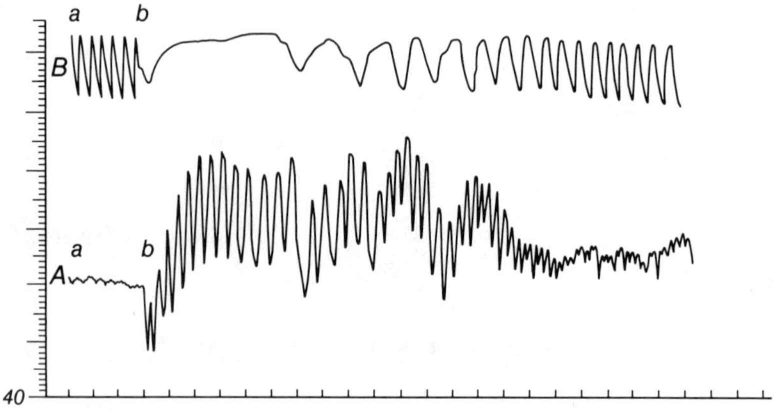

Figure 1 Tracings of blood pressure (bottom) and respiration (top) taken on a rabbit prior to and during inhalation of a sensory irritant. Tracings redrawn from the original (1). Between *a* and *b* recordings taken under normal conditions, exposure to the sensory irritant at *b*.

investigators have further confirmed these observations (2, 6). What is of interest for toxicological investigation of airborne chemicals is that with lower concentrations than those used by Kratschmer (1), the pause during expiration is very well defined when body plethysmography is used to monitor tidal volume and respiratory rate, as shown in Fig. 2. A decrease in respiratory rate due to a

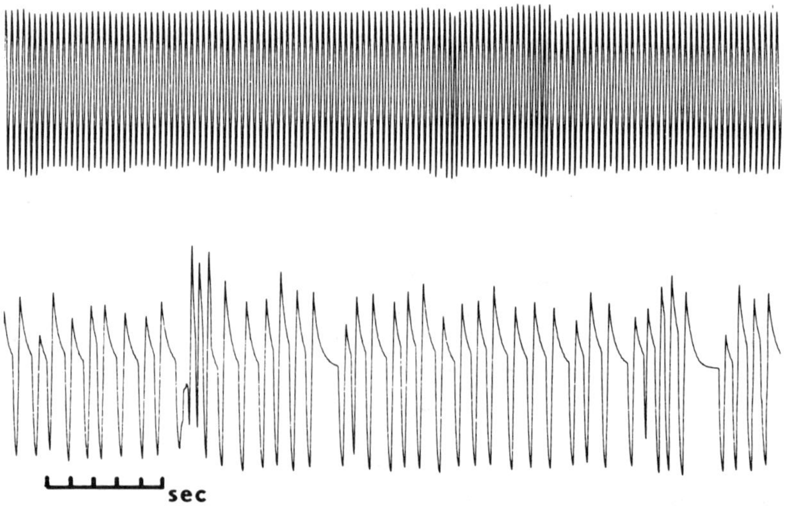

Figure 2 Recording of tidal volume and respiratory rate from a mouse in a body plethysmograph during room air breathing (top) and during inhalation of a sensory irritant (bottom). Inspiration is upward; note the characteristic pause during expiration. [*From Alarie (2).*]

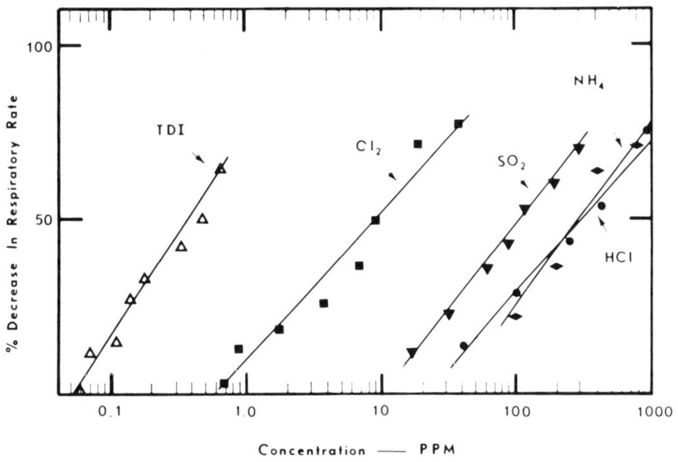

Figure 3 Concentration-response relationships obtained by plotting the percent decrease in respiratory rate, from control condition, versus the logarithm of the exposure concentration of a variety of sensory irritants. [*From Barrow et al. (7).*]

lengthening of this pause, from low to high concentrations, can be shown to be concentration-dependent, as shown in Fig. 3.

METHODS

The method for measuring respiratory rate in mice during exposure to airborne chemicals has been described in detail (7, 9). Briefly, the tidal volume and respiratory rate of each animal are obtained by body plethysmography and recorded on an oscillograph, so that the characteristic pause during expiration can be observed as an indication of the presence of sensory irritation. The average respiratory rate of four mice simultaneously exposed is obtained from this recording. To obtain concentration-response relationships, 5-8 groups of 4 animals are used, each exposed to a different concentration of the chemical being investigated. From the concentration-response relationship, the RD_{50}, i.e., the concentration necessary to decrease the respiratory rate by 50%, is calculated.

Mice are used as experimental animals for practical reasons. First, they are cheap and easy to handle. Second, they can be placed in a body plethysmograph easily and adapt very quickly. Third, they are not too susceptible to bronchoconstriction, which would change the characteristic pause during expiration to a different pattern of breathing and make the evaluation of the effect more difficult (10). Different strains of mice have been tested, and a factor of 10 was found between the least and most sensitive using sulfur dioxide as the sensory irritant (11). Rats can be used, but they are, in general, less sensitive than mice (12, 13). Guinea pigs are about as sensitive as mice (2), but because of possible bronchoconstriction should be avoided in studies of sensory irritation. Rabbits and dogs, as used by Kratschmer (1) and Magne et al. (3, 4), are very sensitive and excellent animals to use. However, dogs are very difficult to handle during exposure to sensory irritants unless anesthesia is used.

Rabbits, although very sensitive (7), do not offer much more advantage than mice, and they too should be used under anesthesia. Cynomolgus monkeys also have been used (Alarie et al., unpublished observations at Hazleton Laboratories). These animals are resistant to sensory irritants. Similarly, baboons have been exposed to high concentrations of irritants and have shown very little effect (Kaplan, unpublished results at Southwest Research Institute). The reasons these animals have higher resistance than mice and humans to sensory irritants remain to be explored.

PREDICTION OF ACCEPTABLE LEVELS

Prior to predicting acceptable levels for humans from the potency found in mice for each chemical, it was necessary to establish that the response measured in mice (i.e., characteristic pause during expiration) is correlated with sensory irritation in humans (i.e., reports of eye, nose, and throat irritation). This was found to be correct for a series of chemicals (2, 14) that has now been extended to include 95 chemicals and 6 mixtures. At the beginning (14), a range of acceptable levels for industrial exposure was given. This was then extended to a more specific prediction when it was found that a good correlation existed between 0.03 RD_{50} and the threshold limit values (TLV) for 26 industrial chemicals (9, 15). This has now been extended to 40 industrial chemicals (16), as presented in Table 1 and Fig. 4. From these results it is reasonable to suggest that 0.03 RD_{50} for a new chemical being tested is likely to be the highest level acceptable for a TLV. However, two restrictions must be imposed. First, if other toxic effects on the respiratory system are observed at exposure concentrations below which sensory irritation occurs, it is obvious that the chemical cannot be classified primarily as a sensory irritant. For example, benzene, when tested in this bioassay, failed to induce sensory irritation but did induce respiratory stimulation (17). Hexamethylene diisocyanate trimer, when tested in this bioassay, induced pulmonary irritation rather than sensory irritation (18). Nitrogen dioxide also induced pulmonary irritation at concentrations similar to those inducing sensory irritation (6). In such cases it is impossible to use this bioassay to predict an acceptable TLV, and other appropriate bioassays must be found (6, 18). Second, 0.03 RD_{50} must be taken only as the highest acceptable level for a TLV. It gives an indication of precautions and engineering controls which will be required for production. Obviously this must be confirmed with further appropriate toxicological evaluations. In designing these toxicological evaluations, we already know that repeated exposure at the RD_{50} will induce histo-

Table 1 The RD_{50} Values, 1983 TLV-TWA Values, TLV-TWA Values Predicted on the Basis of 0.03 RD_{50}, Vapor Pressure, and Activity Coefficient (RD_{50} mm Hg/vapor pressure mm Hg) for 40 Industrial Chemicals

Chemical No. in Fig. 4	Chemical	RD_{50} (ppm)	1983 TLV-TWA (ppm)	0.03 RD_{50} (ppm)	log 1983 TLV-TWA (ppm)	log 0.03 RD_{50} (ppm)	Saturated vapor pressure at 37°C (mm Hg)	RD_{50} (mm Hg)	Activity coefficient	References providing RD_{50} value
1	2, 4-Toluene diisocyanate	0.2	0.005	0.006	−2.30	−2.22	0.048	1.5×10^{-4}	3.1×10^{-3}	21
2	Chlorobenzylidene malononitrile	0.52	0.05	0.016	−1.30	−1.80	—	—	—	14
3	Chloracetophenone	0.96	0.05	0.029	−1.30	−1.54	0.46	7.3×10^{-4}	1.6×10^{-3}	14
4	Acrolein	1.68	0.1	0.05	−1.00	−1.30	439	1.3×10^{-3}	2.9×10^{-6}	22
5	Formaldehyde	3.13	2.0	0.10	0.30	−1.00	5637	2.4×10^{-3}	4.2×10^{-7}	22
6	Benzoquinone	5.0	0.1	0.15	−1.00	−0.82	—	—	—	Y. Alarie, 1979 unpublished
7	Chloropicrin	7.98	0.1	0.24	−1.00	0.62	47	6.1×10^{-3}	1.3×10^{-4}	14
8	Chlorine	9.34	1	0.28	0	−0.55	7.9	7.1×10^{-3}	8.9×10^{-7}	9
9	Benzylchloride	17.0	1	0.51	0	−0.29	2.64	1.3×10^{-2}	4.9×10^{-3}	23
10	Isophorone	27.8	5	0.83	0.69	−0.08	0.94	2.1×10^{-2}	2.2×10^{-2}	23
11	Sulfur dioxide	117	2	3.5	0.30	0.54	4444	8.9×10^{-2}	2.0×10^{-5}	24
12	Acetic acid	163	10	4.9	1.0	0.69	30.4	1.2×10^{-1}	4.1×10^{-3}	23
13	Phenol	166	5	5.0	0.7	0.69	0.95	1.3×10^{-1}	1.3×10^{-1}	23
14	o-Dichlorobenzene	182	50	5.5	1.69	0.74	2.71	1.4×10^{-1}	5.1×10^{-2}	23
15	Ammonia	303	25	9.1	1.40	0.96	10,675	2.3×10^{-1}	2.2×10^{-5}	7
16	Hydrogen chloride	309	5	9.3	0.69	0.97	46,320	2.3×10^{-1}	5.1×10^{-6}	9
17	Ethyl acrylate	315	5	9.5	0.69	0.98	69.8	2.4×10^{-1}	3.4×10^{-3}	23
18	p-tert-Butyltoluene	360	10	11	1.00	1.03	6.5	5.8×10^{-1}	8.8×10^{-1}	17
19	Dimethylamine	511	10	15	1.00	1.19	2,000	3.9×10^{-1}	1.9×10^{-4}	25
20	Ethyl acetate	614	400	18	2.60	1.26	164	4.7×10^{-1}	2.8×10^{-3}	26

Table 1 The RD_{50} Values, 1983 TLV-TWA Values, TLV-TWA Values Predicted on the Basis of 0.03 RD_{50}, Vapor Pressure, and Activity Coefficient (RD_{50} mm Hg/vapor pressure mm Hg) for 40 Industrial Chemicals (*Continued*)

Chemical No. in Fig. 4	Chemical	RD_{50} (ppm)	1983 TLV-TWA (ppm)	0.03 RD_{50} (ppm)	log 1983 TLV-TWA (ppm)	log 0.03 RD_{50} (ppm)	Saturated vapor pressure at 37° C (mm Hg)	RD_{50} (mm Hg)	Activity coefficient	References providing RD_{50} value
21	Epichlorohydrin	687	2	20	0.30	1.31	30.8	5.2×10^{-1}	1.7×10^{-2}	14
22	Cyclohexanone	756	25	23	1.40	1.35	8.2	5.7×10^{-1}	7.0×10^{-2}	23
23	Styrene	980	50	29	1.70	1.47	12.8	7.5×10^{-1}	5.8×10^{-2}	Alarie, 1979 unpublished
24	Chlorobenzene	1054	75	32	1.87	1.50	23	8.0×10^{-1}	3.5×10^{-2}	23
25	o-Xylene	1467	100	44	2.00	1.64	13	1.1	8.5×10^{-2}	23
26	Amylacetate	1531	100	46	2.00	1.66	8.4	1.2	1.4×10^{-1}	26
27	Isopropylbenzene (Cumene)	2490	50	75	1.69	1.87	9.7	1.9	1.9×10^{-1}	17
28	2-Butoxyethanol	2825	25	85	1.40	1.92	2.0	2.1	1.0	26
29	Methylisobutyl ketone	3195	50	96	1.69	1.98	7.5	2.4	3.2×10^{-1}	23
30	Ethylbenzene	4060	100	122	2.00	2.08	22.3	3.1	1.4×10^{-1}	17
31	Isoamyl alcohol	4452	100	134	2.00	2.13	8.9	3.4	3.8×10^{-1}	26
32	n-Butyl alcohol	4785	50	143	1.69	2.15	1.9	3.6	1.9×10^{-1}	26
33	Acetaldehyde	4946	100	148	2.00	2.17	1368	3.8	2.8×10^{-3}	26
34	Toluene	5300	100	159	2.00	2.20	55.5	4.1	7.3×10^{-2}	17
35	Methyl ethylketone	9000	200	270	2.30	2.43	156	8.2	5.2×10^{-2}	27
36	n-Propyl alcohol	12,704	200	381	2.30	2.58	42	9.7	2.3×10^{-1}	26
37	Isopropyl alcohol	17,693	400	531	2.60	2.73	90	13	1.5×10^{-1}	26
38	Ethyl alcohol	27,314	1000	819	3.00	2.91	122	21	1.7×10^{-1}	26
39	Methyl alcohol	41,514	200	1245	2.30	3.10	265	32	1.2×10^{-1}	26
40	Acetone	77,516	750	2345	2.88	3.37	375	58.9	1.6×10^{-1}	26

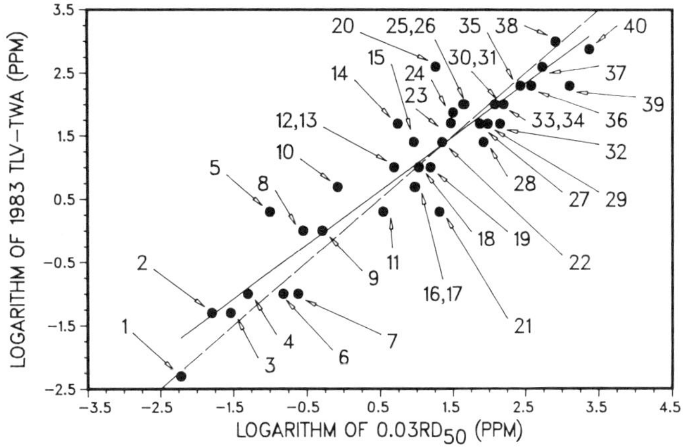

Figure 4 Linear least-squares regression analysis for 40 chemicals, plotting log of 0.03 RD_{50} as the proposed TLV-TWA versus the log of the 1983 TLV-TWA value for each chemical. From the data in Table 1. Regression equation: $Y = 0.302 + 0.81X$. Standard deviation of Y about the regression line = 0.48, $r = 0.92$, $r^2 = 0.85$. The correlation line, slope = 1, is given by the dashed line. Identification of the chemical for each number can be obtained from Table 1. [*From Alarie (16).*]

pathological changes on the nasal mucosa (19). Therefore, the results from this bioassay should also be used as guidelines for selecting levels of exposure in long-term toxicological evaluation, as previously suggested (6).

MECHANISMS OF SENSORY IRRITATION

Inspection of Table 1 and Fig. 4 reveals that a wide variety of chemicals act as sensory irritants and that the range of potency is very large. It has already been shown that among the most potent sensory irritants a good correlation exists between their reactivity toward nucleophilic groups and their biological activity (2). For the moderately potent sensory irritants, cleavage of disulfide bonds has been suggested as a mechanism for their biological activity (2). More recently, a mechanism of action for the weak sensory irritants has been presented (17) following the findings that their biological activity increases as the chain length increases within a homologous series, as shown in Fig. 5. When such relationships are obtained, the biological activity is probably due to a purely physical interaction between the chemical and the receptor, as proposed by Ferguson (20). This concept can be verified in the sense that the potency for each member within a series should be the same if a correction is made for the effect of phase distribution. Such a correction can be made with the RD_{50}, in ppm or mm Hg, divided by the vapor pressure of each chemical to yield an activity coefficient as given in Table 1. It can be seen that the activity coefficients for the weak

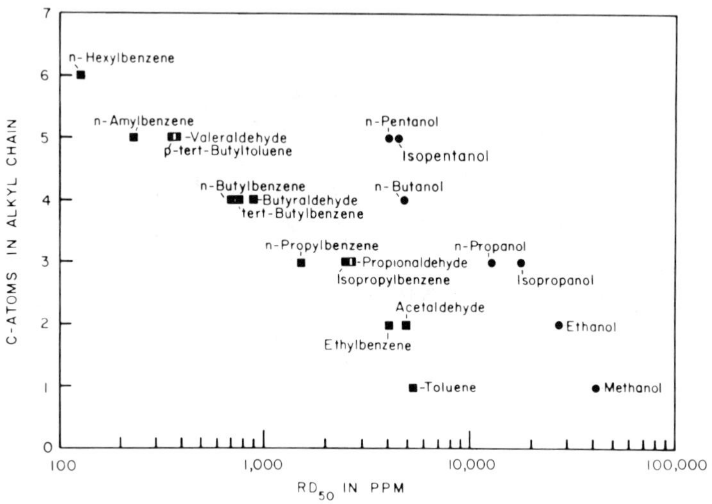

Figure 5 Relationships obtained for alkylbenzenes and aliphatic alcohols according to chain length. [*From Nielsen and Alarie (17) and Luo and Alarie, unpublished.*]

sensory irritants are between 0.1 and 1.0, thus strongly suggesting a purely physical action for aliphatic alcohols and alkylbenzenes. For the aldehydes, the activity coefficients are slightly lower, indicating that a chemical interaction is also involved. A most interesting finding is that the first member in the aliphatic aldehyde series, formaldehyde, has one of the lowest activity coefficients. This indicates a much higher chemical reactivity and specificity of interaction with the receptor than for the other members in the series. Thus, despite the wide variety of chemicals capable of eliciting sensory irritation, it appears that their biological effect can be explained via one of three basic mechanisms.

SUMMARY

Stimulation of trigeminal nerve endings located in the respiratory epithelium of the nasal mucosa by irritating airborne substances causes a variety of reflex reactions. These include inhibition of breathing, bradycardia, and a rise in systemic blood pressure. These reactions to airborne materials are of great interest to toxicologists because they are indicative of a chemical's likelihood to irritate and potentially damage the respiratory tract. In particular, the inhibition of breathing is easy to measure in experimental animals. Using mice, an animal model has been developed based on their characteristic decrease in respiratory rate. Concentration-response relationships can be obtained from the RD_{50}—the concentration necessary to decrease respiratory rate by 50%. It has been found that a good correlation exists between 0.03 RD_{50} and the threshold limit values (TLVs) for 40 industrial chemicals. This finding provides an animal model that can be used to set exposure guidelines for the prevention of sensory irritation in humans. The method is easy to use and requires few animals. These studies have also revealed that a wide variety of chemicals act as sensory irritants. The mechanisms of their effect are reviewed and generally fit three categories: (1) reactivity toward nucleophilic groups, (2) cleavage of disulphide bonds, and (3) a purely physical mechanism involving the thermodynamic and solubility properties of the irritant in a lipid bilayer containing receptor proteins.

REFERENCES

1 Kratschmer, F. Uber reflexe von der nasenschleimhaut auf athmung und kreislauf. In *Sitzungsberichte der Kaiserlichen Akademie der Wissenschaften, Mathematisch-Naturwissenschaftliche Classe,* Vol. 62, *Wein,* pp. 147–170 (1870).
2 Alarie, Y. Sensory irritation by airborne chemicals. *CRC Crit. Rev. Toxicol.* 2:299–366 (1973).
3 Magne, H, A Mayer, and L Plantefol. Recherches sur les actions reflexes produites par l'irritation des voies respiratoires. *Ann. Physiol.* 1:394–427 (1925).
4 Magne, H, A Mayer, and L Plantefol. La mort par inhibition et l'irritation des premieres voies respiratoires. *Ann. Physiol.* 1:428–443 (1925).
5 Allen, WF. Effect of various inhaled vapors on respiration and blood pressure in anesthetized, unanesthetized, sleeping and anosmic subjects. *Am. J. Physiol.* 88:620–632 (1929).
6 Alarie, Y. Toxicological evaluation of airborne chemical irritants and allergens using respiratory reflex reactions. In *Proceedings of the Inhalation Toxicology and Technology Symposium,* edited by BKJ Leong. Ann Arbor, MI: Ann Arbor Science Publishers, pp. 207–231 (1981).
7 Barrow, CS, Y Alarie, and MF Stock. Sensory irritation and incapacitation evoked by thermal decomposition products of polymers and comparisons with known sensory irritants. *Arch. Environ. Health,* Helen Dwight Reid Educational Foundation, 33:79–88 (1978).
8 Alarie, Y. Irritating properties of airborne materials to the upper respiratory tract. *Arch. Environ. Health,* Helen Dwight Reid Educational Foundation, 13:443–449 (1966).
9 Barrow, CS, Y Alarie, JC Warrick, and MF Stock. Comparison of the sensory irritation response in mice to chlorine and hydrogen chloride. *Arch. Environ. Health,* Helen Dwight Reid Educational Foundation, 32:68–76 (1977).
10 Alarie, Y. Bioassay for evaluating the potency of airborne sensory irritants and predicting acceptable levels of exposure in man. *Food Cosmet. Toxicol.* 19:623–626 (1981).
11 Alarie, Y, L Kane, and CS Barrow. Sensory irritation: A basis to establish acceptable exposure to airborne chemical irritants. In *Principles and Practice of Industrial Toxicology,* edited by A Reeves. New York: Wiley (1980).
12 Chang, JCF, WH Steinhagen, and CS Barrow. Effect of single or repeated

formaldehyde exposure on minute volume of B6C3F1 mice and F-344 rats. *Toxicol. Appl. Pharmacol.* 61:541–549 (1981).

13 Barrow, CS, and WH Steinhagen. Sensory irritation tolerance development to chlorine in F-344 rats following repeated inhalation. *Toxicol. Appl. Pharmacol.* 65:383–389 (1982).

14 Kane, LE, CS Barrow, and Y Alarie. A short-term test to predict acceptable levels of exposure to airborne sensory irritants. *Am. Ind. Hyg. Assoc. J.* 40:207–229 (1979).

15 Alarie, Y. Dose-response analysis in animal studies: Prediction of human responses. *Environ. Health Perspect.* 42:9–13 (1981).

16 Alarie, Y. Establishing threshold limit values for airborne sensory irritants from an animal model and the mechanisms of action of sensory irritants. *Adv. Environ. Toxicol.* Vol. 8:153–164 (1984).

17 Nielsen, GD, and Y Alarie. Sensory irritation, pulmonary irritation, and respiratory stimulation by airborne benzene and alkylbenzenes: Prediction of safe industrial exposure levels and correlation with their thermodynamic properties. *Toxicol. Appl. Pharmacol.* 65:459–477 (1982).

18 Weyel, DA, BS Rodney, and Y Alarie. Sensory irritation, pulmonary irritation, and acute lethality of a polymeric isocyanate and sensory irritation of 2,6-toluene diisocyanate. *Toxicol. Appl. Pharmacol.* 64:423–430 (1982).

19 Buckley, LA, XZ Jiang, RA James, KT Morgan, and CS Barrow. Respiratory tract lesions induced by sensory irritants at the RD_{50} concentration. *Toxicol. Appl. Pharmacol.* 74:417–429 (1984).

20 Ferguson, J. The use of chemical potentials as indices of toxicity. *Proc. R. Soc. Lond. Ser. B* 127:387–404 (1939).

21 Sangha, GK, and Y Alarie. Sensory irritation by toluene diisocyanate in single and repeated exposures. *Toxicol. Appl. Pharmacol.* 50:533–547 (1979).

22 Kane, LE, and Y Alarie. Sensory irritation to formaldehyde and acrolein during single and repeated exposures in mice. *Am. Ind. Hyg. Assoc. J.* 38:509–522 (1977).

23 DeCeaurriz, JC, JC Micillino, P Bonnet, and JP Guenier. Sensory irritation caused by various industrial airborne chemicals. *Toxicol. Lett.* 9:137–143 (1981).

24 Alarie, Y, I Wakisaka, and S Oka. Sensory irritation by sulfur dioxide and chlorobenzylidene malononitrile. *Environ. Physiol. Biochem.* 3:53–74 (1973).

25 Steinhagen, WH, J Swenberg, and CS Barrow. Acute inhalation toxicity and sensory irritation of dimethylamine. *Am. Ind. Hyg. Assoc. Meeting Abstr.*, Abstract 297 (1981).

26 Kane, LE, R Dombroske, and Y Alarie. Evaluation of sensory irritation from some common industrial solvents. *Am. Ind. Hyg. Assoc. J.* 41:451–455 (1980).

27 Stone, LC, GT Lawhorn, JC McKinney, and MS McCracken. Upper respiratory tract sensory response to volatile chemicals. *Toxicologist* 1:134. (1981).

Chapter 7

Sensory Irritation: Studies on Correlation to Pathology, Structure-Activity, Tolerance Development, and Prediction of Species Differences to Nasal Injury

Craig S. Barrow, Lorrene A. Buckley, Richard A. James, William H. Steinhagen, and Jane C. F. Chang

INTRODUCTION

The respiratory system is endowed with a variety of defense mechanisms to protect it from injury or to minimize absorption of toxicants of infectious organisms into the body. The components of the respiratory tract defense system include mucociliary clearance, immune responses and antimicrobial defenses, and reflex responses (1). The reflex responses vary depending on the site of the receptor (nasal cavity, larynx, trachea, alveoli). Stimulation of these can result in changes in ventilation, bronchomotor tone, blood pressure, and airway mucus secretion. As summarized by Widdicombe (1), the main functions of these reflex responses are (1) to prevent or minimize penetration of the airborne substance into the respiratory tract, (2) to expel the foreign material by coughing or sneezing, or (3) to make appropriate physiological adjustments for decreasing the action of the stimulus or to prepare the body against the stress (i.e., reflex bradycardia due to decreases in minute ventilation).

The authors thank Ms. J. Quate and Ms. L. Smith for preparation of the manuscript.

Our research has been concerned with one of these reflex responses, specifically the trigeminal nerve or sensory irritation response originating from the nasal epithelium. As discussed in the previous chapter, stimulation of the trigeminal nerve endings results in a painful burning sensation, a desire to withdraw from the contaminated atmosphere, and a decrease in respiratory rate. As a defense mechanism, its importance resides in the fact that inhalation of the noxious agent is minimized while the perception of pain serves as a warning to avoid the contaminated atmosphere (1-3). Our laboratory has conducted a series of different studies on sensory irritation that can be divided into four separate areas.

The first is a comparison of a series of widely differing sensory irritants that induce structural damage to the respiratory system. The animal model described in the preceding chapter uses respiratory rate depression of mice as the endpoint to quantitate the sensory irritation potential of an airborne chemical. This response has been shown to exhibit a concentration-response relationship for a large number of sensory irritants (4). As a point of comparison, the RD_{50} value, or the concentration that causes a 50% decrease in respiratory rate, can be used to conveniently compare the relative potencies of different irritants. Kane et al. (5) have proposed that the RD_{50} concentration of a sensory irritant will cause intolerable sensory irritation and possible respiratory tract injury following extended or repeated exposure and would not be an acceptable occupational exposure level. Although the prediction of pain and intolerable sensory irritation appears to be correct (4, 5), there is little information regarding respiratory tract injury in humans or experimental animals at the RD_{50} concentration. Thus, the objectives of this study were to determine if pathologic changes occur in the respiratory tract of groups of mice after inhalation exposure to various sensory irritants at their respective RD_{50} concentration and to compare any changes with respect to type, distribution, and severity.

In the second study, the renewed interest in formaldehyde toxicity, because of its carcinogenic action on the nasal passages in rats (6, 7), precipitated our investigation of the sensory irritation potential of a series of aldehydes. The purpose of these experiments was (1) to examine the structure-activity of a series of saturated aliphatic, unsaturated aliphatic, and cyclic aldehydes; (2) to compare the sensory irritation potential of the selected aldehydes in male B6C3F1 and Swiss-Webster mice and assess the suitability of using B6C3F1 mice as an alternate strain to study sensory irritation; and (3) to compare the tentative threshold limit values (TLVs) derived from the model to currently published TLVs for aldehydes.

Physiological adaptations to the effects of lower respiratory tract irritants such as ozone have been well documented (8-10), but there are few reports on tolerance and cross tolerance to sensory irritants of the upper respiratory tract. A few studies have been published in animals concerning tolerance to formaldehyde (11, 12) or chlorine (13). Adaptation to the irritating effects of both chlorine (14) and formaldehyde in humans (15) has been published. In general, these reports demonstrated that HCHO or Cl_2 can induce tolerance under different exposure concentrations and exposure times. However, a definitive investigation has not been undertaken. Thus, the third area of study was initiated (1) to provide information on the concentration and duration of exposure required to induce tolerance in F-344 rats to Cl_2 and HCHO, (2) to determine whether tolerance to Cl_2 can lead to cross tolerance to HCHO and vice versa, and (3) to study the persistence of tolerance and cross tolerance after 7 days of recovery.

The fourth and last set of experiments was designed to evaluate the importance of the sensory irritation response in explaining species differences in toxicology of the nasal passages. Data have accumulated that indicate that water-soluble sensory irritants cause varying degrees of toxicity to the nasal passages of mice in comparison to rats after exposure to the same concentrations of each chemical. Three recent examples include formaldehyde (16), acrylic acid (17), and dimethylamine (18). Since the decrease in ventilation to irritants is an important defense mechanism, these species differences may be due, in part, to differences in the sensory irritation response between rats and mice. To evaluate this hypothesis a series of experiments was designed to compare the "dose" available for deposition in the nasal epithelium of mice versus rats for these three chemicals and to correlate nasal cavity toxicity, including tissue damage and cell turnover, with the calculated "dose."

Detailed discussions of the four series of experiments have been previously published (18-20). A summary of each of the studies follows.

COMPARISON OF RESPIRATORY TRACT PATHOLOGY IN MICE

Methods

Male Swiss-Webster mice weighing 25-30 g were used in this study. The compounds studied were selected on the basis of their physical properties (particularly water solubility), chemical reactivity, and sensory irritation potency. Ten chemicals were chosen for comparison (Table 1).

Groups of 16-24 mice were exposed in a whole-body chamber (22) for 5 days, 6 h per day, to the RD_{50} concentration of each sensory irritant. Half of each group of exposed mice, as well as unexposed controls (8-10 per group), were necropsied immediately after the last exposure. All remaining mice were killed and necropsied approximately 72 h after the last exposure. The head, trachea, and lungs were fixed in 10% buffered Formalin. To evaluate the nasal epithelium, blocks were cut at five different levels. All tissues from the respiratory tract were sectioned at 5 μm and stained with hematoxylin and eosin (H&E) for light microscopic examination and grading of lesions.

Table 1 Ten Sensory Irritants Studied with RD_{50} Concentrations, Time-weighted Average Exposure Concentrations, and Water Solubilities

Compound	RD_{50}* (ppm)	TWA (ppm) (range)	Water solubility (25°C) (g/100 g H_2O)
Chloropicrin	7.98	7.9 (7.9–8.0)	0.16
Chlorine	9.34	9.7 (9.5–9.9)	0.50
Epichlorohydrin†	687	697	6.5
Sulfur dioxide	117	117 (116–118)	8.5
Acrolein	1.7	1.7 (1.67–1.73)	25–33
Ammonia	303	305 (298–308)	31
Dimethylamine	511	510 (509–511)	55
Formaldehyde	3.13	3.1 (3.10–3.18)	55
Hydrogen chloride‡	309	304 (298–310)	67.3 (30°C)
Toluene diisocyanate	0.39	0.4 (0.37–0.43)	Decomposes in H_2O

[*From Buckley et al. (18).*]
*Kane et al. (5); Steinhagen et al. (49).
†One exposure.
‡Three exposures.

Results

The time-weighted average (TWA) chamber concentrations for each of the irritants studied are listed in Table 1. Body weights of exposed mice were decreased 10–25 percent compared to controls, but in most cases they returned to normal levels by 3 days postexposure. Only three hydrogen chloride exposures and one epichlorohydrin exposure were performed owing to high mortality.

Control animals showed no histologic evidence of disease or other abnormality in the respiratory tract. The normal anatomy and histologic appearance of the nasal epithelium has been described previously (18, 20). Lesions were found for each of the 10 chemicals studied (18). The anterior respiratory epithelium adjacent to the vestibule and the olfactory epithelium in the dorsal meatus were the most vulnerable areas (Table 2, Fig. 1). Lesions induced in the respiratory epithelium ranged from deciliation, to small areas of epithelial cell damage with exfoliation, to erosions and ulceration, to frank necrosis (Table 2). Chlorine, sulfur dioxide, dimethylamine, and hydrogen chloride caused the most severe effects.

Table 2 Lesions in the Respiratory Tract of Swiss-Webster Mice Exposed to 10 Sensory Irritants at the RD_{50} Concentrations*

Chemical	Squamous epithelium	Respiratory epithelium			Olfactory epithelium				
	(EXF, INF)†	EXF, ERO, ULC, NEC	INF	SQM	ULC, NEC	SQM	DEG of nerves	Serous exudate	Lung
Epichlorohydrin	—	++	+	—	++	—	—	+	+
Chloropicrin	—	++	+	+	++	—	—	+	++
Chlorine	—	+++	+	+	+++	—	+	+	++
Sulfur dioxide	—	+++	++	++	+++	+	—	++	—
Acrolein	—	++	++	+++	++	+	—	+	—
Ammonia	—	+	−+	+/—	—	—	—	—	—
Dimethylamine	—	+++	−/—	+/—	+++	—	++	—	—
Formaldehyde	—	+	+	+	—	—	—	—	—
Hydrogen chloride	+/—	+++	+	—	+	—	—	+	—
Toluene diisocyanate	+/—	++	+	+++	++	—	+	+	—

[*From Buckley et al.* (18).]

*All exposures were carried out for 5 days, 6 h/day, except epichlorohydrin (1 day) and hydrogen chloride (3 days). Lesions are graded with respect to incidence and severity and on a plus-minus scale: —, no change; +/—, slight effect of doubtful significance; +, minimal change; ++, moderate change; +++, severe change.

†Abbreviations used: EXF, exfoliation; INF, inflammation; ERO, erosion; ULC, ulceration, NEC, necrosis; SQM, squamous metaplasia; DEG, degeneration.

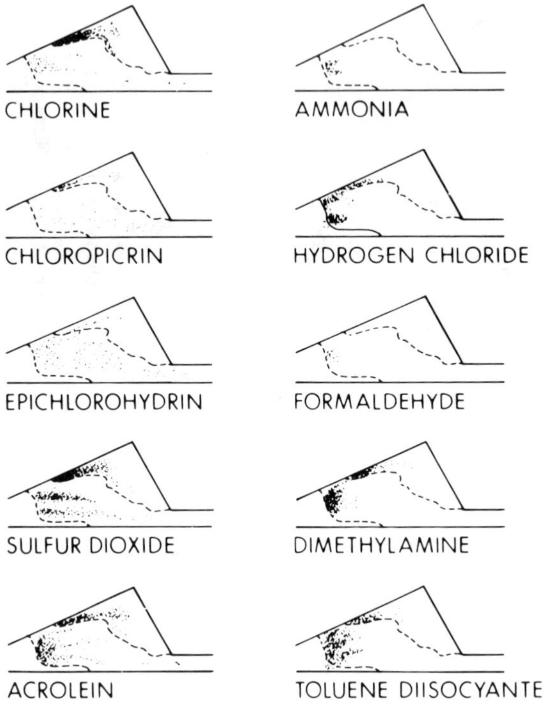

Figure 1 Diagrammatic sketch to show distribution and severity of lesions in the nasal passages. The limits of the squamous, respiratory, and olfactory epithelia are indicated by the broken lines. The density of the stippling gives an indication of severity, with areas having the severest lesions being most densely stippled. [*From Buckley et al. (18).*]

Lesions in the olfactory epithelium varied from a slight loss to more extensive loss of sensory cells including damage to sustentacular cells and underlying olfactory nerves. In severe cases a complete loss of olfactory epithelium occurred, leaving a denuded basement membrane with exudate in the lumen. Chlorine, sulfur dioxide, and dimethylamine caused the most severe olfactory lesions (Fig. 1, Table 2).

Only chlorine, chloropicrin, and epichlorohydrin induced lesions in the lower respiratory tract (Table 2). Chlorine induced a moderately severe, terminal bronchiolitis, with occlusion of affected bronchioles by serocellular exudate. Chloropicrin induced a moderate to severe, fibrosing peribronchitis and peribronchiolitis. With epichlorohydrin, there was only slight exfoliation of bronchial epithelial cells and diffuse infiltration by neutrophils.

Mice sacrificed 72 h after the last exposure exhibited varied recovery. Generally, inflammation and exudation were reduced, but there was little difference in the extent of ulceration or degenerative lesions. Overall, recovery was minimal to moderate, suggesting that the recovery period was insufficient for complete repair of the lesions.

Discussion

Damage to the respiratory epithelium following exposure to the 10 sensory irritants ranged from epithelial hypertrophy or hyperplasia to erosion, ulceration, and necrosis with variable inflammation, and squamous metaplasia. Olfactory epithelium appears to be especially sensitive to injury (17, 23-26). Our study confirmed this, in that 8 of the 10 sensory irritants affected the olfactory epithelium, with the sensory cells being particularly sensitive. The keratinized, squamous epithelium of the vestibule was mostly unaffected, indicating its resistance to these irritants. Lung lesions caused by epichlorohydrin, chlorine, and chloropicrin were similar to those previously reported for the gases (26-30).

Unlike the severity of lesions, which showed considerable variation, the irritants studied caused a very similar pattern of distribution. A distinct anterior-posterior gradient was seen, with the most severe effects found in the anterior respiratory epithelium adjacent to the vestibule and on the free margins of the naso- and maxilloturbinates. Olfactory lesions were largely confined to the dorsal meatus. This type of distribution may be largely determined by airflow patterns, but this remains to be studied. Lesions produced by the most water-soluble irritants were generally restricted to the anterior areas of the nose, whereas only the least water-soluble irritants produced lung lesions.

In conclusion, these studies demonstrated that repeated exposure to the RD_{50} concentration is associated with respiratory tract damage in mice and is not an acceptable concentration for occupational exposure. This provides support to the validity of the sensory irritation model for prediction of injury from exposure to airborne sensory irritants.

STRUCTURE-ACTIVITY STUDY OF ALDEHYDES

Methods

Male B6C3F1 mice weighing 19-27 g and male Swiss-Webster mice weighing 20-32 g were used. Aldehydes studied included acetaldehyde, propionaldehyde, butyraldehyde, isobutyraldehyde, valeraldehyde, isovaleraldehyde, caproaldehyde, 2-ethylbutyraldehyde, acrolein, crotonaldehyde, 2-furaldehyde, cyclohexanecarboxaldehyde, 3-cyclohexene-1-carboxaldehyde, and benzaldehyde. The inhalation exposure techniques used to generate and analyze these test atmospheres have been described previously (31).

Sensory irritation was quantitated by measuring respiratory rate depression in the test animals during exposure to varying concentrations of each aldehyde. The animals were sealed in airtight body plethysmographs attached to the head-only exposure chamber and allowed to acclimate for ~10 min. Respiratory rates were recorded during a 5-min preexposure, 10-min exposure, and 5-min recovery period. The average maximum decrease in respiratory rate for a 1-min period was computed from the response of each group of animals and plotted versus the logarithm of the exposure concentration. This was performed using various concentrations of each aldehyde, and a concentration-response curve plotted from which the RD_{50} value was determined. Comparisons were then made between the various aldehydes tested.

Results

The 14 aldehydes studied had RD_{50} values that spanned three orders of magnitude (Fig. 2). Acetaldehyde (RD_{50} 2845 ppm) had an irritation potential three orders of magnitude less than formaldehyde (RD_{50} 3.1 ppm), demonstrating irritancy reduction by methyl group addition. However, if a carbon double bond was also present–i.e., acrolein or crotonaldehyde (RD_{50} values of 1.03 and 3.53 ppm, respectively)–the relative potency was similar to formaldehyde (RD_{50} 3.13 ppm). Saturated aliphatic aldehydes with 3-6 carbon atoms had RD_{50} values similar to acetaldehyde. Cyclic aldehydes produced RD_{50} values intermediate between the saturated aliphatic aldehydes and formaldehyde. Thus, the relative potencies of these aldehydes fall into three groups as follows: unsaturated aliphatics and formaldehyde (RD_{50}s 1-3 ppm), cyclics (RD_{50}s 100-300 ppm), and saturated aliphatics (RD_{50}s 1000-3000 ppm).

No statistically significant differences in slope were found between Swiss-Webster and B6C3F1 mice for any of the aldehydes tested. When differences

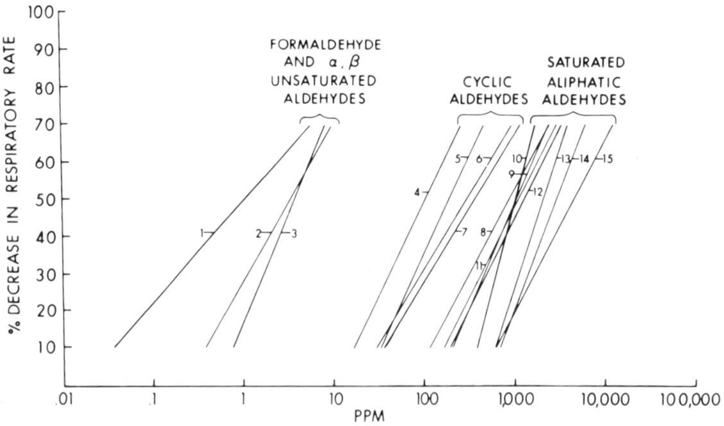

Figure 2 Concentration-response curves of Swiss-Webster mice exposed to aldehydes: (1) acrolein, (2) formaldehyde (11), (3) crotonaldehyde, (4) 3-cyclohexene-1-carboxaldehyde, (5) cyclohexanecarboxaldehyde, (6) 2-furaldehyde, (7) benzaldehyde, (8) 2-ethylbutyraldehyde, (9) isovaleraldehyde, (10) butyraldehyde, (11) caproaldehyde, (12) valeraldehyde, (13) propionaldehyde, (14) acetaldehyde, and (15) isobutyraldehyde. [*From Steinhagen and Barrow (31).*]

in elevation were compared, it was determined that butyraldehyde, crotonaldehyde, 2-ethylbutyraldehyde, and 3-cyclohexene-1-carboxaldehyde were statistically different between the two strains. However, these represented a factor of only 1.2 to 1.6, indicating little, if any, biological significance.

Discussion

Clear conclusions regarding the mechanisms involved in the large potency differences seen between the aldehydes cannot be made at this time because it is not known how airborne chemical irritants stimulate the trigeminal nerve endings in the nasal mucosa. Several theories have been proposed, such as reaction with SH groups, NH_2 groups, and/or the amide nitrogen of receptor proteins associated with free trigeminal nerve endings (32). Aldehydes are known to react with these functional groups, and the differences in relative potencies reported here would be expected to coincide with their ability to react with SH or NH_2 groups (33). The sensory irritation response of the saturated aliphatic aldehydes may also be a function of their ability to undergo hydration (31). Addition reactions with SH, NH_2, and OH groups in receptor proteins by acrolein and crotonaldehyde have also been proposed as a possible mechanism (31). Recently, it has been proposed that some airborne chemicals (i.e., alkylbenzenes) may have a physical mechanism of stimulation related to certain thermodynamic characteristics of the molecule (34). Additionally, molecular conformation and receptor binding may contribute to potency differences for these chemicals.

Tentative TLVs for human exposure to sensory irritants have been extrapolated from the RD_{50} value for Swiss-Webster mice, based on the reflex decrease in respiratory rate (5, 35). Based on this animal model, TLVs for sensory irritation of airborne chemicals have been proposed to be 0.01-0.1. These are the RD_{50} values where the expected human responses would range from minimal or no sensory irritation to slight, but tolerable, irritation (Table 3). The 0.1 RD_{50} is also recommended as the ceiling value. As discussed in the previous chapter, 0.03 RD_{50} has also been recommended as a tentative TLV because of the strong correlation to current TLVs. Either approach provides useful information for establishing TLVs for prevention of sensory irritation.

The suggested TLVs for acetaldehyde, acrolein, valeraldehyde, and furfural are in good agreement with those currently established (Table 3). Two notable exceptions are crotonaldehyde and formaldehyde. Each has a current TLV of 2 ppm, approximately an order of magnitude higher than suggested from the sensory irritation animal model. In reviewing human exposure data for crotonaldehyde, the threshold for highly irritating concentrations is reported to range from 4.1 to 45 ppm. It is possible that these conflicting results may result from errors in accurately measuring the air concentration of crotonaldehyde (36).

Table 3 List of Recommended TLVs for Aldehydes Studied

Aldehyde tested	RD_{50} (ppm)	Recommended TLV based on prevention of sensory irritation (0.01–$0.1\ RD_{50}$)	Current TLV (ppm)*
Acetaldehyde	2845	29-285	100
Propionaldehyde	2052	21-205	–†
Acrolein	1.03	0.01-0.1	0.1
Butyraldehyde	1015	10-100	–
Isobutyraldehyde	4167	42-417	–
Crotonaldehyde	3.53	0.04-0.4	2
Valeraldehyde	1121	11-112	50
Isovaleraldehyde	1008	10-101	–
Caproaldehyde	1029	10-103	–
2-Ethylbutyraldehyde	843	8-84	–
2-Furaldehyde	287	3-29	2
Cyclohexanecarboxaldehyde	183	2-18	–
3-Cyclohexene-1-carboxaldehyde	95	1-10	–
Benzaldehyde	333	3-33	–
Formaldehyde‡	3.13	0.03-0.3	2

[*From Steinhagen and Barrow (31).*]

*From threshold limit values for chemical substances in workroom air adopted by ACGIH for 1982.

†Indicates no TLV has been published.

‡Kane and Alarie, 1977 (11).

For formaldehyde, there is evidence from human studies that sensory irritation occurs between 1 and 2 ppm and perhaps at lower concentrations (37–41). The current 2-ppm TLV is defended by stating "rapid inurement to such concentrations develops, and there is a general absence of complaints from workers exposed at levels below 2 or 3 ppm" (36). The present studies suggest, however, the necessity of further research for crotonaldehyde and formaldehyde to provide a perspective on the current TLVs of 2 ppm for the prevention of sensory irritation.

TOLERANCE AND CROSS-TOLERANCE BETWEEN Cl_2 AND HCHO

Methods

For these studies, male F-344 rats weighing 150–200 g were used. To investigate tolerance to Cl_2 rats were exposed to 10 ppm Cl_2 6 h/day for 1, 4, or 10 days or to 2.5 ppm for 4 or 10 days. Sensory irritation was quantitated by constructing concentration-response curves in these animals as described in the aldehyde study and compared to naive animals exposed to Cl_2. Cross tolerance to HCHO was also investigated in Cl_2-pretreated animals. The reversibility of tolerance to Cl_2 or cross tolerance to HCHO was also studied in animals given a 7-day recovery period following pretreatment to Cl_2.

Experiments were also undertaken to investigate sensory irritation tolerance development in HCHO-pretreated rats exposed to 15 ppm HCHO, 6 h/day for 4 or 10 days, or 28 ppm HCHO for 4 days. Similar to the experiments with rats pretreated to Cl_2, cross-tolerance studies were performed in HCHO-pretreated rats challenged to Cl_2. Investigations to assess reversibility were also done.

Results

Rats pretreated to 10 ppm Cl_2 for 1, 4, or 10 days showed tolerance development when compared to naive animals (Fig. 3). The RD_{50} values were 10.9, 35.9, 206, and 242 ppm for naive, 1, 4, and 10 days of pretreatment, respectively (19). Animals pretreated to 2.5 ppm Cl_2 also showed tolerance development, but only in the 10-day exposure group. These results revealed both time and concentration dependence for Cl_2 tolerance development. The RD_{50} increased less than twofold compared to naive animals in the group exposed to 2.5 ppm for 10 days, but a 20-fold increase occurred in the groups pretreated to 10 ppm for 4 or 10 days.

Rats exposed to 15 ppm HCHO 6 h/day for up to 10 days did not show tolerance to HCHO. However, a pretreatment to 28 ppm for 4 days did result in a shifted concentration-response curve, with an increase in RD_{50} from 31.7 to 70.2 ppm (19).

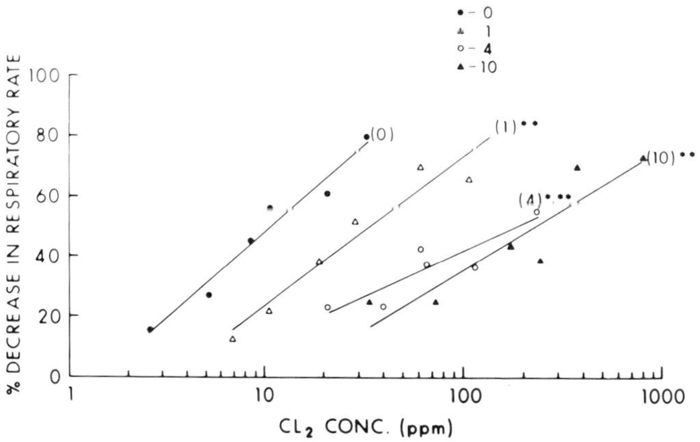

Figure 3 Concentration-response curves for Cl_2 for naive rats (0) and rats preexposed to 10 ppm Cl_2 (6 h/day) for 1, 4, or 10 days. Single and double asterisks indicate significant differences in slope and elevation compared to the naive group, respectively. [*From Chang and Barrow (19).*]

Rats pretreated to Cl_2 and found to be tolerant were also cross-tolerant to HCHO (Fig. 4). The RD_{50} for HCHO at 10 days (115 ppm) was increased twofold over the 1-day (64.5 ppm) and 4-day (66 ppm) groups, and fourfold over the naive animals (31.7 ppm).

Exposure to 15 ppm HCHO, although failing to induce tolerance to HCHO, did result in cross tolerance to Cl_2 (Fig. 4). The effect was significant after a single 6-h exposure and was most pronounced in the 10-day group. Compared to the Cl_2 RD_{50} in naive animals (10.9 ppm), this was increased to 22.6, 16.8, and 64.5 ppm following 1, 4, or 10 days' pretreatment, respectively.

Experiments designed to study the degree of recovery in rats tolerant to Cl_2 demonstrated a considerable loss of tolerance in rats exposed to 10 ppm Cl_2 for 4 days followed by 7 days of recovery. The RD_{50} following recovery was approximately threefold higher than in naive animals (10.9 ppm) compared to 20-fold higher RD_{50} in the group with no recovery period. After 7 days of recovery only slight reductions were seen in cross tolerance to HCHO in rats pretreated to Cl_2 or vice versa (19).

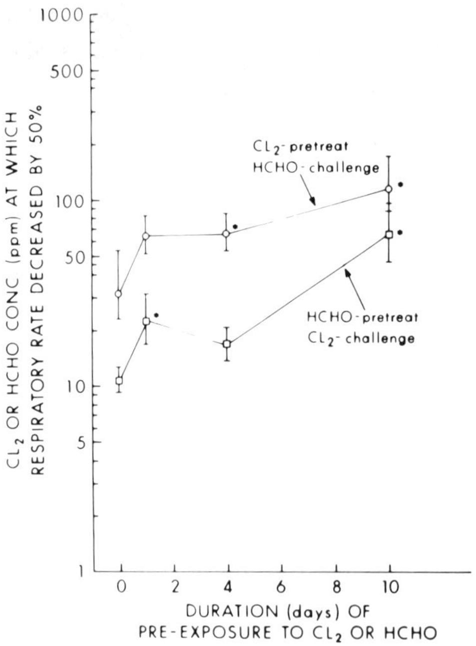

Figure 4 Time-course development of cross tolerance to Cl_2 in rats preexposed to HCHO and vice versa. The preexposure concentration was 15 ppm for the HCHO group and 10 ppm for the Cl_2 group. Each data point represents the RD_{50} and its 95 percent confidence interval. An asterisk indicates a significant difference compared to the RD_{50} value of the naive group. [*From Chang and Barrow (19).*]

Discussion

The occurrence of tolerance to Cl_2 and cross tolerance between HCHO and Cl_2 suggests that a common mechanism exists whereby these chemicals react with the trigeminal nerve endings. Different reactive sites for Cl_2 and HCHO may help explain the finding of cross tolerance to Cl_2 in HCHO-pretreated rats even though no tolerance to HCHO was seen. Pretreatment to Cl_2 may have destroyed or desensitized both Cl_2 and HCHO reactive sites thereby accounting for the simultaneous development of tolerance to Cl_2 and cross tolerance to HCHO. On the other hand, pretreatment to HCHO may have desensitized or destroyed more Cl_2 reactive sites than those of HCHO, resulting only in cross tolerance to Cl_2.

The actual mechanism of this effect is obscure. Reactions with sulfhydryl (SH) groups may be involved (32). The trigeminal nerve endings are cholinergic (42), and cholinergic receptor proteins possess SH groups (43). It is possible that pretreatment to Cl_2 or HCHO could change the SH concentration of the receptor, resulting in tolerance and/or cross-tolerance. Damage of the trigeminal nerve as a mechanism responsible for tolerance and cross-tolerance development is also possible. The partial return to a normal state following the 7-day recovery suggests the occurrence of neuronal repair. Such damage is known to be slowly reversible (44). However, similar to the SH hypothesis, no direct evidence is currently available to either prove or disprove these theories.

In summary, these studies have demonstrated that tolerance and cross tolerance can be induced under various exposure conditions. As stated earlier, the reflex apnea response evoked by sensory irritants is an important respiratory tract defense mechanism (1, 32). Tolerance or cross tolerance compromises this and may place the animals at greater risk to respiratory tract injury from inhaled chemicals.

QUANTITATION OF NASAL "DOSE" WITH FORMALDEHYDE, ACRYLIC ACID, AND DIMETHYLAMINE

Methods

Male F-344 rats (180–280 g) and male B6C3F1 mice (20–30 g) were used in these studies. The animals were first pretreated by whole-body exposure to a target concentration of 15 ppm formaldehyde (HCHO), 75 ppm acrylic acid (AA), or 175 ppm dimethylamine (DMA) 6 h/day for 4 days. On the fifth day, groups of two rats or two mice were exposed to these same target concentrations of HCHO, AA, or DMA for 6 h in a glass, head-only chamber. Respiratory rates and tidal volumes were measured before and during exposure to HCHO, AA, or DMA by a body plethysmograph technique (45). Twenty minutes after groups of two animals entered the head-only chamber, a 10-min preexposure period of baseline tidal volume and respiratory rate was recorded. This was followed by a 6-h exposure to HCHO, AA, or DMA, during which a recording was made the first 10 min of the first hour, followed by the last 10 min of each hour until the exposure ended. Since this study was designed to quantify the amount of chemical inhaled, only the inspiratory tidal volume was recorded. From the tidal volume and respiratory rate recordings, minute volume was calculated. A total of 7-10 rats or mice were studied for each chemical.

The "dose" to the nasal epithelium was derived from normalization of the amount of HCHO, AA, or DMA inhaled over the nasal cavity surface area as described by Chang et al. (20):

$$\text{"dose"} = \frac{\text{HCHO, AA, or DMA concentration } (\mu\text{g/liter}) \times \text{ minute volume (liter/min)}}{\text{nasal cavity surface area } (\text{cm}^2)}$$

Nasal cavity surface area has been reported to be 13.44 cm^2 for 288-g rats and 2.77 cm^2 for 30-g mice, respectively (46).

Species differences in delivered "dose" were further assessed by comparative histopathology and cell turnover studies. Eighteen hours after 5 days of exposure to either HCHO, AA, or DMA, mice and rats were administered 2 μCi/g body weight of [^{3}H]thymidine by intraperitoneal injection. Two hours later the animals were anesthetized with methoxyflurane and killed by exsanguination. The head was skinned and the lower jaw removed. With HCHO the tissue was processed into four paraffin blocks per animal. Sections 4-6 μm thick were obtained from levels 1, 2, 3, and 4 of the nasal cavity (20), mounted on slides, deparaffinized, and dipped in Kodak NTB-2 emulsion. For AA or DMA, the tissue was mounted in glycol methacrylate (GMA) and sections cut 2 μm thick. For histopathology, sections were prepared in a similar manner, but were not dipped in emulsions. After determination of the principal location of the lesion, the rate of cell replication was quantitated. For AA, the total number of cells lining the olfactory epithelium from the dorsal meatus of level 3 were counted. For HCHO, the total number of cells lining the respiratory epithelium from the nasal and maxillary turbinates and lateral wall were counted. The number of cells with five or more silver grains over the nucleus, divided by the total number of cells, was expressed as a percentage of replicating cells. Cell turnover data for DMA have not been completed.

Results

Exposure of F-344 rats and B6C3F1 mice to 15 ppm HCHO for 6 h following the 4-day pretreatment resulted in an immediate decrease in respiratory rate and minute volume (20). Tidal volume was unchanged. During the 6-h exposure, minute volume in mice was depressed by 50 percent of preexposure values or greater. On the other hand, rats had only a 15 percent decrease in minute volume (20). When these data were used to calculate the dose of HCHO to the nasal cavity, it was found that mice had significantly less intake than rats (Fig. 5). Integrated over the entire 6 h this was found to be ~75 percent greater in rats than mice.

Cell proliferation results indicated that rats had a 13-fold increase compared to an eightfold increase in mice after 1 day of exposure (20). With repeated daily exposure to 15 ppm HCHO for 5 days, the increase above control labeling in mice was 13-fold, not significantly different from that of the 1-day exposure. However, rats showed an increase that was 23-fold greater than that of the control animals, which was statistically significant compared to the 1-day group.

Histopathologic examination of the nasal epithelium of rats and mice exposed to 15 ppm HCHO after 5 days of exposure revealed that rats had more severe lesions (20). Characteristic lesions in the rat nasal cavity included severe ulcerative rhinitis, inflammatory infiltrates, epithelial hyperplasia, increased numbers of mitoses, and early karyomegaly. Mice showed only mild to moderate hyperplasia and focal areas of ulceration.

Exposure of F-344 rats to 75 ppm AA after 4 days of pretreatment resulted in a 17 percent decrease in respiratory rate within the first 10 minutes of exposure. This decrease remained constant for the 6-h exposure, ranging

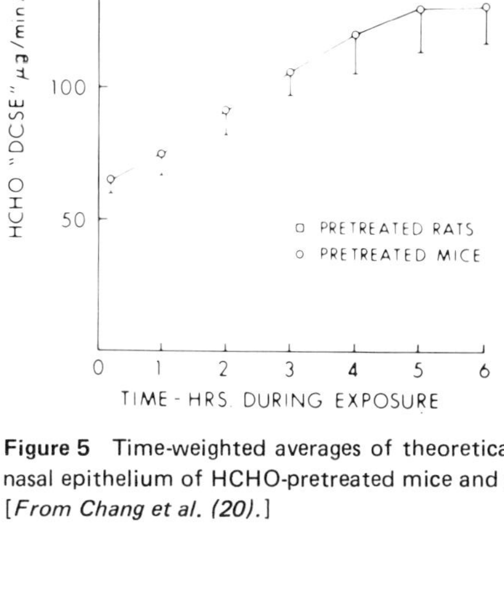

Figure 5 Time-weighted averages of theoretical HCHO dose available for deposition on the nasal epithelium of HCHO-pretreated mice and rats during a 6-h exposure to 15 ppm HCHO. [*From Chang et al. (20).*]

between 16 percent and 23 percent. There was very little effect on tidal volume, with the percent change varying between 93 percent and 103 percent of control values. Because of this failure to compensate for the decrease in respiratory rate, the decrease in minute volume essentially paralleled that of respiratory frequency, and averaged approximately 23 percent during the entire exposure.

The changes in respiratory frequency, tidal volume, and minute volume of B6C3F1 mice exposed to 75 ppm AA following pretreatment were similar to those found in F-344 rats. The decrease in respiratory rate ranged from 32 percent to 37 percent, with only slight effects on tidal volume. The decrease in minute volume ranged from 27 percent to 34 percent and averaged 31 percent.

Exposure to AA resulted in significantly more predicted intake of AA in the nasal passages of mice than rats (Fig. 6). The "dose" in mice ranged from 3.5 to 3.8 $\mu g/min/cm^2$ compared to 1.8-2.1 $\mu g/min/cm^2$ in rats. Averaged over the 6-h exposure period, mice were predicted to receive 88 percent more acrylic acid to the nasal cavity epithelium than rats.

This predicted dose difference was supported by the histopathology and cell proliferation studies. The pathology was characterized by severe lesions in both species. Respiratory tract lesions were confined to the nasal passages and particularly the olfactory epithelium of the dorsal meatus. Mice had more severe lesions, as seen by the presence of more cellular exudate in the lumen of the nose and a much greater loss of sensory cells. In the dorsal meatus of level 3, total epithelial cell counts indicated a 50 percent decrease in mice versus 15 percent in rats. Cell proliferation studies showed a statistically significant increase in cell turnover of the olfactory epithelium in the dorsal meatus of

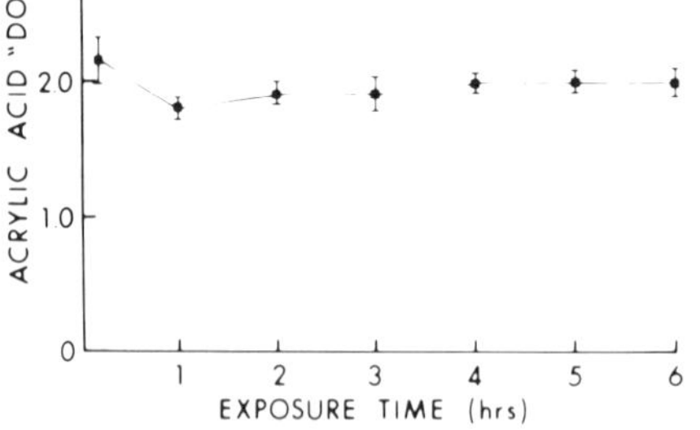

Figure 6 Calculated amounts of acrylic acid available for deposition on the nasal epithelium of mice and rats during a 6-h exposure to 75 ppm of acrylic acid. Animals were pretreated to 75 ppm of acrylic acid 6 h/day for 4 days.

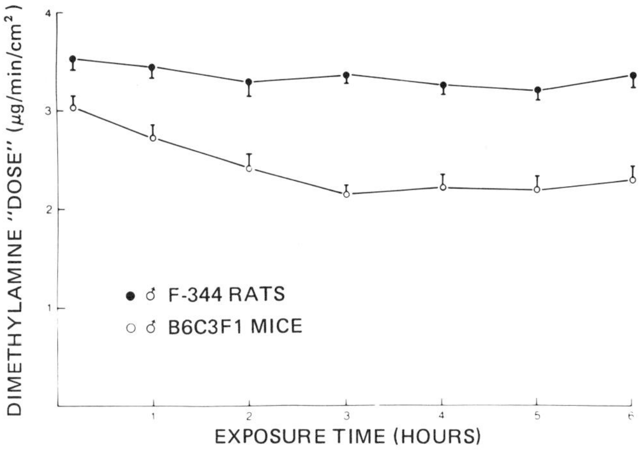

Figure 7 Calculated amounts of dimethylamine available for deposition on the nasal epithelium of mice and rats during a 6-h exposure to 175 ppm of dimethylamine. Animals were pretreated to 175 ppm of dimethylamine 6 h/day for 4 days.

both species. Control rats had a turnover rate of 0.9 percent versus 4.0 percent in AA-exposed animals, representing a fourfold increase. Mice, on the other hand, had a 0.1 percent rate in controls versus 1.7 percent in treated animals, or a 17-fold increase.

Exposure of F-344 rats to 175 ppm DMA resulted in a minute volume decrease of approximately 20 percent during the 6-h exposure, which closely paralleled the respiratory rate decrease. No change occurred in tidal volume. Mice had a larger decrease in minute volume (~60 percent). As with rats, there was virtually no change in tidal volume, and changes in the respiratory rate were very similar to changes in minute volume.

From these results, the predicted dose of DMA to the nasal epithelium was calculated (Fig. 7). In rats the dose ranged from approximately 3.15 to 3.40 μg/min/cm^2. Mice ranged from 2.10 to 3.00 μg/min/cm^2. Averaged over the 6-h exposure, rats were predicted to receive ~33 percent more DMA to the nasal epithelium than mice on a μg/min/cm^2 basis.

Histopathological examination of the respiratory tracts of mice and rats following 5 days of exposure to DMA revealed a similar distribution of lesions in both species. Lesions included focal necrosis of the free margins of the naso- and maxilloturbinates. Also present was a mild inflammatory response with variable amounts of serocellular exudate. These lesions were confined to the most anterior regions of the respiratory epithelium, adjacent to the vestibule. Degeneration of olfactory sensory cells in the anterior dorsal meatus also occurred. The severity of the lesions in rats and mice was nearly identical. Results of the DMA cell proliferation study have not been completed.

Discussion

The quantitation of dose to the nasal cavity (μg/min/cm^2) for very water-soluble irritants gives a more appropriate comparison between species for the concentration-response relationship. For example, the conventional expression of dose (μg/min/kg) in the HCHO study predicts that mice would receive twofold more HCHO on a per-kilogram body weight basis than rats. Since HCHO is almost totally absorbed by the nasal epithelium (47), producing its main toxicity in the nasal cavity, it is clear such a conclusion is misleading. Computation of the "dose" to the actual target tissue is a more legitimate means of comparing species. With this approach, mice exposed to 15 ppm HCHO had approximately half as much formaldehyde delivered to the surface of the nasal epithelium as rats. This may account, in part, for the apparently different sensitivities of rats and mice to inhaled HCHO.

Histopathology and cell proliferation correlated well with the dose difference in mice and rats. Pretreated mice had far less tissue damage and cell turnover than rats. Thus, the local concentration of HCHO available for deposition over the nasal mucosa is critical in determining toxicity.

Mice exposed to 75 ppm AA were predicted to receive nearly a twofold increase in dose compared to rats. Mice also have been found to be more sensitive to AA than rats (17). Histopathology results and cell proliferation studies, as reported here, confirm this difference in sensitivity. The results of the DMA study are not as clear. After 5 days of exposure to 175 ppm DMA, there was no difference in response between rats and mice. This was also the case after 6 months of exposure (48). However, after 12 months of exposure, rats appear to have slightly more severe lesions of the nasal epithelium than mice (24). It is worth noting, however, that rats exposed to DMA were predicted to receive only 33 percent more DMA than mice. This is much less than the nearly twofold differences seen with HCHO or AA. With DMA, much longer exposures may be required to see any differences in species sensitivity. It is also important to consider that an actual species difference to the cytotoxic effects of an irritant might exist. For instance, mice and rats exposed to 6 ppm HCHO are predicted to receive similar doses to the nasal mucosa, but rats are more sensitive (20).

Although these studies point to the need to examine species differences based on pulmonary ventilation and nasal cavity surface area, it is important to recognize that the responses of these species will also be influenced by a variety of other factors. For example, the dose calculations described here assume that the chemical is evenly distributed over the entire nasal surface area. Since this may not represent the actual surface area during in vivo exposure (49), the dose calculated here must be regarded as theoretical. Other important considerations may include differences in metabolism, mucociliary clearance, nasal blood flow, and cellular repair mechanisms.

In summary, the differences in ventilation described here are very important in the overall defense of the respiratory tract, but represent only one factor of many when attempting to understand species differences to highly water-soluble airborne sensory irritants.

SUMMARY

The respiratory tract possesses a wide variety of sensory nerve endings which respond to chemical and/or physical stimuli. The predominant nerve endings in the nasal epithelium are those associated with the trigeminal nerve. Airborne chemical irritants capable of causing their stimulation will result in the sensation of pain which, if great enough, will compel the organism to flee from the contaminated atmosphere. Physiological adjustments also occur, the most important of which is a decrease in respiratory rate. Sensory irritants, substances which cause this response, are potentially damaging to the respiratory tract. Thus, these reflex actions represent an important respiratory tract defense mechanism. In recent years, our laboratory has conducted a number of studies concerning sensory irritation from airborne chemicals. These have included (1) evaluation of the mouse sensory irritation model, (2) a sensory irritation structure-activity study of various aldehydes, (3) the examination of tolerance and cross tolerance from exposure to the sensory irritants chlorine (Cl_2) and formaldehyde (HCHO), and (4) the quantitation of nasal epithelium dose of some selected sensory irritants. In the first study, mice were exposed to the RD_{50} concentration (that concentration causing a 50 percent decrease in respiratory rate) of 10 sensory irritants. All produced unequivocal lesions in the respiratory tract. These findings provide additional support for the usefulness of the mouse sensory irritation model for setting occupational exposure guidelines. The structure-activity study of inhaled aldehydes demonstrated that α,β-unsaturated aliphatic aldehydes had RD_{50} values approximately 3 orders of magnitude less than saturated aliphatic aldehydes. Cyclic aldehydes produced intermediate RD_{50} values. Several hypotheses are discussed that may help explain the differences seen in this study. Investigations of tolerance and cross tolerance with Cl_2 and HCHO revealed that rats pretreated to Cl_2 were tolerant to Cl_2 or cross-tolerant to HCHO. On the other hand, rats pretreated to HCHO were not tolerant to HCHO but were cross-tolerant to Cl_2. These results suggest a common mechanism for tolerance and cross-tolerance development, but different reactive sites may exist for Cl_2 and HCHO at the trigeminal nerve endings. In the fourth and final investigation, differences in toxicity to the nasal passages between rats and mice exposed to highly water-soluble airborne irritants (i.e., HCHO) were found to be correlated to the calculated deposition ($\mu g/min/cm^2$) of the material on the nasal epithelium. By utilizing this approach, species differences in nasal toxicity may be better understood.

REFERENCES

1 Widdicombe, JG. Defense mechanisms of the respiratory tract and lungs. In *Respiratory Physiology II,* edited by JG Widdicombe. Baltimore: University Park Press, pp. 291–315 (1977).

2 Alarie, Y. Irritating properties of airborne materials to the upper respiratory tract. *Arch. Environ. Health* 13:433–449 (1966).

3 Comroe, JH, Jr. Defense mechanisms of the lungs. In *Physiology of Respiration,* edited by JH Comroe Jr. Chicago: Year Book, 2d ed., pp. 220–228 (1974).

4 Alarie, Y. Bioassay for evaluating the potency of airborne sensory irritants and predicting acceptable levels of exposure in man. *Food Cosmet. Toxicol.* 19:623–626 (1981).

5 Kane, LE, CS Barrow, and Y Alarie. A short-term test to predict acceptable levels of exposure to airborne sensory irritants. *Am. Ind. Hyg. Assoc. J.* 40: 207–229 (1979).

6 Swenberg, JA, WD Kerns, RI Mitchell, EJ Gralla, and KL Pavkov. Induction of squamous cell carcinoma of the rat nasal cavity by inhalation exposure to formaldehyde vapor. *Cancer Res.* 40:3398–4402 (1980).

7 Albert, RE, AR Sellakumar, S Laskin, M Kuschner, N Nelson, and C Snyder. Gaseous formaldehyde and hydrogen chloride induction of nasal cancer in the rat. *JNCI* 68:597–603 (1982).

8 Horvath, SM, JA Gliner, and LJ Folinsbee. Adaptation to ozone: Duration of effect. *Am. Rev. Respir. Dis.* 123:496–499 (1981).

9 Hackney, JD, WS Linn, JG Mohler, and CR Collier. Adaptation to short-term respiratory effects of ozone in men exposed repeatedly. *J. Appl. Physiol.* 43:82–85 (1977).

10 Farrel, BP, HD Kerr, TJ Kulle, LR Sander, and JL Young. Adaptation in human subjects to the effects of inhaled ozone after repeated exposure. *Am. Rev. Respir. Dis.* 119:725–730 (1979).

11 Kane, LE, and Y Alarie. Sensory irritation to formaldehyde and acrolein during single and repeated exposures in mice. *Am. Ind. Hyg. Assoc. J.* 38: 509–522 (1977).

12 Chang, JCF, WH Steinhagen, and CS Barrow. Effect of single or repeated formaldehyde exposure on minute volume of B6C3F1 mice and F-344 rats. *Toxicol. Appl. Pharmacol.* 61:451–459 (1981).

13 Barrow, CS and WH Steinhagen. Sensory irritation tolerance development to chlorine in F-344 rats following repeated inhalation. *Toxicol. Appl. Pharmacol.* 65:383–389 (1982).

14 Dixon, WM, and D Drew. Fatal chlorine poisoning. *J. Occup. Med.* 10:249–251 (1968).

15 Weber-Tschopp, A, T Fischer, and E Grandjean. Reizwirkungun des formaldehyde (HCHO) auf den Menschen. [Irritating effects of formaldehyde on man.] *Int. Arch. Occup. Environ. Health* 39:207–218 (1977).

16 Kerns, WD, KL Pavkov, DJ Donofrio, EJ Gralla, and JA Swenberg. Carcinogenicity of formaldehyde in rats and mice after long-term inhalation exposure. *Cancer Res.* 43:4382–4392 (1983).

17 Miller, RR, JA Ayres, GC Jersey, and MJ McKenna. Inhalation toxicity of acrylic acid. *Fund. Appl. Toxicol.* 1:271–277 (1981).
18 Buckley, LA, XZ Jiang, RA James, KT Morgan, and CS Barrow. Respiratory tract lesions induced by sensory irritants at the RD_{50} concentration. *Toxicol. Appl. Pharmacol.* 74:417–429 (1984).
19 Chang, JCF, and CS Barrow. Sensory irritation tolerance and cross-tolerance in F-344 rats exposed to chlorine or formaldehyde gas. *Toxicol. Appl. Pharmacol.* 76:319–327 (1984).
20 Chang, JCF, EA Gross, JA Swenberg, and CS Barrow. Nasal cavity deposition, histopathology, and cell proliferation after single or repeated formaldehyde exposures in B6C3F1 mice and F-344 rats. *Toxicol. Appl. Pharmacol.* 68:161–176 (1983).
21 Steinhagen, WH, JA Swenberg, and CS Barrow. Acute inhalation toxicity and sensory irritation of dimethylamine. *Am. Ind. Hyg. Assoc. J.* 43:411–417 (1982).
22 Barrow, CS, and WH Steinhagen. Design, construction and operation of a simple inhalation exposure system. *Fund. Appl. Toxicol.* 2:33–37 (1982).
23 Giddens, WE, and GA Fairchild. Effects of sulfur dioxide on the nasal mucosa of mice. *Arch. Environ. Health* 25:166–173 (1972).
24 Buckley, LA, KT Morgan, JA Swenberg, RA James, TE Hamm Jr, and CS Barrow. The toxicity of dimethylamine in F-344 rats and B6C3F1 mice following a 1-year inhalation exposure. *Fund. Appl. Toxicol.* 5(2):341–352 (1985).
25 Appleman, LM, RA Woutersen, and VJ Feron. Inhalation toxicity of acetaldehyde in rats. I. Acute and subacute studies. *Toxicology* 23:293–307 (1982).
26 Jiang, XZ, LA Buckley, and KT Morgan. Pathology of toxic responses to the RD_{50} concentration of chlorine gas in the nasal passages of rats and mice. *Toxicol. Appl. Pharmacol.* 71:225–236 (1983).
27 Barrow, CS, RJ Kociba, LW Rampy, DG Keyes, and RR Albee. An inhalation toxicity study of chlorine in Fischer 344 rats following 30 days of exposure. *Toxicol. Appl. Pharmacol.* 49:77–88 (1979).
28 Fomin, AP. Biological effects of epichlorohydrin and its hygienic significance as an atmospheric pollutant. In *NIOSH Criteria for a Recommended Standard—Occupational Exposure to Epichlorohydrin.* Washington: U.S. Government Printing Office, HEW Publ. No. (NIOSH) 76-206 (1966).
29 Gage, JC. The toxicity of epichlorohydrin vapour. *Br. J. Ind. Med.* 16: 11–14 (1959).
30 Clayton, GD, and FE Clayton (Eds.). *Patty's Industrial Hygiene and Toxicology,* Vol. II, *Industrial Hygiene and Toxicology,* 3d ed. New York: Wiley, pp. 2242–2247 (1981).
31 Steinhagen, WH, and CS Barrow. Sensory irritation structure-activity study of inhaled aldehydes in B6C3F1 and Swiss-Webster mice. *Toxicol. Appl. Pharmacol.* 72:495–503 (1984).
32 Alarie, Y. Sensory irritation by airborne chemicals. *CRC Crit. Rev. Toxicol.* 2:299–363 (1973).
33 Schauenstein, E, H Esterbauer, and H Zollner. *Aldehydes in Biological Systems.* London: Pion Limited (1977).

34 Nielsen, GD, and Y Alarie. Sensory irritation, pulmonary irritation and respiratory stimulation by airborne benzene and alkylbenzenes. Prediction of safe industrial exposure levels and correlation with their thermodynamic properties. *Toxicol. Appl. Pharmacol.* 65:459–477 (1982).

35 Barrow, CS, Y Alarie, JC Warrick, and MF Stock. A comparison of the sensory irritation response to chlorine and hydrogen chloride in mice. *Arch. Environ. Health* 32:68–76 (1977).

36 Documentation of the Threshold Limit Values. American Conference of Governmental Industrial Hygienists, Inc., Cincinnati, Ohio, pp. 107 and 197–199 (1982).

37 National Institute for Occupational Safety and Health (NIOSH). *Criteria for a Recommended Standard–Occupational Exposure to Formaldehyde.* Washington: U.S. Government Printing Office DHEW, NIOSH Publ. No. 77-126 (1976).

38 Loomis, TA. Formaldehyde toxicity. *Arch. Pathol. Lab. Med.* 103:321–324 (1979).

39 National Research Council. *Formaldehyde–An Assessment of Its Health Effects.* Washington: National Academy of Sciences (1980).

40 European Chemical Industry Ecology and Toxicology Center. Assessment of data on the effects of formaldehyde on humans. Tech. Report No. 1, Brussels (1981).

41 Andersen, I, and L Malhave. Controlled human studies with formaldehyde. In *Formaldehyde Toxicity,* edited by JE Gibson. New York: Hemisphere (1983).

42 Cauna, N, KH Hinderer, and RT Wentges. Sensory receptor organs of the human nasal mucosa. *Am. J. Anat.* 124:187-210 (1969).

43 Karlin, A, and M Winnik. Reduction and specific alkylation of the receptor for acetylcholine. *Proc. Natl. Acad. Sci. USA* 60:668–674 (1968).

44 Grote, JJ, W Kinjpers, and PL Huygen. Selective denervation of the automatic nerve supply of the nasal mucosa. *Acta Otolaryngol.* 79:124–132 (1975).

45 Barrow, CS, and WH Steinhagen. NH_3 concentrations in the expired air of the rat: Importance to inhalation toxicology. *Toxicol. Appl. Pharmacol.* 53:116–121 (1980).

46 Gross, EA, JA Swenberg, S Fields, and JA Popp. Comparative morphometry of the nasal cavity in rats and mice. *J. Anat.* 135:83–88 (1982).

47 Egle, JL Jr. Retention of inhaled formaldehyde, propionaldehyde and acrolein in the dog. *Arch. Environ. Health* 25:119–124 (1972).

48 Chemical Industry Institute of Toxicology (CIIT). *Inhalation Toxicity of Dimethylamine in F-344 Rats and B6C3F1 Mice.* Research Triangle Park, NC: CIIT, Docket 10413 (1983).

49 Proctor, DF, and JCF Chang. Comparative anatomy and physiology of the nasal cavity. In *Nasal Tumors in Animals and Man,* edited by G Reznik, SF Stinson. Boca Raton, FL: CRC Press, Vol. 1, Chapter 1 (1983).

Chapter 8

Responses of the Nasal Mucociliary Apparatus to Airborne Irritants

Kevin T. Morgan, Daniel L. Patterson, and Elizabeth A. Gross

INTRODUCTION

The mucociliary apparatus, which lines much of the upper and lower respiratory tract (1-3), consists of a ciliated epithelium (4) and complex secretions (5) that are swept over the surface by the action of the cilia (6). There is a voluminous literature on the mucociliary apparatus, and the effects of air pollutants, including a number of detailed reviews (1-3, 7). However, much of the available literature concerns the lower airways, whereas the nasal mucociliary apparatus has received less attention (1). Furthermore, we could find only one review (8) that specifically addressed the state of knowledge concerning mechanisms of toxicity of air pollutants on the mucociliary apparatus.

The constant flow of watery secretions over the surface of the delicate epithelial lining of the airways provides a protective layer in which particles, such as dust and bacteria, become entrapped and are then carried to the glottis to be swallowed (1). Whether the mucociliary apparatus can protect the nasal

We thank Dr. Craig Barrow and Dr. James Swenberg for their help and encouragement and Dr. Ray David for assistance with studies of acetaldehyde.

epithelium against gases or vapors in a similar manner has yet to be established, but theoretical considerations for such protection have been discussed (9, 10). However, the mucociliary apparatus represents an important component of the airway defense mechanisms (11), and inspired gaseous irritants can both stimulate (12) and inhibit (13) nasal mucociliary function. The possible mechanisms responsible for these effects will be discussed after a brief description of the structure and physiology of the nasal mucociliary apparatus with special reference to the rat because of its wide use in inhalation toxicology.

STRUCTURE AND FUNCTION

The nasal passages vary considerably in size and shape between species, and detailed comparative descriptions have been published (14, 15). The nasal airway is lined by three principal epithelial types–squamous, respiratory and olfactory–and the proportion of each varies considerably between different species (14, 15). The extent of each epithelial type has been determined morphometrically for rats and mice (16), and their distribution in the nose of the rat is shown in Fig. 1. The mucociliary apparatus is present in regions of the nose that are lined

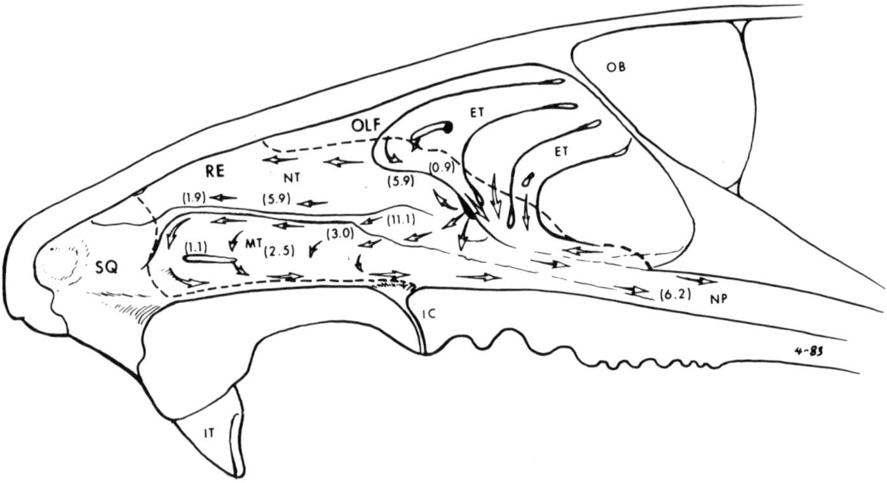

Figure 1 Diagram of rat nasal passages opened adjacent to the midline, with the septum removed to show the turbinates. The limits of the squamous (SQ), respiratory (RE), and olfactory (OLF) epithelia are indicated by the broken lines. Arrows indicate the direction of mucus flow, and numbers in parentheses show mucus flow rates derived from previously reported procedures (10, 18). Note that mucus flows anteriorly in the anterodorsal nasal passages; it reaches the ventral meati via the lateral wall or nasal septum, to eventually flow out of the nose through the nasopharynx. Key: IT, incisor tooth, OB, olfactory bulb; IC, incisive canal; NP, nasopharynx; NT, nasoturbinate; MT, maxilloturbinate; ET, ethmoid turbinate.

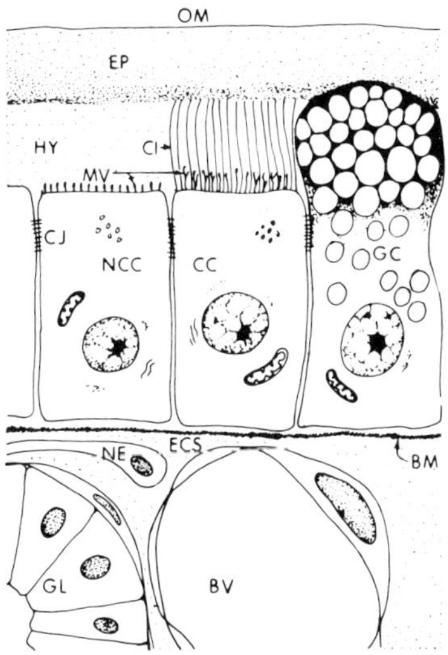

Figure 2 Diagrammatic representation of the nasal respiratory epithelium to show the main components. The thickness of the mucus and the epithelium vary considerably throughout the nose, as do the relative proportions of the different cell types. The nerves present in the subepithelial region often extend through the basement membrane, and lie both beneath and between the epithelial cells. Key: OM, osmiophilic membrane; EP, epiphase; HY, hypophase; CI, cilia; MV, microvilli; CJ, cell junction; CC, ciliated cell; NCC, nonciliated cell; GC, goblet cell; NE, nerve; GL, gland; BV, blood vessel; ECS, extracellular space; BM, basement membrane.

by respiratory epithelium, but the olfactory mucosa also contributes to the surface secretions. The structure of the respiratory epithelium, including the nasal mucociliary apparatus, has been described previously by other workers (4, 17, 18) and is shown diagrammatically in Fig. 2.

In histologic sections or electron micrographs the mucous coat lying on the surface of the respiratory epithelium appears as a layer of amorphous or fibrous, variably stained or variably electron-dense material. This gives a very false impression of the nature of respiratory tract mucus, which in the functioning system looks more like a "river or series of streams" of glistening mucoid or watery material, that is best demonstrated by direct observation or with movie film.* For descriptions of nasal mucus flow patterns in several animal species, the reader is referred to an article by Lucas and Douglas (19) and the flow diagrams from that article which have recently been reprinted (15). Mucus flow patterns in certain regions of the nasal passages of the rat are shown in Fig. 1. The mucus ultimately flows toward the nasopharynx and leaves the nose to be swallowed.

*A short film, *The Mucociliary Apparatus,* has been made demonstrating this point and is available for loan from CIIT, on film (16 mm) or videotape.

A procedure developed by Lucas and Douglas (19) for determination of nasal mucus flow patterns was used extensively by Bang and Bang (20) for studies of the nasal mucociliary apparatus of chickens, and was recently applied to rats using video analysis techniques (18). These studies in rats revealed that different regions of the nose have characteristic mucus flow rates, ciliary beat frequencies, ciliary length, and ciliated cell density. These findings demonstrated the complexity of the nasal mucociliary apparatus of the rat. This study also resulted in observations that supported the proposal of Lucas and Douglas (19) that the airway secretions are present as two distinct phases, with a more viscous surface layer (epiphase) floating on a less viscous fluid (hypophase or periciliary fluid). There has been debate for many years concerning the continuity or discontinuity of the more viscous superficial mucus (1). This is an important question when considering the potential of the mucus to protect the underlying epithelium against inhaled gaseous irritants (9). It was concluded by Morgan et al. (18) on the basis of direct observation, microprobe studies, and light and electron microscopy of fixed material, that nasal mucus is present as a continuous layer over the respiratory epithelium in the nasal passages of the rat. Whether this is also true for other species and for the mucociliary apparatus of the lower airways has yet to be established. The significance of the osmiophilic membrane (Fig. 2), which has been observed on the surface of the mucous blanket in several mucociliary systems, including that of the frog palate (21) and the rat nose (18), is unknown.

The hypophase, or periciliary fluid, represents an important component of the mucociliary apparatus, but the exact source and control mechanisms involved in its regulation are unknown (1). The movement of water from the subepithelial region to the airway lumen is influenced in part by the movement of ions across the epithelium. The mechanisms involved have been reviewed with special reference to the lower airways by Boucher (8). Much remains to be learned about the hypophase and whether there are important differences between the nasal passages and the lower airways in the control mechanisms involved in its production. The proposal that the superficial layer of the hypophase moves in the same direction as the epiphase (1) was supported by recent studies in frogs and rats (18, 21).

The cilia, which beat in the hypophase, provide a major part of the driving force which propels the surface secretions over the epithelial surface. Cilia have a characteristic movement, being straight for the forward or effector stroke, and bending closer to the cell during the recovery stroke (6). The beat frequency of cilia varies considerably, ranging from 5 to > 20 beats per second in the lower respiratory tract of the rat (6). In recent studies by Morgan et al. (18) of the nasal passages of the rat, cilia were found to vary in length (4-6.4 μm) and beat frequency (6-18 beats per second), and there was a wide range of ciliated cell density (0 to >90 percent) in different regions of the nose. However, mucus flow rate was considered to be related more to the nature of the surface secretions than to local ciliary activity. For a detailed review of the complex structure and mode of action of respiratory tract cilia, the reader is referred to Sleigh (6).

RESPONSES TO AIRBORNE IRRITANTS AND MECHANISMS OF TOXICITY

It is evident that the nasal mucociliary apparatus is complex; however, effects of airborne irritants on the function of this system are essentially limited to local or general alteration of mucus flow rate (or flow patterns) and changes in the nature and amount of the secretions. Most of these responses have been described in the lower airways of experimental animals exposed to cigarette smoke (22), a material that has probably stimulated more studies on toxic effects involving the airway mucociliary apparatus than any other air contaminant. However, the fact that humans do not smoke through their nose and that nasal disease is rarely life-threatening has probably contributed to the paucity of information on responses of the nasal mucociliary apparatus to airborne irritants. Furthermore, the mucociliary apparatus of the nose appears to be more resistant than that of the trachea to cigarette smoke (23) and to formaldehyde gas (10), and thus studies that have been carried out on the trachea and more distal airways might not be directly applicable to prediction of responses by the nose.

In spite of the limited range of functional effects that inhaled irritants induce on mucociliary clearance, many different mechanisms may be responsible for the same end result. For instance, slowing of mucus flow may be induced by (a) altered viscoelastic properties of the mucus (24) due to crosslinking of the mucous glycoproteins, or as a result of contamination with albumin (25) or DNA (24); (b) tethering of the mucus to goblet cells (26); (c) defective ciliary function due to direct toxic effects on cilia (8) or interference with ciliated cell metabolism (8); or (d) alteration of the depth of the hypophase (Reid, cited by Proctor et al. [27]). In spite of very different mechanisms, the functional deficit is the same—reduced airway clearance.

As in any tissue, an important step in the determination of mechanisms of action of a toxic substance is the identification of its site(s) of action. On the basis of the main components of the mucociliary ciliary apparatus shown in Fig. 2, a brief list of potential mechanisms of toxicity for each, with examples where available, is presented in Table 1. The paucity of work on the nasal mucociliary apparatus necessitated the use in Table 1 of examples from the lower airways and other mucociliary systems in both disease states and exposure to air contaminants. It is evident from Table 1 that many different mechanisms may account for defective airway clearance. However, of the mechanisms proposed in Table 1, very few have been demonstrated experimentally.

The frog palate has been used extensively for studies of mucociliary

Table 1 Mucociliary Apparatus: Potential Mechanisms Proposed for Defective Mucociliary Function in Airway Diseases or Following Exposure to Air Pollutants

Structural component*	Proposed toxic modification	Example: known or postulated as mechanism of action**
1. Osmiophilic membrane	Altered surface tension	NF†
2. Epiphase	a. Altered viscoelasticity	Chronic bronchitis; cigarette smoke; formaldehyde
	b. Excessive quantity	Chronic bronchitis; cystic fibrosis; asthma
	c. Tethering to goblet cells	Dehydration
3. Hypophase	a. Altered viscoelasticity	NF
	b. Increased amount	Postulated
	c. Altered composition	Cystic fibrosis
	d. Altered pH	Sulfuric acid mist (29)
4. Cilia	a. Decreased or no activity or loss of cilia	Numerous gaseous irritants; cigarette smoke
	b. Reduced beat frequency	Cadmium salts; acetaldehyde
	c. Reduced amplitude of beat	Dimethylamine
	d. Incoordinated beating	Cigarette smoke (22)
	e. Reversed direction of beat	Cigarette smoke (22); dimethylamine
5. Microvilli	Impairment of function	NF
6. Cell junctions	Leakage of macromolecules and/or small ions	Cigarette smoke; antigen challenge; diethyl ether
7. Epithelial cells	a. Defective ion transport	Cystic fibrosis; physical trauma
	b. Altered intracellular pH	Ammonium and sulphate ions
	c. Defective energy metabolism	Cadmium
	d. Cell death	Many irritants at high enough concentration
8. Blood vessels	Increased permeability	Allergy
9. Mucoserous glands	Reduced, excessive, or altered secretions	NF
10. Nerves	a. Increased goblet cell or glandular secretions	Pharmacologic agents
	b. Modified ciliary activity	NF for mammalian system.

*See Fig. 2.

**Where this is not discussed in the cited reviews or the text, the appropriate reference is present in parentheses.

†NF = No example was found in the available literature.

function, and combined with video analysis this model can provide useful information on mechanisms of toxicity (21). Following a procedure reported previously for formaldehyde (21), with appropriate modifications to the analytical procedures (unpublished studies), we examined four gaseous irritants in the frog palate preparation. Each of the four gases produced both an initial phase of stimulation, followed by inhibition of mucociliary function, and a clear concentration response, as has been reported for formaldehyde (21). Observations during the inhibitory phase revealed characteristic effects for each gas, which are summarized in Table 2. For these gases, with the exception of chlorine, cessation of mucus flow clearly preceded ciliastasis, and each gas had distinct, but different effects on the mucous blanket and ciliary beat characteristics. Studies such as these, combined with determination of specific effects of these gases on individual components of the mucociliary apparatus, may indicate possible mechanisms of action for gaseous air pollutants.

Ideally, studies of mucociliary function should be carried out with mammalian tissues whenever possible, as significant differences may exist between the frog palate and the mammalian airway mucociliary apparatus. A wide range of techniques have been developed to study in vivo mucociliary function (1-3). However, the majority of these techniques do not demonstrate the specific locations in the nasal passages that are affected, or the nature of changes responsible for the alteration of mucus clearance rate. A simple procedure was developed in rats to address these questions, and this has been reported previously (10, 28). Briefly, this technique involves exposure of rats to gaseous irritants in standard exposure systems, and at the end of the last exposure the animals are killed by decapitation, the nasal passages are rapidly

Table 2 Gaseous Irritants and In Vitro Mucociliary Responses by the Frog Palate Preparation*

Gas (ppm)**	Ciliary beat† decreased: Freq.	Ciliary beat† decreased: Amp.	Mucostasis before ciliastasis	Increased opacity	Mucus appears rigid
Formaldehyde (15)	—	—	+++	+++	+++
Chlorine (9)	—	—	±	+	±
Dimethylamine (200)	—	++	+++	++	+
Acetaldehyde (1500)	+++	—	+++	++	++

*Features of the inhibitory phase only.

**Nominal gas concentrations.

†Ciliary beat characteristics were based on visual interpretation of events, not on video analysis.

Key: —, not a feature; +, slight effect; ++, moderate effect; +++, distinct effect.

dissected to expose the nasal mucosa, the specimen is placed in a humid, controlled environment, and mucociliary function is observed by light microscopy using long working-distance objectives and a fiber-optics lighting system. Defects in mucociliary function are recorded on maps, and video analysis is used to determine mucus flow rate and ciliary beat frequency. A map showing examples of the distribution and nature of lesions induced by exposure of rats to formaldehyde, chlorine, and dimethylamine is shown in Fig. 3.

This procedure revealed the nature and location of both small and more extensive defects in the nasal mucociliary apparatus of rats, and the effect of exposure concentration for formaldehyde has been reported using this system (10, 30). Studies such as these, combined with work using the frog palate and other preparations, and where possible in vivo studies, preferably in humans, should demonstrate mechanisms of toxicity, and may also clarify normal mechanisms of action of this complex but very important airway defense system.

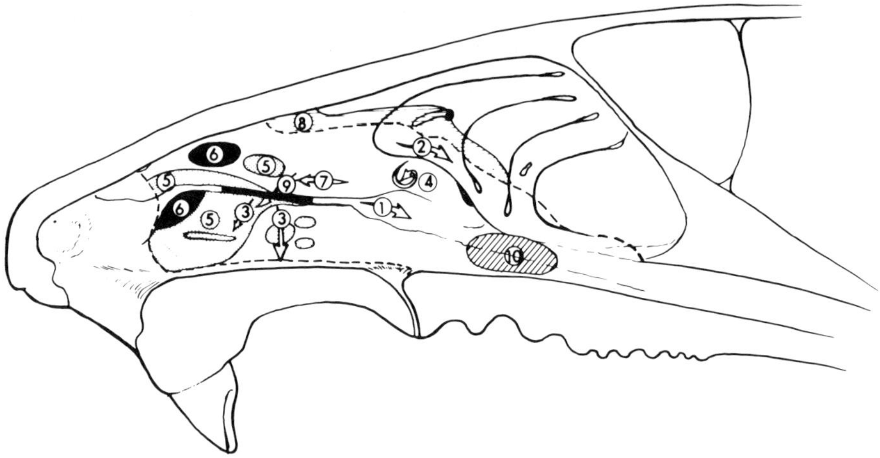

Figure 3 Diagram of rat nasal passages to show location and nature of some lesions of interest seen in the nasal passages of rats following acute and/or chronic in vivo exposure to gaseous irritants (10, 28, 30, 31 and unpublished observations). Key: 1, reversal of direction of mucus flow and ciliary beat (dimethylamine); 2, increased flow rate in some areas, in some animals (formaldehyde); 3, mucus flow over areas exhibiting no ciliary activity (chlorine); 4, disorganized flow, "whirlpools," (formaldehyde); 5, small patches of ciliastasis (formaldehyde); 6, fenestration of the naso- and maxilloturbinates with loss of the mucociliary apparatus in these areas (dimethylamine); 7, reduced mucus flow rate (formaldehyde); 8, posterior extension of the ciliated respiratory epithelium, replacing the normal olfactory epithelium in this area (respiratory metaplasia) (dimethylamine); 9, fusion of the margins of the naso- with the maxilloturbinates with mucus flow across the "bridge" (dimethylamine); 10, accumulation of large quantities of viscid mucus (chlorine, dimethylamine).

SUMMARY

The nasal mucociliary apparatus is a complex and extremely effective airway defense system, but little is known about its ability to protect the nasal epithelium against inspired gases and vapors. A great many materials have been studied for their effects on the mucociliary apparatus, but much less is known about responses in the nose compared to the trachea and more distal airways. Very little is known about the mechanisms responsible for toxic effects of inhaled irritants that impair mucociliary function, and we have a great deal to learn about the normal function of this system, especially with respect to production and control of the hypophase. Localized defects induced by gaseous irritants in the nasal mucociliary apparatus of rats are described. Methods for the detection of similar lesions in humans could provide a valuable tool in human occupational health assessment in relation to determination of risks associated with air pollutants.

REFERENCES

1 Proctor DF. The mucociliary system. In *The Nose, Upper Airway Physiology and the Atmospheric Environment,* edited by DF Proctor, I Anderson. Amsterdam: Elsevier, pp. 245–278 (1982).
2 Wanner A. Clinical aspects of mucociliary transport. *Am. Rev. Resp. Dis.* 116:73–125 (1977)
3 Asmundsson T, KH Kilburn. Mechanisms of respiratory tract clearance. In *Sputum, Fundamentals and Clinical Pathology,* edited by MJ Dulfano. Springfield, Ill.: Charles C Thomas, pp. 107–180 (1973).
4 Jeffery PK, and LM Reid. The respiratory mucous membrane. In *Lung Biology in Health and Disease,* Vol. 5, *Respiratory Defense Mechanisms,* edited by JD Brain, DF Proctor, LM Reid. New York: Marcel Dekker, pp. 193–245 (1977).
5 Widdicombe JG, and UM Wells. The airway secretions. In *The Nose, Upper Airway Physiology and the Atmospheric Environment,* edited by DF Proctor, I Anderson. Amsterdam: Elsevier, pp. 215–237 (1982).
6 Sleigh MA. The nature and action of respiratory tract cilia. In *Lung Biology in Health and Disease,* Vol. 5, *Respiratory Defense Mechanisms,* edited by JD Brain, DF Proctor, LM Reid. New York: Marcel Dekker, pp. 247–288 (1977).
7 Phipps RJ. The airway mucociliary system. *International Review of Physiology, Respiratory Physiology III,* Vol. 23, edited by JD Widdicombe. Baltimore, MD: University Park Press, pp. 213–260 (1981).
8 Boucher RC. Mechanisms of pollutant-induced airways toxicity. *Clin. Chest Med.* 2:377–392 (1981).
9 National Research Council, Committee on Medical and Biologic Effects of Environmental Pollutants. Ozone and other photochemical oxidants. In *Medical and Biologic Effects of Environmental Pollutants.* Washington: National Academy of Sciences, p. 301 (1977).
10 Morgan KT, DL Patterson, and EA Gross. Formaldehyde and the nasal

mucociliary apparatus. In *Formaldehyde: Toxicology, Epidemiology and Mechanisms,* edited by JJ Clary, JE Gibson, RS Waritz. New York: Marcel Dekker (1983).

11 Widdicombe JG. Defense mechanisms of the respiratory system. In *International Review of Physiology, Respiratory Physiology II,* Vol. 14, edited by JG Widdicombe. Baltimore, MD: University Park Press, pp. 291-315 (1977).

12 Marshall TC, FF Hahn, RF Henderson, SA Silbaugh, and CH Hobbs. Subchronic inhalation exposure of guinea pigs to formaldehyde. In *The Inhalation Toxicology Research Institute Annual Report of 1981-1982.* Albuquerque, NM: Lovelace Biomedical and Environmental Research Institute (1982).

13 Mannix RC, RF Phalen, RB Walters, and TT Kurosaki. Effects of sulfur dioxide and formaldehyde on particle clearance in the rat. *J. Toxicol. Environ. Health* 12:429-440 (1983).

14 Negus V. *The Comparative Anatomy and Physiology of the Nose and Paranasal Sinuses.* Edinburgh and London: Livingstone (1958).

15 Proctor DF, and JCF Chang. Comparative anatomy and physiology of the nasal cavity. In *Nasal Tumors in Animals and Man,* Vol. 1, edited by G Reznik, SF Stinson. Boca Raton, FL: CRC Press, pp. 1-33 (1984).

16 Gross EA, JA Swenberg, S Fields, and JA Popp. Comparative morphometry of the nasal cavity in rats and mice. *J. Anat.* 135:83-88 (1982).

17 Monteiro-Riviere N, and JA Popp. Ultrastructural characterization of the nasal respiratory epithelium in the rat. *Am. J. Anat.* 169:31-43 (1984).

18 Morgan KT, XZ Jiang, DL Patterson, and EA Gross. The nasal mucociliary apparatus: Correlation of structure and function in the rat. *Am. Rev. Resp. Dis.* 130:275-281 (1984).

19 Lucas AM, and LC Douglas. Principles underlying ciliary activity in the respiratory tract. II. A comparison of nasal clearance in man, monkey and other animals. *Arch. Otolaryngol.* 20:518-541 (1934).

20 Bang BG, and FB Bang. Nasal mucociliary systems. In *Respiratory Defense Mechanisms,* Part 1. *Lung Biology in Health and Disease,* Vol. 5, edited by JD Brain, DF Proctor, LM Reid. New York: Marcel Dekker, pp. 405-426 (1977).

21 Morgan KT, DL Patterson, and EA Gross. Frog palate mucociliary apparatus: Structure, function and response to formaldehyde gas. *Fund. Appl. Toxicol.* 4:58-68 (1984).

22 Iravani J, and GN Melville. Long-term effect of cigarette smoke on mucociliary function in animals. *Respiration* 31:358-366 (1974).

23 Frances R, D Alessandro, M Lippmann, DF Proctor, and RE Albert. Effect of cigarette smoke on particle transport on nasociliary mucosa of donkeys. *Arch. Environ. Health.* 21:25-31 (1970).

24 Lutz RJ, M Litt, and LW Chakrin. Physical-chemical factors in mucus rheology. In *Rheology of Biological Systems,* edited by HL Gabelnick, M Litt. Springfield, IL: Charles C Thomas, pp. 119-157 (1973).

25 Boucher RC. Chemical modulation of airway epithelial permeability. *Environ. Health Perspect.* 35:3-12 (1980).

26 Anderson I, and DF Proctor. The fate and effects of inhaled materials. In *The Nose, Upper Airway Physiology and the Atmospheric Environment,* edited by DF Proctor, I Anderson. New York: Elsevier, p. 430 (1982).

27 Proctor DF, I Anderson, and G Lundqvist. Nasal mucociliary function in humans. In *Respiratory Defense Mechanisms,* Part 1, *Lung Biology in Health and Disease,* Vol. 5, edited by JD Brain, DF Proctor, LM Reid. New York: Marcel Dekker, p. 447 (1977).

28 Morgan KT, XZ Jiang, EA Gross, and DL Patterson. A procedure for the study of effects of irritant gases on the nasal mucociliary apparatus of rats. *Acta Pharmacologica Sinica.* 6:111-114 (1985).

29 Chen LC, and RB Schlesinger. Response of the bronchial mucociliary clearance system in rabbits to inhaled sulfite and sulfuric acid aerosols. *Toxicol. Appl. Pharmacol.* 71:123-131 (1983).

30 Morgan KT, DL Patterson, and EA Gross. Localization of areas of inhibition of nasal mucociliary function in rats following in vivo exposure to formaldehyde. *Am. Rev. Resp. Dis. (Suppl.)* 127:166 (1983) (abstract).

31 Gross EA, DL Patterson, and KT Morgan. The effect of acute and chronic inhalation exposure dimethylamine on the rat nasal mucociliary apparatus. *Pharmacologist* 23:224 (1983) (abstract).

Chapter 9

Epidemiology of Nasal Cancer

E. D. Acheson

DESCRIPTIVE EPIDEMIOLOGY

Malignant tumors of the interior of the human nose and accessory air sinuses are rare. Examination of data from cancer registers throughout the world shows a variation in incidence of about tenfold (1). The highest rates in both sexes have been reported from Japan (50 per million per annum in males; 30 per million per annum in females). High rates have also been reported among Nigerians, Jamaicans, and, in U.S. and South African blacks of both sexes. In many European countries and in the United States, typical annual incidence rates approximate to 10 per million in men and 5 per million in women. The frequency of these tumors is placed in perspective when it is considered that the incidence in both sexes is about one one-hundredth that of the most common malignant tumors in most developed countries–i.e., carcinoma of the bronchus in men and carcinoma of the breast in women. In England and Wales no definite upward or downward trend in incidence of nasal tumors has been noted since it was first possible to separate them from tumors of other parts of the respiratory tract 30 years ago (2). In most series, squamous cell tumors account for more than three-quarters of all malignant tumors of this area. Adenocarcinomas account for about 10 percent and anaplastic tumors about the same proportion.

MUCOCILIARY MECHANISM OF THE NOSE

The majority of the nasal mucus membrane in man is lined with pseudostratified columnar ciliated epithelium interspersed with mucus-secreting glands and islands of squamous epithelium. Particles of dust and dyes deposited on this epithelium are transported by ciliary action in a stream of nasal mucus into the nasopharynx. Physiological studies with dyes, sweetening agents, and radioactive labeled resin beads have demonstrated the rate of removal of substances by ciliary action in normal adults (3-5). The average rate of movement is about 5 mm per minute.

NASAL CANCER AND OCCUPATION

Six occupational groups have a definite association with nasal cancer: chromate workers, nickel refiners and workers, isopropyl alcohol makers (by the strong-acid process), mustard gas makers, makers of wooden furniture and certain other woodworkers, and boot and shoe operatives and repairers exposed to leather dust.

Workers in the chromate production industry and the chromate pigment industry, who experience an increased risk of lung cancer, also experience an increased risk of cancer of the accessory nasal sinuses (6, 7). The human data do not allow an evaluation of the relative contributions of the various chromium compounds to the incidence of respiratory cancer, but the highest risk appears to be associated with exposure to a mixture of hexavalent chromium compounds of different solubilities, as occurs in the chromate production industry. Animal work incriminates certain hexavalent chromium compounds as definite carcinogens (8).

Striking increases in risk of both nasal and lung cancer have also been described in nickel refiners in several countries (9-11). Relative risks of more than 100 and in one study of more than 500 for nasal cancer and of 10 or more for lung cancer have been reported (12). Nickel-containing dusts from sintering and roasting processes seem to contain the carcinogen. Animal experiments have shown that metallic nickel, nickel oxide, and nickel subsulfide are all carcinogenic, and all of these may be involved in the occurrence of respiratory cancer in these workers (13). As workers employed in both the electrolytic and nickel carbonyl processes have been at risk, the early hypothesis that the cancers were attributable to nickel carbonyl has not been substantiated. Hernberg and his colleagues, in a study of nasal cancer in Denmark, Sweden, and Finland, have shown that welders, flame-cutters, and solderers have an increased risk of nasal cancer and have attributed this to exposure to nickel and chromium metallic fumes (14).

An excess risk of nasal cancer (and possibly of laryngeal cancer) has been found in three factories in which isopropyl alcohol was manufactured by the strong-acid process (15). The nature of the carcinogen is unknown. A group of Japanese workers who manufactured mustard gas before and during World War II developed a high risk of nasal, laryngeal, and lung cancer (16).

FURNITURE MAKERS

The occurrence of an increased risk of nasal cancer in makers of wooden furniture has now been described in most European countries and within the United States and Australia (17). The tumors that occur in these workers are almost exclusively adenocarcinomas. An incidence of approximately one in 2000 per annum (i.e., a relative risk of about 500) has been found in furniture makers in England, Denmark, Norway, and Tasmania (18-21).

In 1970 Hadfield noted that intranasal examination of furniture workers revealed deposits of dust at the anterior and end of the middle turbinate (22). Such deposits did not occur in men who had recently joined the industry. The presence of dust deposits was associated with squamous metaplasia. Subsequent work has confirmed that the mucociliary transport system breaks down more frequently in furniture makers than in men of similar age from outside the industry, and that nasal epithelial dysplasia is commoner in furniture workers than in age-matched volunteer controls (23). According to Hadfield, the inhalation of wood dust in the furniture industry over an extended period of time depressed mucociliary clearance. This phenomenon, which may be due to loss of cilia, leads to stasis and retention of wood dusts at the anterior end of the middle turbinate. This in turn may lead to penetration of the mucus glands by a carcinogen and to the occurrence of the adenocarcinomas. Other work has shown that the prevalence of mucociliary stasis in woodworkers is related to the concentration of the wood dust inhaled (20).

THE NATURE OF THE CARCINOGEN

The epidemiological evidence shows that the incidence of adenocarcinoma is similar in machinists who cut timber with high-speed machines and in men who assemble and sand pieces of wood into cabinets and chairs. However, the tumor is rare in persons who apply stains, polishes, and varnishes to the assembled furniture. Analysis shows that the only factor that is a common exposure to machinists and cabinet and chair makers is hardwood dust (18). The tumors also occur in other occupations exposed to hardwood dusts—for example, men who sand and fit wooden parquet floors, coopers, patternmakers, and wheelwrights (14, 24, 25). Analysis of individual occupational histories shows that the factor is certainly present in beech and in oak (18). It may also be present in many other woods. The chemical nature of the factor is unknown. However, as cases of adenocarcinoma have occurred in men who left the British furniture industry prior to 1930 (24), it is most unlikely to be a chlorophenol as these were not used in this industry prior to 1940 in the United Kingdom (17, and Furniture Industry Research Association, personal communication).

Nasal adenocarcinoma rarely occurs in carpenters or joiners who work principally in the construction industry usually with soft woods. The reason for this is unknown. There is, however, evidence from Scandinavia, Canada, and Britain of an increased risk of squamous cell carcinoma of the nasal mucosa in carpenters and sawmill workers (14, 18, 26). The question must arise whether different carcinogens are involved in adenocarcinoma in hardwood workers and squamous carcinoma in softwood workers.

The epidemiological evidence suggests strongly that the carcinogen responsible for adenocarcinoma of the nasal cavity in hardwood workers is in the wood dust itself. The substance may be a naturally occurring agent or an agent produced by pyrolysis during the action of high-speed grinding and cutting machines. It is worth noting that timber, notably hardwoods, contains biologically active compounds that act as repellants and insecticides. The flavonoids, quercitin and dihydroquercitin, which are highly mutagenic, are present in the bark of oak but not in beech or oak sawdust (Harborne, personal communication). They cannot therefore be incriminated.

There are many other complex compounds in wood dust of which the condensed tannins are one class. There are also a number of complex aldehydes. This is of particular interest in view of the carcinogenic action of formaldehyde and acetaldehyde in rats (27-29).

BOOT AND SHOE WORKERS

Nasal cancer has been described and accepted as an occupational risk in the makers and repairers of leather boots and shoes both in England and Wales and in Italy (30-32). Most of the information comes from studies of the boot and shoe industry in Northamptonshire, England, where since the 17th century men's boots and shoes have been made in large quantities (33). In men working in this industry it is possible to demonstrate increased risks of adenocarcinoma and of other histological types of nasal tumor. The occurrence of these tumors is concentrated in two small areas in the factories. These are the areas where dusty work is done with leather used to make heels and soles. Most of the cases occur in the preparation or press rooms, where the leather hides used for heels and soles are sorted and cut, and in the finishing room, where high-speed machines are used to trim and scour these parts of the shoe (32). It is important to point out that the hard, durable leather used for soles and heels is tanned exclusively by vegetable extracts and not by chrome. These vegetable extracts contain a number of complex compounds also found in wood dust. The question must therefore arise whether there may be a link between adenocarcinoma in furniture makers and similar tumors in persons who are exposed to vegetable-tanned dust from leather in the boot and shoe trade.

FORMALDEHYDE AND NASAL CANCER IN MAN

A number of epidemiological studies have now been reported of men exposed to formaldehyde in industry and in the preservation of human tissues (31, 34-36). In none has a case of nasal cancer been described. However, even considered together, the studies have not yet followed a sufficient number of heavily exposed men a sufficient period of time to exclude an increase in risk of nasal cancer occurring after an extended induction period, say 20 years. It is worth noting that in other occupational nasal cancers the induction period usually approximates or exceeds two decades (17). All that can be said safely at this point is that the evidence so far is negative.

It is worth considering whether formaldehyde can be held responsible for the occurrence of nasal cancer in the furniture, boot, and shoe industries. At the present time it is used extensively in both, principally in adhesives. However, in the United Kingdom formaldehyde was not used prior to World War II in either industry. And yet it is known that a number of men who subsequently developed the disease had left the industry prior to 1930 in the furniture industry (24) and before 1920 in the boot and shoe industry (25, 32). It therefore seems very unlikely that formaldehyde can be incriminated in these industries. There may, however, be a role for other aldehydes.

SUMMARY

Malignant tumors of the human nose and accessory air sinuses are very rare. This fact is placed in perspective when one considers that the incidence of such nasal tumors is about one one-hundredth that of bronchogenic carcinoma in men and of breast cancer in women. However, six occupational groups have an unequivocal association with nasal cancer. These include chromate workers, nickel refiners and workers, makers of isopropyl alcohol, mustard gas manufacturers, makers of wooden furniture, and boot and shoe workers. The epidemiological findings in these exposure groups are reviewed. The reason for this conference is undoubtedly the discovery by Swenberg and Albert and colleagues that rats exposed to 15 ppm formaldehyde for up to 2 years develop a high incidence of nasal cancer (27, 28). In recent years a number of epidemiological studies have been completed on this widely used and very important chemical. The results of these are reviewed.

REFERENCES

1 IARC Scientific Publication 42. *Cancer Incidence in Five Continents,* Vol. 4. Geneva: WHO (1982).

2 Osmond C, MJ Gardner, ED Acheson, and AM Adelstein. Trends in cancer mortality analyses by period of birth and death. England and Wales 1951–1980. *HMSO Lond. OPCS Ser. DH1* 11 (1983).

3 Proctor DF, and NH Wagner. Clearance of particles from the human nose. *Arch. Environ. Health* 11:366–371 (1956).

4 Quinlan MF, SD Salman, DL Swift, HN Wagner, and DF Proctor. Measurement of mucociliary function in man. *Am. Rev. Resp. Dis.* 99:13–23 (1969).

5 Andersen I, GR Lundqvist, and DF Proctor. Human nasal mucosal function in a controlled climate. *Arch. Environ. Health* 23:408–420 (1971).

6 Bidsrup PL, and RAM Case. Carcinoma of the lung in workmen in the biochromates-producing industry in Great Britain. *Br. J. Ind. Med.* 13:260–264 (1956).

7 Enterline PE. Respiratory cancer amongst chromate workers. *J. Occup. Med.* 16:523–526 (1974).

8 IARC Monographs. *Evaluation of the Carcinogenic Risk of Chemicals to Humans. Some Metals and Metallic Compounds,* Vol. 23. Geneva: WHO (1980).

9 Doll R. Cancer of the lung and nose in nickel workers. *Br. J. Ind. Med.* 15: 217–223 (1958).

10 Virtue JA. The relationship between the refining of nickel and cancer of thin nasal cavity. *Can. J. Otolaryngol.* 1:37–42 (1972).

11 Predersen E, AC Hogetveit, and A Andersen. Cancer of respiratory organs among workers at a nickel refinery in Norway. *Int. J. Cancer* 12:32–41 (1973).

12 Doll R, LG Morgan, and FE Speizer. Cancers of the lung and nasal sinuses in nickel workers. *Br. J. Cancer* 24:623–632 (1970).

13 IARC Monographs. *Evaluation of Carcinogenic Risk of Chemicals to Man. Cadmium, Nickel, Some Epoxides, Miscellaneous Industrial Chemicals and General Considerations on Volatile Anaesthetics,* Vol. 11. Geneva: WHO (1976).

14 Hernberg S, P Westerhold, K Schultz-Larsen, R Degerth, E Kuosma, A Englund, U Engzell, HS Hansen, and P Mutanen. Nasal and sinonasal cancer. Connection with occupational exposures in Denmark, Finland and Sweden. *Scand. J. Work. Environ. Health* 9:315–326 (1983).

15 Hueper WC. Occupational and environmental cancer of the respiratory system. *Recent Results Cancer Res.* 3:105–107, 183 (1966).

16 Yamada A. On the late injuries following occupational inhalation of mustard gas, with special reference to carcinoma of the respiratory tract. *Acta Pathol. Jpn.* 13:131–155 (1963).

17 IARC Monographs. *Evaluation of the Carcinogenic Risk of Chemicals to Humans. Wood, Leather and Some Associated Industries,* Vol. 25. Geneva: WHO (1981).

18 Acheson ED. Nasal cancer in the furniture and boot and shoe manufacturing industries. *Prev. Med.* 5:295–315 (1976).
19 Andersen HC. Eksogene ar sagar til cancer cavi nasi. *Ugeskr. Laeg.* 137: 2567–2570 (1974).
20 Boysen M, and LA Solberg. Changes in the nasal mucosa of furniture workers a pilot study. *Scand. J. Work Environ. Health* 8:273–282 (1982).
21 Franklin CIV. Adenocarcinoma of the paransal sinuses in Tasmania. *Australas. Radiol.* 26:49–52 (1982).
22 Hadfield EH. A study of adenocarcinoma of the paranasal sinues in woodworkers in the furniture industry. *Ann. R. Coll. Surg. Engl.* 46:301–319 (1970).
23 Black A, JC Evans, EH Hadfield, RG Macbeth, A Morgan, and M Walsh. Impairment of nasal mucociliary clearance in woodworkers in the furniture industry. *Br. J. Ind. Med.* 31:10–17 (1974).
24 Acheson ED, RH Cowdell, E Hadfield, and RG Macbeth. Nasal cancer in woodworkers in the furniture industry. *Br. Med. J.* 2:587–596 (1968).
25 Acheson ED, RH Cowdell, and E. Rang. Adenocarcinoma of the nasal cavity and sinuses in England and Wales. *Br. J. Ind. Med.* 29:21–30 (1972).
26 Elwood JM. Wood exposure and smoking: Association with cancer of the nasal cavity and paranasal sinuses in British Columbia. *Can. Med. Assoc. J.* 124:1573–1577 (1981).
27 Swenberg JA, WD Kerns, RI Mitchell, EJ Gralla, and KL Pavkov. Induction of squamous cell carcinomas of the rat nasal cavity by inhalation exposure to formaldehyde. *Cancer Res.* 40:3398–3401 (1980).
28 Albert RE, AR Sellakumar, S Laskin, M Kuschner, N Nelson, and CA Snyder. Gaseous formaldehyde and hydrogen chloride induction of nasal cancer in the rat. *JNCI* 68:597–603 (1982).
29 Appelman LM, RA Woutersen, and VJ Feron. Inhalation toxicity of acetaldehyde in rats. I. Acute and subacute studies. *Toxicology* 23:293–307 (1982).
30 Acheson ED, RH Cowdell, and B Jolles. Nasal cancer in the Northamptonshire boot and shoe industry. *Br. Med. J.* 1:385–393 (1970).
31 Cecchi F, E Buiatti, D Kriebel, L Nastasi, and M Santucci. Adenocarcinoma of the nose and paranasal sinuses in shoe makers and woodworkers in the province of Florence Italy (1963–1977). *Br. J. Ind. Med.* 37:222–225 (1980).
32 Acheson ED, EC Pippard, and PD Winter. Nasal cancer in the Northamptonshire boot and shoe industry: Is it declining? *Br. J. Cancer* 46:940–946 (1982).
33 Baynes K, and K Baynes. *Shoe Show: British Shoes Since 1790.* London: Crafts Council. (1979).
34 Marsh GM. Proportional mortality patterns among chemical plant workers exposed to formaldehyde. *Br. J. Ind. Med.* 39:313–322 (1982).
35 Walrath J, and JF Fraumeni. Mortality patterns among embalmers. *Int. J. Cancer* 31:407–411 (1983).
36 Acheson ED, HR Barnes, MJ Gardner, C Osmond, B Pannett, and CP Taylor. Formaldehyde in the British chemical industry, and occupational cohort study. *Lancet* 1:611–616 (1984).

Chapter 10

Effects of Airborne Substances on Nasal Function in Human Volunteers

Ib Andersen

INTRODUCTION

Studies of human subjects exposed under controlled conditions allow conclusions about cause-effect relationships. For that reason they are useful supplements to epidemiological studies and to studies in the workplace, both of which are troubled by a multitude of uncontrollable variables.

The exposures may be performed as (1) mouthpiece or face mask inhalation; (2) "head-only" exposure, where the airways, the eyes, and the skin of the head are exposed to the pollutant by means of a "diver's helmet" arrangement; and (3) exposure chamber studies where the whole body is exposed to the pollutant.

Only the last type of exposure resembles real-life situations, as for example in the workplace, and is to be preferred for such studies. An exposure chamber able to house one or several subjects is therefore needed for such studies. An exposure chamber consists of a technical facility to maintain the basic climatic conditions (temperature, humidity, etc.), a pollution-generating and monitoring system, and a data-acquisition system for physiological and performance measurements and for subjective responses (statements about severity of nasal irritation, odor, etc.).

One important drawback for exposure chamber studies on subjects sampled from the general population is the short duration of such studies–normally 8 hours or less. Only highly motivated people can be kept for 1 to 2 weeks. For this reason only acute and subacute exposure effects can be studied under controlled conditions in chambers.

Studies of subchronic or chronic effects will have to be performed either at the workplace, where the workers are exposed for long periods to the substance in question, or by taking these workers to an exposure chamber and exposing them during one or more working days to the substance in question.

Because of the legal situation with a tradition for huge compensations for damages inflicted upon a person in an exposure study, few human exposure studies are performed in the United States. Provided the exposure concentrations are at or below the threshold limit value (TLV), such obstacles are not prominent in western Europe and Japan. As a result, most human exposure studies are performed in these countries.

A transatlantic collaboration group, consisting of Dr. Proctor and his staff at the Johns Hopkins School of Public Health, Baltimore, Maryland, and our group in Denmark, started its investigations on the human nose in 1969 as we considered the basic knowledge about the normal function and the effects of the environment on this part of the airways to be out of proportion to its importance for the respiratory system. The lack of interest in the upper airways at this time was not well advised, as it is the most easily accessible part of the human airway system, and furthermore it is the first target of and the first line of defense against the ambient air. The main reason for this lack of interest in the upper airways was probably its physiological designation as "the dead space." Who wants to study a "dead space"? Today it is common knowledge that this part of the airways is far from dead, and the interest in studying its functions is growing rapidly.

The effects of inhaled substances on nasal functions may include impairment of mucociliary nasal flow, changes in nasal airflow resistance, and irritation of the nasal mucous membranes. Another effect is damage to the epithelial cells including development of nasal cancer, but this aspect is covered in other chapters.

NASAL MUCOCILIARY FLOW

The nasal mucociliary flow may be impaired either by changes in airway secretions, by impairment of ciliary activity, or by combinations of these. Techniques for studying the motility of ciliated cells obtained from the nasal cavity using a curette have been developed, primarily for the diagnosis of Kartagener's syndrome (1) and for the study of mucus composition and mucus properties. However, studies of the effects of airborne substances are normally restricted to the nasal mucociliary flow.

All methods for measuring human nasal mucociliary flow employ a marker substance–a tracer–that is placed by means of a probe, a syringe, or a spray on a small area of the mucus. The time taken for the tracer to travel a known distance or the distance traveled in a known time is measured, and from these data the velocity of the tracer is calculated.

Two types of methods exist: one where *visible* tracers are directly observed and one where *invisible* tracers are used, the detection of which requires special techniques.

The size and weight of the tracer particle is not critical. Small steel balls and pieces of paper have been used with equal success, but of course they should be kept as small as possible. Particles as small as 0.5 to 1 mm in diameter are still easy to handle and can be gently placed on the superior surface of the inferior turbinate approximately 5 cm from the tip of the nose or 1 to 2.5 cm posterior to the anterior turbinate tip, which is situated in the path of the main stream of inspiratory air flow. If a particle is placed more anteriorly, it may be deposited in the unciliated part of the nose or in the first part of the ciliated area where the ciliary current moves forward (2).

Several types of visible tracers have been used (3) but a particle consisting of a blend of a strong-tasting chemical (saccharin) and a dye is preferred. The saccharin-dye particle dissolves almost immediately in the mucus and moves backward as a colored spot. At the arrival in the pharynx a sweet taste is reported, and when the colored spot appears the transit time is noted. In normal subjects it is from 12 to 15 min. Anything exceeding 30 min is considered abnormal.

Invisible tracers are primarily radioactive substances, whose movements with the mucus are followed by a gamma camera, by scanning apparatus, or by fixed slit-collimated scintillation detectors (3). Radiopaque material in combination with X-ray techniques has also been used. In our group we developed a technique using a 0.5-mm resin particle tagged with 1 μc technetium-99m and an external detection system. This method is suitable for determination of the effects of inhaled pollutants on nasal mucus flow in different parts of the nasal cavity. In Fig. 1 are shown the position of the collimated areas in the nose, the record taken, and the calculated mucus flow rates on the five different positions in the nose. It appears that the mucus flow velocity varies in the different parts of the nose, with the fastest flow in the middle third and slower flow in the anterior and posterior thirds.

The average flow varies from under 1 to over 20 mm/min, but the majority lies between 2 and 10 mm/min. Because of this wide interindividual variation, it is advantageous to use subjects as their own controls. In the same individual the nasal mucociliary flow does not vary much over a period of some days' duration. The variation over longer periods of time is not known. The nasal

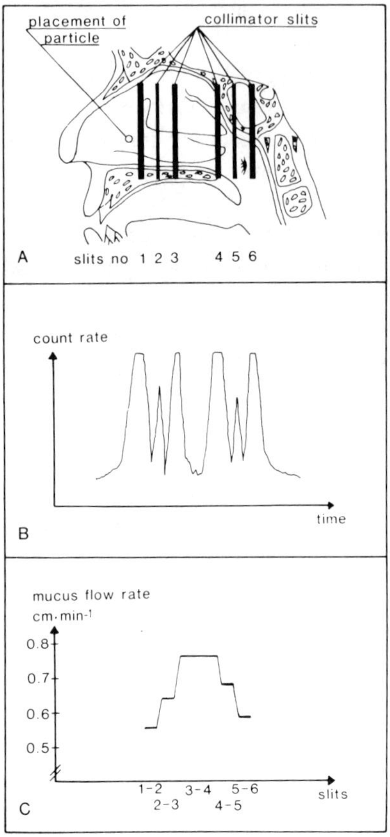

Figure 1 (*A*) A sagittal view of the right side of the nose. The projection of the collimator slits is superimposed. (*B*) A record from a subject with normal clearance rate. When the radioactive particle passes a slit, the count rate is increased. (*C*) The mucus flow rate of five different positions in the nose calculated from measurements of time (from *B*) and from the distances between the slits (from *A*).

mucociliary flow is not affected by temperature and humidity in the range we find in normal indoor environments (2).

EFFECTS OF AIRBORNE SUBSTANCES

Only a few studies of the effects of airborne substances on human nasal mucociliary flow have been performed. In our own studies we have exposed healthy subjects to different pollutants during 6 h at controlled conditions. We have so far studied SO_2, formaldehyde, toluene, inert plastic dust, wood dust, rhinovirus, SO_2 and plastic dust together, and SO_2 and rhinovirus together (Table 1).

Nasal mucus flow is reduced significantly by SO_2 at 65 and 13 mg m^{-3} (25 and 5 ppm) but is not affected by 2.6 mg m^{-3} (1 ppm). The decrease in mucus flow is greatest in the anterior part of the nose, but the affected area increases at higher concentrations and with longer exposure periods. Mucostasis is found in the anterior part of the nose at 4-6 h exposure to 65 mg m^{-3} (25 ppm). SO_2 is highly soluble in water (39 liters SO_2 per liter H_2O at 20°C and normal pressure) and is probably fully absorbed in the affected area, as less than 1 percent can be found in pharyngeal air (4).

For formaldehyde, which is even more water-soluble than SO_2, a similar picture is seen, as the mucus flow rate decreases in the anterior two-thirds of the nose during exposures from 0.3 to 2.0 mg m^{-3} (0.24, 1.63 ppm) whereas no effects are found in the posterior third. There is no further reduction when the exposure period is increased from 1-3 to 4-6 h. Mucostasis is never found (5).

Toluene in concentrations of 37.5, 150, and 375 mg m^{-3} (10, 40, and 100 ppm) during 6 h exposure does not affect nasal mucus flow. Toluene is almost insoluble in water, and we have not been able to detect any absorption of toluene during the passage of the inspiration air through the nose (6).

Also, 43 male printers exposed from 9 to 25 years to solvents during employment in printing plants and controls with no history of solvent exposure have been studied. There was no difference in nasal mucus flow in the printers and the controls, and exposure to 375 mg m^{-3} (100 ppm) toluene in the climate chamber caused no effects in any of the groups (7). Thus chronic exposure to toluene does not affect the nasal mucociliary flow.

We have also studied dust, a commercially available, fully polymerized plastic dust containing carbon black (Rank Xerox toner 6R 90005). The concentrations studied were 2, 10, and 25 mg m^{-3}, and the aerodynamic equivalent diameter (AED) was from 1.8 to 12.5 μm. The nose removed approximately 45 percent of the smallest particles, 55 percent of those with an AED of 1.9 to 5.3

Table 1 Acute Effects of Airborne Pollutants on Human Nasal Mucus Flow

	Pollutant (6-h exposure)	Effect	No. subjects
Gases and vapors	SO_2	Decrease of mucus flow at 65 and 13, but not at 2.6 mg m^{-3}	15
	HCHO	Decrease of mucus flow in the anterior part of nose at 2, 1, 0.5, and 0.3 mg m^{-3}	16
	Toluene	No effect of 375 mg m^{-3}	
Particles	Plastic dust*	No effect of 25 mg m^{-3}	16
	Wood dust	No effect of 10 mg m^{-3}	16
	Common cold	Decrease of mucus flow rate for 3-8 weeks	60
Combinations	SO_2 + rhinovirus	As SO_2 but fewer symptoms and lower virus shedding	32
	SO_2 + plastic dust*	As SO_2	16

*Rank Xerox toner 6R 90005.

μm, 65 percent of those with an AED between 5.4 and 8.9 μm, and 80-100 percent of larger particles. The proportion of particles deposited in the nose did not seem to be related to their concentration in inspired air. At the highest level of exposure, 25 mg m^{-3}, approximately 9.5 mg of dust was deposited in the upper airways per hour. No effect was found on nasal mucus flow of inhalation of the dust during 5 hours, for which reason the purely mechanical effect of the dust seems to be of minor importance in comparison to the chemical effect of soluble substances in the dust (8).

A similar study has been done with wood dust with exposures to either dust from pine, beech, oak, mahogany, or chipboard in a concentration of 10 mg m^{-3} and a size distribution from $\leqslant 1.6$ to $\leqslant 14.9$ μm with maxima of approximately 30 percent from 4.9 to 8.0 μm. Here no effect of a 5-h exposure was found (Andersen, in preparation). This showed us that an exposure chamber study of the acute effects of an airborne substance on young healthy subjects not always can be used for prediction of the effects of the substance in the workplace. Therefore, both kinds of studies should be performed when the effects of a substance are studied.

Earlier (9), we studied the chronic effects of wood dust exposure in 68 workers employed on average 16 years (range 1-51 years) in the furniture industry. The dust concentrations in the workplace were measured at the same time as the concentrations were performed, and we found that the proportion of workers with mucostasis increased in direct proportion to the dust concentration. In the group with the highest wood dust concentration (25.5 mg m^{-3}) 63 percent had mucostasis, whereas this was found in only 11 percent at 2.2 mg m^{-3}. Nine subjects with mucostasis were reexamined in their homes at the end of a weekend after 48 h without wood dust exposure. Three subjects were still mucostatic, whereas 6 had normal mucus transit times. A similar study among grain silo workers who are also heavily exposed to dust showed a similar reduction in nasal clearance (B. Bach, 1984, personal communication). The mucostatic factor in wood dust may be of importance for the development of nasal cancers and for susceptibility to airborne disease. The latter hypothesis is supported by the fact that workers at high dust concentrations had more upper-airway infections than workers at low dust concentrations (9).

Interaction between two substances has only been studied for SO_2 and a common-cold virus (rhinovirus) and for SO_2 and plastic particles. The hypothesis behind the SO_2-rhinovirus study was that subjects exposed to SO_2 owing to the consequent decrease in the nasal mucus flow rate would be more susceptible to an experimentally induced virus infection than would nonexposed subjects. Thirty-two subjects were divided into two groups balanced with respect to age, antibody levels, and nasal mucus flow rates. One group was exposed to 5 ppm SO_2 during 4 hours, which caused a 50 percent reduction of the mucus flow rate in the anterior part of the nose, and the other was exposed to clean air. We found no difference in the number of colds developed in the two groups, but there were fewer symptoms and the virus shedding was at a lower level but more persistent in the SO_2 group than in the control group. We concluded that the rhinovirus and the mucous membrane in the nose both were adversely affected by the SO_2 and that the virus probably was more affected than the mucous membrane (10).

The rhinovirus infection in the control group caused a gradual decrease in nasal mucus flow rate starting 2 days after the virus instillation, and after 5 days the rate was less than half of its initial value. It is our experience from this and the other studies that it takes about 3 weeks after the start of a common cold before the mucous membrane has fully recovered. This has also been found by Sakakura et al. (11). In other studies the nasal clearance in some subjects first returned to normal after more than 5 weeks (12, 13).

Finally a study of the combined effects of SO_2 and plastic particles showed that the reduction in nasal mucus flow rate was related principally to the SO_2 concentration. There was no indication of potentiation (14).

NASAL AIRFLOW RESISTANCE

Resistance is a pressure-flow ratio that can be obtained by plotting respiratory airflow against pressure. These measurements have been performed for almost a century, but relatively few studies have been directed at measuring nasal airflow resistance during exposure to air pollutants. Exercise decreases nasal airflow resistance, cold air increases it, whereas moderate changes in ambient temperature have no influence.

At 5 ppm SO_2 there is a distinct increase in the airflow resistance, but at 1 ppm there is little or no effect (4). Formaldehyde, toluene, and plastic dust do not affect the nasal airflow resistance (5, 6, 8).

NASAL IRRITATION

Eye and airway irritation are common complaints in the occupational environment, and about one half of the compounds for which TLVs are set are sensory irritants. Nasal and eye irritation due to exposure to airborne substances can be measured by questionnaire methods or by a comfort meter. When using a comfort meter the subject is asked to move the pointer whenever he (or she) becomes aware of a change in nasal irritation. We use no graduation on the scale, which is divided into three equal zones—"slight discomfort," "discomfort," and "strong discomfort." The response is recorded in percent of full scale. The subjects sometimes adjust their dial setting by as little as 5 percent of full scale (4).

We have during our studies of nasal mucociliary clearance also investigated the irritation effect on the eyes and upper airways of the subjects. In all our studies the subjects first have been exposed to clean air for about 2 h, and after this control period the concentration of the pollutant has slowly increased during 1 h or so to a concentration that has been kept constant during the rest of the experiment–that is, an exposure period of about 6 h duration. For SO_2 there was no discomfort at 2.6 mg m^{-3} (1 ppm), whereas the 65- and 13-mg m^{-3} (25- and 5-ppm) exposures caused slight discomfort (4) (Fig. 2).

For formaldehyde a similar picture is seen, but only the 1.0- and 2.0-mg m^{-3} (0.8- and 1.63-ppm) exposure increases the discomfort during the first 2 h of exposure. This effect was not seen at the 0.3- and 0.5-mg m^{-3} (0.24- and 0.41-ppm) exposure (5). At identical concentrations formaldehyde is more irritating than SO_2 (Fig. 2).

During exposures to toluene the average eye and airway irritation was 13 percent (slight irritation) during the 375-mg m^{-3} (100-ppm) exposure. Also here the irritation was felt just after the beginning of the exposure, and it was constant throughout the exposure. At the lower concentrations (40 and 10 ppm), the irritation response was also proportionately lower. During acute exposures to toluene, there is no difference in the irritation response of printers exposed for many years to organic solvents and of control subjects not occupationally exposed to toluene (7). At identical concentrations toluene is less irritating than SO_2 (Fig. 2).

Exposure to plastic dust causes only slight discomfort even at concentrations above the TLV (8). In the combination exposure to SO_2 and dust, the response followed the SO_2 concentration (14).

Wood dust was almost four times as irritating at 10 mg m^{-3} as plastic dust in the same concentration (Andersen, in preparation) (Fig. 2).

There is a wide interindividual variation in the votings of the subjects. During exposure to SO_2 at the TLV value 13 mg m^{-3} (5 ppm), the mean

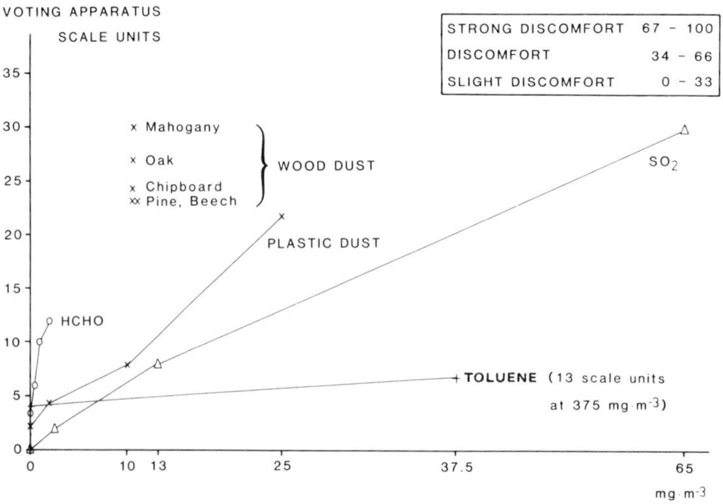

Figure 2 The average discomfort votings in the upper airways in groups of subjects (N = 16) exposed to the different concentrations of the pollutants for 4 h.

discomfort was about 8 percent of full scale, but the range of votings was from 0 to 40. Seven subjects experienced no irritation during the whole exposure, and two exceeded the bottom third of the scale (4). During the toluene exposure at TLV 375 mg m^{-3} (100 ppm) where the average response was 13 percent of full scale, six subjects did not report any irritation, whereas one individual voted 64 percent of full scale (6).

Irrespective of the exposure substance, the description was similar—irritation and a feeling of dryness. The investigators, who occasionally had to enter the chamber, experienced at the higher concentrations a very strong irritation just after entering the chamber. The irritation disappeared after a few minutes despite the continual exposure. After a period in clean air, this acute irritation was again experienced at the same magnitude. Because of the slow increase in concentration during 1 h, the subjects in the chamber did not experience this very strong irritation.

In most of our studies human subjects have only been exposed to pure gases and vapors. This situation is hardly ever encountered in daily-life situations, so a series of exposure studies with mixtures of the solvents found in indoor air of offices in the so-called sick buildings (15) have recently been performed. In these studies 62 subjects were exposed to either 0, 5, or 25 mg m^{-3} of a mixture of 21 organic solvents. The irritation response at both 5 and 25 mg m^{-3} was significantly different from the clean-air exposure, and increased throughout the exposure period (16). Five mg m^{-3} of organic solvent may be encountered in many new buildings with low ventilation rates, and this study indicates that irritation is now an important problem not only in the industrial environment but also in the nonindustrial occupational environment and in the home.

DISCUSSION

An important task for toxicologists and medical doctors is to provide an adequate description of the effects on human health and well-being due to changes in the function of any organ.

Impairment of mucociliary flow in the form of decreased nasal mucus flow or even mucostasis is seen during any common cold. Normally this causes no adverse effects, but now and then a secondary infection of the sinuses or the middle ear develops.

An acquired and chronic impairment of the nasal mucociliary flow is seen in patients with primary ciliary dyskinesia—a disease due to a congenital abnormal ciliary ultrastructure, also found in Kartagener's syndrome (the clinical triad of bronchiectasis, sinusitis, and situs inversus). Such patients have airway problems from early childhood. They suffer from chronic nasal stuffiness or discharge and chronic infection of the paranasal sinuses, recurrent otitis, bronchitis, and bronchiectasis. The frequency of common colds is not increased in these patients, and they live a surprisingly normal life and have a virtually normal life expectancy in spite of complete absence of mucociliary transport, provided their respiratory infections are vigorously and promptly treated. Thus even complete absence of mucociliary transport is not life-threatening, but impaired mucociliary transport causes retention of the mucus and infection. It probably also increases the subject's susceptibility to any airborne pollutant.

The experience from studies of workers occupationally exposed to wood dust or grain dust is that middle-ear and upper-airway infections are more frequent at high dust concentrations, where nasal mucociliary flow is impaired or stopped (9). This experience is in accordance with the results of the studies of the primary ciliary dryskinesia.

Any increase of the airflow resistance in the nose due to inhalation of an irritant is to be considered as harmful, as mouth breathing then occurs at a lower respiration volume. During mouth breathing, the lower airways are less protected against inhaled air pollutants than during nasal breathing.

Nasal irritation causes annoyance and decreased respiratory rate, decreased heart rate, peripheral vasoconstriction, closure of the glottis, increased nasal flow resistance, and possibly changes in the resistance of the lower respiratory tract (17).

An animal model to evaluate sensory irritation properties of airborne chemicals has been developed (18). From the concentration-response curve with response expressed as decrease in breathing frequency, an RD_{50} (the concentration required for a decrease in respiratory rate of 50 percent from control) is calculated. After this a 0.03 RD_{50} can be obtained, which has been shown to be highly correlated to the TLV of most irritant substances. This generally good agreement between the animal data and the TLV is strong but indirect proof of the predictive value of the model. We have compared our human irritation measurements after an exposure period of 4 h duration with results from the published animal data. Predictions of TLV for formaldehyde, SO_2, and toluene from the animal data are 0.1, 3.8, and 159 ppm, respectively, for 0.03 RD_{50}, and 3, 117, and 5300 ppm, respectively, for RD_{50}. This means that the animal model predicts SO_2 about 40 times more irritating than toluene, and formaldehyde about 40 times more irritating than SO_2. Exactly the same ranking order is seen in our data from human subjects (Fig. 2). Nasal irritation in man therefore seems to be predicted very well by the animal model developed by Alarie and his co-workers.

Because of the great interindividual variations in nasal functions, it is suggested that future exposure studies of human subjects in chambers should include an adequate number of subjects, that is, at least 16 but preferably 25 subjects or more. This will decrease the risk for type 2 errors; acceptance of a null hypothesis even if it is wrong. Furthermore, subjects occupationally exposed over many years to the substance in question should be studied as well as the young healthy subjects (students) normally used for such studies. Both groups should be included, since their response may be very different.

There is a need for a test battery generally agreed upon for chamber studies of human nasal function. This applies to methods for registration of subjective irritation, for classification of the appearance of the mucous membrane, and for measurement of nasal mucociliary flow and nasal resistance.

For acute cases as well as long-term studies, a questionnaire for upper-airway symptoms and diseases should be developed to enable international comparison of studies. The use through several decades of the British Medical Research Council's questionnaire on respiratory symptoms has proved to be of immense value as a standardized research tool.

SUMMARY

Only a few studies of the effects of inhaled substances on nasal functions have been performed in human volunteers under controlled conditions in climate chambers. The acute effects studied are impairment of nasal mucociliary flow, changes in nasal airflow resistance, and irritation of the nasal mucous membrane. The interindividual variations for these parameters are great, so it is preferable in such studies to use subjects as their own controls.

Nasal mucus flow is studied by means of visible or invisible tracers placed on and transported by the mucus. In 6-h exposures at the threshold limit value (TLV), the mucus flow rate is reduced by SO_2 and formaldehyde, but not by toluene, plastic dust, or wood dust. A common cold reduces the nasal mucus flow for 3-5 weeks. A chronic decrease of nasal mucus flow causes retention of mucus and recurrent infections of the paranasal sinuses and of the middle ear.

Nasal airflow resistance is a pressure-flow ratio obtained by plotting respiratory airflow against pressure. At 6-h exposures at the TLV, SO_2 causes an increase in nasal airflow resistance whereas no effects are seen due to formaldehyde, toluene, or plastic-dust exposure at their TLVs.

Nasal irritation can be measured by questionnaire methods or by a voting apparatus. For the above-mentioned substances abrupt changes in concentrations cause more irritation than constant exposures, but the effect fades off after some minutes. During 6-h exposures at the TLV, toluene was the least irritating substance whereas SO_2, plastic dust, wood dust, and formaldehyde had increasing irritation potency in the order mentioned. A comparison of these human data of nasal irritation with similar exposure data from the animal model of Alarie (18) shows that the animal model predicts nasal irritation in man very well.

REFERENCES

1 Pedersen M. Specific types of abnormal ciliary motility in Kartagener's syndrome and analogous respiratory disorders. *Eur. J. Respir. Dis.* 64 (Suppl. 127):78–90 (1982).

2 Proctor DF, and I Andersen. (eds). *The Nose.* Amsterdam: Elsevier (1982).

3 Andersen I, and DF Proctor. Measurement of nasal mucociliar clearance. *Eur. J. Respir. Dis.* 64(Suppl. 127):37–40 (1983).

4 Andersen, I, GR Lundquist, PL Jensen, and DF Proctor. Human response to controlled levels of sulfur dioxide. *Arch. Environ. Health* 28:31–39 (1974).

5 Andersen I, and L Mølhave. Controlled human studies with formaldehyde. In *Formaldehyde Toxicity,* edited by JE Gibson, pp. 154–165. Washington: Hemisphere (1983).

6 Andersen I, GR Lundquist, L Mølhave, OF Pedersen, DF Proctor, M Voeth, and DP Wyon. Human response to controlled levels of toluene in six-hour exposures. *Scand. J. Work Environ. Health* 9:405–418 (1983).

7 Baelum J, I Andersen, GR Lundquist, L Mølhave, OF Pedersen, M Voeth, and DP Wyon. The response of solvent-exposed printers and non-exposed controls to toluene in six-hour exposures. *Scand. J. Work Environ. Health* (in print).

8 Andersen I, GR Lundquist, DF Proctor, and DL Swift. Human response to controlled levels of inert dust. *Am. Rev. Respir. Dis.* 119:619–627 (1979).

9 Andersen HC, I Andersen, and J Solgaard. Nasal cancers, symptoms and upper airway function in wood workers. *Br. J. Ind. Med.* 34:201–207 (1977).

10 Andersen I, PL Jensen, SE Reed, JW Craig, DF Proctor, and GK Adams Induced rhinovirus infection under controlled exposure to sulfur dioxide. *Arch. Environ. Health* 32:120–125 (1977).

11 Sakakura Y, Y Sasaki, Y Togo, HN Wagner, RB Horwick, AR Schwartz, and DF Proctor. Mucociliary function during experimentally induced rhinovirus infection in man. *Ann. Otol. Rhinol. Laryngol.* 82:203–211 (1973).

12 Ginzel A, and P Illum. Messung des Schleimtransportes in der Nase an Gesunden und am Anschluss an die Erkältung mittels des Saccharin-Sky-blue-tests. *HNO-Praxis (Leipzig)* 6:31–37 (1981).

13 Pedersen M, Y Sakakura, B Winther, S Brofeldt, and N Mygind. Nasal mucociliary transport, number of ciliated cells, and beating pattern in naturally acquired colds. *Eur. J. Respir. Dis.* 64 (Suppl. 128):355–364 (1983).

14 Andersen I, L Mølhave, and DF Proctor. Human response to controlled levels of combinations of sulfur dioxide and inert dust. *Scand. J. Work Environ. Health* 7:1–7 (1981).

15 World Health Organization. *Indoor Air Pollutants: Exposure and Health Effects.* Copenhagen: Euro Reports and Studies 78, WHO (1983).

16 Bach B, L Mølhave, and OF Pedersen. Human reactions during controlled exposures to low concentrations of organic gases and vapours known as normal indoor air pollutants: Performance tests. *Proc. Third Int. Conf. Indoor Air Quality and Climate,* Stockholm, Vol. 3, pp. 397–402 (1984).

17 Widdicombe J (ed). *Respiratory Pharmacology.* Oxford, England: Pergamon (1980).

18 Alarie Y. Irritating properties of airborne materials to the upper respiratory tract. *Arch. Environ. Health* 13:433–449 (1966).

Chapter 11

Effects of Chemical Exposure on Olfaction in Humans

John E. Amoore

INTRODUCTION

One very important function of the nose is that of providing our sense of smell. The nose is vital to the enjoyment of some of the good things of life, such as fragrances, beverages, and especially food flavor. There is very little pleasure in eating if your sense of smell is suppressed by a cold. Also the nose can help to protect us from some of the bad things in life: the smell of fire, the smell of leaking gas, the smell of spoiled foodstuffs.

Anosmia is defined as a loss of the sense of smell, whereas hyposmia is a diminished sense of smell. If a factory worker is anosmic or hyposmic and believes that this was due to chemical exposure, he or she may seek disability or other compensation (1). Also, he will be at greater risk on the job because he has lost a useful early warning system (2).

I am most grateful to Lorrene Buckley of the Chemical Industry Institute of Toxicology, Research Triangle Park, North Carolina, for contributing the results of her initial literature review on this subject. Librarians Willanna Griffin and Beth Williamson of CIIT, and Levon Megrian at the University of California, Berkeley, did an excellent job of data base and library searching. Final typing of the manuscript was provided by Ms. Cathy Ghee.

It has recently been demonstrated that rats and mice exposed to dimethylamine, on a simulated work shift schedule (6 h/day, 5 days/week for 12 months), developed lesions of the olfactory epithelium (3). At 175 ppm, there was extensive loss of olfactory sensory cells and olfactory nerves. Less damage was seen at 50 ppm, and still detectable focal degeneration of the olfactory epithelium at 10 ppm dimethylamine, which is the currently recommended threshold limit value (TLV) for this substance (4). The same authors cited other recent studies that have demonstrated similar susceptibility of the olfactory epithelium to acetaldehyde, acrylic acid, chlorine, ethyl acrylate, furfural, and *N*-methylformimino-methylester in rats, mice, or hamsters.

Such extensive damage to structure implies a loss of function but, owing to the difficulties in performing olfactory evaluations with animals, sensitivity loss has rarely been established (for an exception, see Rehn et al. [5], using the last-named compound above). Instead, Buckley et al. (3) drew attention to the large but diffuse literature on reductions of smell sensitivity (hyposmia, anosmia) occurring in workers exposed to various industrial chemicals. They cited several representative papers, and two reviews (6, 7).

The present chapter was derived from the likely references in the above two reviews, as well as from articles or reviews by Koelsch (8), Schwab (9), Lehnhardt and Rollin (10), Zenk (11), Herberhold (1), Emmett (12), and Sahli (13). Bibliographies of odor and olfaction by Paschal (14) and by Michels et al. (15) were also helpful, and *Chemoreception Abstracts* covers the literature from 1973. Computer searches on MEDLINE from 1966 and TOXLINE from 1974 caught some more references, especially in the Eastern European literature of occupational medicine. The resulting compilation is believed to be the first quantitative review of olfactory effects associated with chemical exposure.

METHODS

Normal Range of Smell Sensitivity

Many methods have been described for measuring the sensitivity of olfaction (6), but no widely recognized standard has emerged. Several methods in current clinical use are refinements and variations on the liquid dilution procedure introduced by Proetz (16). After two decades of measuring human olfactory thresholds for research purposes, the current author has recommended glass flasks containing serial dilutions of pyridine in water (17) or plastic squeeze bottles containing pyridine in mineral oil (18). Each successive solution of the odorant is one-half the concentration of the preceding step. This provides a geometric ($\log_2$) concentration series. The use of a logarithmic scale is appropriate because, as with all the senses, the intensity of the sensation is proportional to the logarithm of the strength of the stimulus (Fechner's Law). At each binary step, the person being tested is asked to distinguish the odorous bottle from one or two otherwise identical blank bottles containing only the diluent, water, or oil. The lowest concentration reliably selected represents that person's detection threshold for pyridine.

Normal Distribution This pyridine odor threshold test has been applied to 205 healthy adults ages 18-65, having no known nasal pathology, and not exposed to any significant industrial chemicals (Fig. 1). The serial dilution numbers represent the number of binary dilution steps from pure pyridine, step 0; 50 percent pyridine + 50 percent water, step 1; 25 percent pyridine, step 2, etc. On this scale, the individual olfactory thresholds ranged from step 13 for the least sensitive person, to step 22 for the most sensitive. The corresponding threshold concentrations of pyridine vapor in air, calculated from the air/liquid partition coefficient, range from 20 down to 0.04 ppm, v/v. The sensitivities constitute a very nearly normal (Gaussian) distribution, wih a mean threshold at step 18.07, and standard deviation (SD) of ± 1.76 steps. In earlier work on inborn olfactory deficiencies, sensitivities below the − 2 SD limit were arbitrarily defined as abnormal (19)–i.e., hyposmic–and it may be justifiable to adopt the same criterion for deficiencies of external origin. Theoretically, 2 percent of a normal distribution lies below the − 2 SD level.

Rating Scale Fortunately, most other odorants that have been tested show approximately the same standard deviation of odor detection thresholds, averaging close to ± 2.0 binary steps (20). This means that comparable results could be obtained with more or less any odorant, apart from the restrictions that it should not be too similar to any odors encountered in the workplace, and that it should not exhibit the relatively rare phenomenon of inborn smell-blindness (21). These considerations lend some support to the idea that an individual's olfactory threshold can be designated by reference to the normal

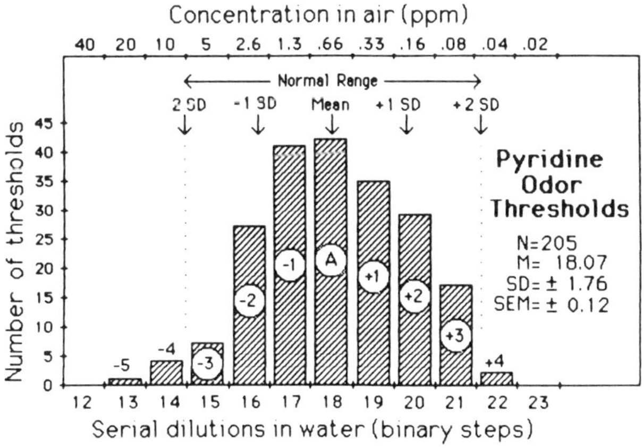

Figure 1 Distribution of individual olfactory thresholds to pyridine among 205 healthy adults. The circled numbers indicate sensitivity ratings relative to the normal average of step 18.

mean threshold. Thus, a person whose threshold is the same as the group mean (step 18 in Fig. 1) for a given odorant would be designated "A" for average. Thresholds one or two steps higher than average sensitivity would be indicated by +1 and +2, respectively, and low sensitivities by −3, −4, etc. These proposed sensitivity ratings are entered in the columns of the bar graph (Fig. 1).

Factors Affecting Normal Sensitivity There are negligible systematic differences between the olfactory sensitivities of men and women, or between moderate tobacco smokers and nonsmokers, so long as the groups tested have approximately the same average age (22). The distribution and mean in Fig. 1 are for average age about 40 years. People averaging 18 years old are about one binary step more sensitive than this mean, and those about 62 years old are one step less sensitive. The age effect should be taken into consideration when reviewing measured thresholds.

Smoking, eating, chewing candy, or drinking a beverage during the test or within the 15 min beforehand should be avoided, because the apparent olfactory sensitivity will be lowered about two steps. Persons suffering from a head cold or nasal allergy should not be tested until they recover, as a spurious two-step deficit is also likely to be found. Persons wearing perfume, scented cosmetics, or hand lotion should be excluded from the test until they wash off the fragrance, which could contaminate the test bottles. Observing these precautions, a person's olfactory threshold measurement should be reproducible within ± 1 step.

Olfactory Abnormalities

Descriptive assessments for the commonly encountered range of olfactory sensitivities are suggested in Table 1. The term hyposmia is appropriate for persons who have an abnormally weak (−5 or lower), but nevertheless functional, sense of smell. The term anosmia should be reserved for people who have no true olfactory (first cranial) nerve sensitivity–i.e., no sense of smell at all. Such persons usually retain the ability to detect irritants of the common chemical sense, registered as a tingling or stinging sensation in the nasal cavity by the trigeminal (fifth cranial) nerve. Pyridine, at scale step 9 and below, exhibits this irritant property. Some rare persons lack also the irritant sensibility of the IX and X cranial nerves as well as the trigeminal. Henkin (23) described this condition as "complete anosmia." Approximate frequencies to be expected in the population for each olfactory sensitivity are given in the right column of Table 1. In the clinical literature, anosmia and hyposmia are sometimes called hyposmia I and hyposmia II, respectively, terms introduced by Henkin (24).

Nonchemical Causes for Hyposmia There are many pathological conditions, unrelated to chemical exposure, that can lead to hyposmia or anosmia.

Table 1 Proposed Rating and Assessment of Individual Olfactory Threshold Sensitivities, Using the Pyridine Scale for Illustrative Purposes

Pyridine scale step	Sensitivity rating	Sensitivity assessment	Approximate frequency (percent)*
23 and above	⩾ +5	Hyperosmia	2
22	+4	High normal	14
21	+3		
20	+2	Above average	68
19	+1		
18	A	Average	
17	−1	Below average	
16	−2		
15	−3	Low normal	14
14	−4		
13	−5	Hyposmia	2
12	−6		
11	−7		
10	−8		
9 and below	⩽ −9	Anosmia	~ 0.2
< 0	< −18	Complete anosmia	~ 0.02

*Calculated for a normal distribution, assuming SD ± 2 binary steps.

The subject has recently been reviewed by Alter and Seltzer (25), Herberhold (1), Van den Eeckhaut (26), Doty (7), and Schiffman (27). Therefore, if just one chemical factory worker is found to be hyposmic (with no acute causative incident), then an extensive clinical work-up would be necessary to eliminate all other possible causes for the hyposmia before one could justifiably indict the work environment. Nevertheless, hyposmia is an uncommon condition in a normal population, with incidence of only about 2 percent, as defined above. Anosmia is distinctly rare, with incidence of only about 0.2 percent of the population (28). Complete anosmia (no trigeminal sensitivity either) afflicts perhaps one-tenth of anosmic individuals (17). Therefore if, among a group or class of workers exposed to the same chemicals, there should be a more frequent incidence of hyposmia or anosmia than expected on the basis of probability, one may suspect an environmental etiology.

Preferably, enough similarly exposed workers should be evaluated olfactometrically to prepare a bar chart or histogram resembling Fig. 1. If the mean threshold of the group deviates significantly from the mean threshold of an otherwise matching group of unexposed workers, then there is evidence for an effect of chemical exposure on the sense of smell. The literature, summarized in Tables 3-9, includes both clinical reports of single cases and group studies by industrial hygiene methods.

Drugs Two other forms of chemical exposure can affect the sense of smell and should not be forgotten. Many prescription drugs have been reported to cause hyposmia as a side effect; see reviews by Herberhold (1) and Schiffman (27). Common social drugs such as alcohol, nicotine, and cocaine consumed to excess may lead to a chronic hyposmia (29). Instead of a simple hyposmia, occasionally complex distortions of the sense of smell have been reported. Henkin (30) gave definitions for dysosmia, cacosmia, phantosmia, and heterosmia.

Methods of Olfactometry in Occupational Medicine

The presence of hyposmia or anosmia is frequently first detected as a medical symptom, either complained of by the patient or elicited by questions from the physician, and sometimes supplemented by some informal tests with coffee, tobacco, ammonia, etc. More elaborate odor recognition tests, using a battery of familiar substances, have been described by Mancioli (31) and Naus (32). From the results of symptom and recognition tests, either the original authors or the present reviewer could form an approximate assessment of the degree of hyposmia. Standardized odor recognition tests have recently been described by Cain et al. (33) and Doty et al. (34), the latter using convenient Microfragrance "Scratch 'n Sniff" tapes. Both have developed quantitative scales that can be correlated with threshold test results, and can reveal qualitative distortions of the sense of smell.

Liquid Dilution Tests These are generally conducted with serial dilutions of the odorant in vials, bottles, or flasks that are opened to permit sniffing the contents directly. Two current versions of odor threshold test were described at the beginning of the Methods section (17, 18). The thresholds are expressed directly in binary dilution steps. Earlier forms of the test (16, 35) give results quoted in "olfacts," where 1 olfact is the average normal threshold concentration of the odorant in the liquid (mineral oil). An olfactory defect of 50 olfacts means simply that the test threshold is at 50 times higher concentration than the normal threshold. This may be converted to binary steps deficiency by taking the $\log_{10}$ and dividing by 0.301 (the $\log_{10}$ of 2). Thus, 50 olfacts corresponds with 5.6 binary-steps deficiency (−5.6 binary-steps rating).

A slight variation on this procedure involves dipping a disposable filter-paper strip into the odorant solution, and holding it close to the subject's nostrils for sniffing. Roseburg et al. (36) used this method with six odorants in binary dilution series in diethyl phthalate. They suggested that an average deficiency of four binary steps indicates hyposmia and that eight steps or greater defect means anosmia. This is concordant with the proposed ratings in Table 1. The T&T olfactometer, described by Zusho et al. (37) uses five odors in decadic dilution steps in Nujol oil, which are likewise tested in filter-paper strips. An olfactory defect measured in decadic ($\log_{10}$) steps is readily converted to binary ($\log_2$) steps by dividing by 0.301.

Blast Injection Tests This method, introduced in the United States by Elsberg and Levy (38), uses a 500-ml bottle and attachments to deliver measured volumes of odorized air to the nostrils. The bottle typically contains 30 ml of an odorous chemical which rapidly odorizes the air inside. It is fitted with a double-bored bung and two tubes. The exit tube is closed by a stopcock or pinchcock, leading to a Y-piece bearing two olive-shaped beads for insertion in the nostrils of the subject. The entry tube is fitted with a calibrated syringe and three-way stopcock, so that a known volume of air can be injected into the bottle to produce a slight overpressure. While the patient holds his breath, the opening of the delivery cock permits a calibrated puff ("blast") of air to enter the nostrils.

Starting with very small injections, the volume of odorized air delivered is increased at each successive trial, until the subject detects the odor. When this happens, the effective volume of air delivered is regarded as the threshold, in milliliters. A separate bottle and attachments are prepared for each odorous substance. Elsberg et al. (39) recommended seven suitable odorants, but concluded that for most purposes just coffee and citral would give the required information. Elsberg et al. (40) and Jerome (41) demonstrated that air pressure, rather than air volume, was the effective variable in the test. This does not matter in practice, since the volume is proportional to the pressure (Boyle's law).

The Elsberg method was studied thoroughly by Strauss (42), who tested 300 healthy people with phenylethyl alcohol. There were 100 each of three age groups: 8-10 years, 16-18 years, and 21-39 years. Each group showed a nearly normal distribution of individual thresholds, with SD approximately equal to half the value of the mean threshold in ml. The decrease of sensitivity with increasing age, which may be calculated to be about one binary step in 13 years, is in general agreement with an estimate by liquid dilution threshold tests (one binary step in 22 years; Venstrom and Amoore [22]). On the basis of this rather indirect justification, the present reviewer decided to use the Elsberg thresholds in ml for relative sensitivity estimates. For example, if normal observers had thresholds averaging 4 ml for a given odorant, and exposed workers average 18 ml for the same odorant in the same apparatus, their threshold deficit is 18/4, or 4.5-fold. Taking the $\log_{10}$ and dividing by 0.301, this leads to a -2.2 binary-steps rating.

An evaluation of the Elsberg method by Jones (43) demonstrated that there could be no justification for attempting to convert the threshold ml readings and known vapor pressures into threshold concentrations. His criticisms, and those of Jerome (41), may have resulted in the Elsberg method being disregarded for purposes of occupational health testing in the United States and the United Kingdom. Nevertheless, the method was originally intended for testing the sensitivities of different people to the same odor, *not* the sensitivities of the same people to different odors. The Elsberg method has been used extensively, through the present, for occupational health research in Germany, Italy, Eastern Europe, and the Soviet Union.

In some of these countries, the modified apparatus of Fortunato and Niccolini (44) is used, which has six Elsberg bottles on a lazy Susan, rotating around a single axial turret valve and syringe. A hybrid method was proposed by Naus et al. (45). It uses an assembly of syringes, connected by stopcocks, for diluting the odorant vapor, e.g., benzene. It allows the concentration of benzene to be adjusted *and* the air volume delivered to be altered. For the smaller odor volumes, makeup air was added to bring the volume injected up to 20 ml and thus equalize the velocity of the injection. The results appear very similar to those obtained with the regular Elsberg method.

Detection of Malingering

The tests for hyposmia depend on the cooperation and honesty of the subject. For considerations related to disability, damages, etc., a subject may be motivated to deny an olfactory sensation, even when it is actually perceived. Several strategies have been suggested for the detection of a malingerer. The simplest may be to present an irritant or other strong, unpleasant odor (ammonia, asafetida) and watch for interrupted breathing, hesitation, or surprise. Unsophisticated subjects may not know the distinction between olfactory and trigeminal nerve sensitivities and may try to deny both. Repeated forced-choice threshold testing with pyridine solutions may reveal malingering, because the subject may not be able to show a consistent olfactory or irritation threshold or may mistakenly pick the blank bottles more frequently than expected statistically.

The act of perceiving odor, and especially irritation, may give rise to uncontrollable autonomic nervous reflexes, particularly in the sympathetic system. Woelk (29) suggested kymography, and Faleg et al. (46) the psychogalvanic reflex, to check on doubtful cases. Van den Eeckhaut (26) uses a polygraph for this purpose, measuring various circulatory, respiratory, and sudomotor reflexes. Nevertheless, as shown by Okhnyanskaya and Ginzburg (47) with a finger plethysmograph, the act of perceiving a weak, purely olfactory stimulus may have no effect whatsoever on these distal reflexes. Other Russian work has demonstrated, however, several more proximal neurological reflexes (ophthalmologic and encephalographic) in response to odorants, which occur at the same, or even lower, concentrations than the odor detection threshold (48, 49).

Of course, genuine complete anosmics do occur in the population, who give no reaction even to sniffing pure pyridine vapor, 30 percent formaldehyde, concentrated hydrochloric acid, or ammonium hydroxide (23). Such elaborate or heroic tests as those described above may not be necessary, as Doty et al. (34) describe a stratagem with Scratch 'n Sniff tapes that reliably identifies malingerers.

RESULTS

General Explanation of the Tables

The literature on chemically induced hyposmias is surprisingly extensive, with wide ranges of reported exposure times and severities of defect. Nevertheless, certain broad classes emerge, which are summarized in Table 2 as an aid to analyzing the data. Hyposmia has been reported to result from acute exposure to a noxious chemical vapor for a few hours or minutes, and sometimes even following a single inhalation. The consequent hyposmia may be temporary, recuperable, or permanent. Chronic exposure, usually measured in years of factory work, can result in a recuperable hyposmia, but more often a permanent hyposmia or anosmia develops. Although some illustrative examples are cited, the same chemical can appear in several classes, depending on its concentration and the duration of exposure (8).

Many of the reports include a quantitative measure of the degree of hyposmia in terms of olfactory thresholds, or else enough qualitative information to permit a confident assessment. Data from these systematic papers are assembled in Tables 3-9. Reports without sufficient data are summarized in Table 10. The data tables all have the same basic layout (with gaps where the information was not provided by the original authors). The concentration of the chemical(s) in the air was recalculated, if necessary, as ppm, v/v for gases and vapors, and as mg/m^3 for dusts, using the mean of the measured concentrations or, if these were unavailable, half the maximum recorded value. The approximate duration of the exposure is listed, which is the mean of the individual worker's exposure years, if provided, or the middle of the given range. Many authors provided the ages or age groups of the workers and their sex, but these

Table 2 A Classification of Chemically Induced Hyposmias, According to the Extent of the Exposure and the Duration of the Resulting Hyposmia

Exposure	Hyposmia	Duration	Examples	Table
ACUTE (sec/min/h)	Temporary	min	H_2S HCN	3A
	Recuperable	weeks	H_2Se $ZnSO_4$	3B
	Permanent	years	$POCl_3$ SO_2	3C
CHRONIC (month/year)	Recuperable	weeks	Acetone	3D
	Permanent	years	$ZnCrO_4$ Cl_2	4-9

Table 3 Substances Reported to Cause Acute Olfactory Injury in Man, Resulting in Temporary, Recuperable, or Permanent Hyposmias, as Defined in Methods. (See general explanation of Tables 3-9 at the beginning of Results. The table concludes with one case of chronic, but recuperable, hyposmia.)

	Exposure			Incidence of hyposmia		
Substance	Conc.	Time	Olfactometric method	Frequency (percent)	Assessment	Reference
A. Acute exposure; temporary hyposmia						
Formaldehyde		min	symptom		hyposmia	(78)
Hydrogen cyanide		sec	symptom		anosmia	(79)
Hydrogen selenide	0.3 ppm	min	symptom		hyposmia	(80)
Hydrogen sulfide	100 ppm	sec	symptom		anosmia	(81)
B. Acute exposure; recuperable hyposmia						
Hydrogen selenide	gas	2 sec§	symptom	1 case	anosmia	(82)
N-Methylformimino-methylester	sat. vap.	2 sec	symptom	1 case	anosmia‖	(83)
Sulfuric acid	5% soln.*	2 sec	symptom	1 case	anosmia	(29)
Zinc sulfate	1% soln.†	sec	symptom	25	anosmia	(58)
C. Acute exposure; permanent hyposmia						
Cesspool		h	symptom	1 case	anosmia	(84)
Decomp. cadaver		h	symptom	1 case	anosmia	(29)

C. Acute exposure; permanent hyposmia (*continued*)						
Pepper, Cresol	powder	2 sec	symptom	1 case	hyposmia, cacosmia#	(10)
Phosphorus oxychloride		sec	symptom	1 case	anosmia	(85)
Sulfur dioxide	270 ppm‡	2 sec	symptom	1 case	anosmia	(55)
D. Chronic exposure; recuperable hyposmia						
Acetone, Tetrahydrofuran, Cyclohexanone		3 mo	recognition	1 case	hyposmia, phantosmia#	(12)

*Patient fell into a disinfectant bath; the anosmia may have been an indirect consequence of the resultant chronic rhinitis.

†Nasal spray intended as a prophylactic against poliomyelitis.

‡Concentration seems underestimated. This was the head-space of a 6 percent solution of sulfurous acid, which is nearly saturated with sulfur dioxide

§"Two-sec exposure" indicates a single sniff or inhalation.

||Confirmed in tests with mice (5). After 0.5-sec exposure to the saturated vapor, an anosmia of — 20 binary steps severity resulted, which persisted for 3 weeks.

#Terms for olfactory perceptual abnormalities (30); cacosmia, obnoxious smell sensation caused by normally pleasant or neutral odorants; phantosmia, persistent odor sensation, even when no odorant is inhaled.

Table 4 Metallurgical Processes Considered Responsible, on Chronic Exposure, for Permanent Hyposmia in Man

			Incidence of hyposmia			
Substance	Exposure time (years)	Olfactometric method	Frequency (percent)	Rating (steps)	Assessment	Reference
Chromium	1.5	Elsberg	17	(−0.7)	below average	(86)
Chromium plating	4	recognition	cohort		low normal	(87)
Lead	8	Elsberg	33	(−0.6)†	below average	(86)
Lead (severe intox.)		Elsberg	cohort	−1.2	below average	(88)
Lead (severe intox.)		Elsberg	cohort	−1.3	below average	(73)
Magnet production*	10	recognition	10 cases		hyposmia	(89)
Mercury (chronic intox.)	29	Elsberg	55	−3.6	low normal	(46)
Nickel plating	4	recognition	cohort		low normal	(87)
Nickel refining (electrolytic)	> 5	recognition	33		anosmia	(90)
Silver plating	6	recognition	cohort		below average	(87)
Steel production	4	Elsberg	6	< −3.3	low normal	(91)
Zinc production	> 5	Elsberg	3	< −2.7	low normal	(92)

*Iron, aluminum, nickel, cobalt, and chromium powders.

†Just one worker was affected, and he had a unilateral hyposmia.

Table 5 Metallic Compounds Considered Responsible, on Chronic Exposure, for Permanent Hyposmia in Man

	Exposure			Incidence of Hyposmia			
Substance	Conc. (mg/m^3)	Time (years)	Olfactometric method	Frequency (percent)	Rating (steps)	Assessment	Reference
Cadmium compounds			Elsberg	13		anosmia	(11)
Cadmium compounds*	1.3	7	Elsberg	66		hyposmia §	(93)
Cadmium oxide		3	recognition	1 case		anosmia	(94)
Cadmium oxide } Nickel hydroxide }	9† 80	20	symptom	44		anosmia	(95)
Cadmium oxide } Nickel hydroxide }	0.5‡ 0.01	15	Proetz	27	< -7.6	hyposmia	(96)
Chromate salts		18	T&T	27	< -18	anosmia	(97)
Zinc chromate	10	10	Roseburg	30	~ -7	hyposmia‖	(98)

*Oxide, sulfate, carbonate, nitrate, sulfide, selenide, stearate.

†Before dust control.

‡After installation of industrial hygiene equipment.

§The hyposmia was ameliorated by giving caffeine.

‖A follow-up study on 11 of the same workers 4 years later (after reducing the chrome-dust exposure in the factory) showed no recovery of olfactory performance (99).

Table 6 Dusts Considered Responsible, on Chronic Exposure, for Permanent Hyposmia in Man

			Incidence of Hyposmia			
Substance	Exposure time (years)	Olfactometric method	Frequency (percent)	Rating (steps)	Assessment	Reference
Cement		Proetz	2		hyposmia	(100)
Chemicals	6	Proetz	8	< -6.6	hyposmia	(101)
Hardwoods		symptom	5		anosmia	(8)
Hardwoods		symptom			anosmia	(102)
Lime		Proetz	6		hyposmia†	(100)
Printing		Naus	24	-3.0	low normal	(45)
Silicosis (first stage)*		Elsberg	cohort	-1.2	below average	(88)

*First-, second-, and third-stage silicosis cohorts all showed about the same olfactory deficit.

†Damage to the olfactory epithelium, sensory cells, and bulbar fibers was observed in rats exposed 2 months in the dustiest locations in the factory (64).

Table 7 Nonmetallic Inorganic Compounds Considered Responsible, on Chronic Exposure, for Permanent Hyposmia in Man

	Exposure			Incidence of Hyposmia			
Substance	Conc. (ppm)	Time (years)	Olfactometric method	Frequency (percent)	Rating (steps)	Assessment	Reference
Carbon disulfide		15	Elsberg	22	−3.4	low normal	(86)
Carbon disulfide (average intox.)			Elsberg	cohort	−2.0§	low normal	(74)
Carbon disulfide (intox.)	62‡	20	Elsberg‡	14		hyposmia	(56)
Carbon monoxide		13	recognition	1 case		anosmia	(103)
Carbon monoxide (intox.)*	> 100		Elsberg	6		anosmia	(59)
Chlorine		3	Froetz	70	< −6.6	hyposmia	(101)
Hydrazine			Elsberg	cohort	−0.8	below average	(104)
Nitrogen dioxide (NO_x) Ammonia	3 30	5	Elsberg	cohort	−0.7	below average	(105)
Nitrogen dioxide (NO_x) Sulfur dioxide (SO_x)		8	Proetz	60	< −6.6	hyposmia	(101)
Sulfur dioxide	90	4	symptom	14		hyposmia	(106)
Sulfur dioxide	155	20	Elsberg	cohort	−3.4	low normal	(107)
Sulfur dioxide Ammonia†	80	32	T&T	cohort	−4.4	hyposmia	(108)
Sulfur dioxide (SO_x) Nitrogen dioxide (NO_x) Fluorides (HF?)		> 5	Elsberg	cohort	−1.2	below average	(109)

*Includes both acute and chronic intoxications.

†Workers exposed to ammonia alone showed no significant olfactory deficit.

‡Information given by Zenk (11).

§The hyposmia could be partially or completely reversed, for 1 or 2 h, by injections of caffeine or eserine.

Table 8 Organic Compounds Considered Responsible, on Chronic Exposure, for Permanent Hyposmia in Man

Substance	Exposure			Incidence of hyposmia			
	Conc. (ppm)	Time (years)	Olfactometric method	Frequency (percent)	Rating (steps)	Assessment	Reference
Acetone		8	recognition	1 case		hyposmia	(94)
Acetophenone		6	Elsberg	12	(< −2.3)	low normal	(110)
Benzene		10	Elsberg	cohort	−0.8	below average	(111)
Benzine	400	5	Proetz	37	−6	hyposmia	(112)
Benzine, Ethyl acetate, Butyl acetate (combined)	60	8	Elsberg	30	< −3.1	low normal	(113)
Chloromethanes*			Elsberg	44	−2.7	low normal	(114)
Menthol			recognition	cohort		hyposmia	(32)
Menthol		45	symptom	1 case		hyposmia	(10)
Pentachlorophenol			symptom	1 case		anosmia‡	(115)
Trichloroethylene	380	10	Naus	cohort	−3.1†	low normal	(116)
Trichloroethylene (intermittent abuse)	sat. vap.	9	symptom	1 case		complete anosmia	(117)

*CH_3Cl, CH_2Cl_2, $CHCl_3$, CCl_4.

†Tested at beginning of shift, i.e., a permanent hyposmia. When tested at the end of the shift, an additional −2.1 steps of temporary hyposmia was demonstrated.

‡May have been due to upper respiratory tract infection, not occupational exposure.

Table 9 Manufacturing Processes Considered Responsible, on Chronic Exposure, for Permanent Hyposmia in Man

Substance	Exposure time (years)	Olfactometric method	Incidence of Hyposmia: Frequency (percent)	Rating (steps)	Assessment	Reference
Acids (organic and inorganic)	7	Proetz	5	< -6.6	hyposmia	(101)
Asphalt (oxidized)	6	Elsberg	18	< -2.3	low normal	(110)
Cutting oils (machining)		Elsberg	cohort	-0.8	below average	(104)
Fragrances	4	recognition	50		below average	(118)
Paint (lead)		Naus	56	-2.9	low normal	(45)
Paprika	14	Elsberg	4		hyposmia	(119)
"Pavinol" (sewing)*		Elsberg	55	< -2.3	low normal	(120)
Spices	11	Naus	cohort	-1.0†	below average	(121)
Tobacco	12	Elsberg	1		hyposmia	(122)
Varnishes	10	recognition	78		low normal	(31)
Varnishes	5	Elsberg	1		hyposmia	(123)
Waste water (refinery)	7	Elsberg	18	< -2.3	low normal	(110)

*A synthetic leather. The material contains a slightly volatile plasticizer, dibutyl phthalate, which may be responsible for the hyposmic effect.

†Tested at the beginning of the shift, i.e., a permanent hyposmia. When tested at the end of the shift, an additional -1.6 steps of temporary hyposmia was demonstrated.

Table 10 Incidental Reports of Industrial Substances Suspected of an Association with Hyposmia in Man, but with Insufficient Detail for Inclusion in Tables 3-9. (The reference for each substance is the earliest citation that could be traced with reasonable bibliographic effort.)

Substance	Type of hyposmia	Reference
Metallurgical processes		
Aluminum fumes	Chronic	(11)
Arsenic	Chronic	(9)
Chromium fumes	Chronic	(11)
Copper fumes	Chronic	(11)
Manganese fumes	Chronic	(11)
Tin fumes	Chronic	(11)
Vanadium fumes	Chronic	(11)
Zinc fumes	Chronic	(11)
Metallic compounds		
Alum	Acute, recuperable	(8)
Arsenic compounds	Chronic	(1)
Bis-(diethyldithiocarbamato)-cadmium		(13)
Chlorovinylarsine chlorides	Acute, permanent	(8)
Chromic acid	Chronic, permanent	(8)
Copper arsenite	Chronic, permanent	(8)
Dichromates	Chronic	(11)
Lye	Chronic	(9)
Osmium tetroxide	Chronic, permanent	(8)
Potassium sulfide		(13)
Silver nitrate	Acute, recuperable	(8)
Strontium sulfide		(13)
Dusts		
Cotton	Chronic	(89)
Cyanides	Chronic, permanent	(104)
Flax	Chronic	(89)
Flour	Chronic	(115)
Potash	Chronic	(9)
Nonmetallic inorganic compounds		
Ammonia	Chronic, permanent	(8)
Bromine	Acute, temporary	(11)
Flue gas (CO/SO_2?)	Chronic, permanent	(8)
Hydrazine	Chronic, permanent	(124)
Hydrogen chloride	Chronic, permanent	(8)
Hydrogen fluoride	Chronic, permanent	(8)
Nitric acid	Chronic, permanent	(8)
Nitrogen dioxide (NO_X)	Chronic, permanent	(8)
Phosgene	Acute, temporary	(8)
Selenium dioxide	Chronic	(9)
Sewer gas (H_2S?)	Chronic, permanent	(8)
Sulfuric acid	Chronic, permanent	(8)

Table 10 (*Continued*) **Incidental Reports of Industrial Substances Suspected of an Association with Hyposmia in Man, but with Insufficient Detail for Inclusion in Tables 3-9. (The reference for each substance is the earliest citation that could be traced with reasonable bibliographic effort.)**

Organic compounds		
Acetaldehyde	Chronic, permanent	(8)
Acetic acid	Chronic, permanent	(8)
Acetonitrile		(13)
Acid chlorides	Acute, temporary	(8)
Benzaldehyde	Chronic, permanent	(8)
Benzoic acid	Acute, permanent	(8)
Butylene glycol	Acute, permanent	(8)
Carbon tetrachloride	Chronic, permanent	(8)
Chloroform		(29)
Dimethyl sulfate		(13)
Ethyl ether	Acute, permanent	(8)
Fluorine compounds	Acute, temporary	(8)
Formaldehyde	Chronic, permanent	(8)
Furfural	Chronic, permanent	(8)
Halogen compounds	Chronic	(11)
Iodoform	Chronic	(9)
Isocyanates (TDI, etc.)	Chronic	(11)
Nitro compounds	Chronic	(11)
Phenylene diamine	Chronic	(11)
Selenium compounds (volatile)	Acute, temporary	(8)
Sulfur compounds	Chronic	(11)
Tetrachloroethane	Chronic	(1)
Trichloroethane	Chronic	(1)
War gases (WW I)	Acute, permanent	(8)
m-Xylene		(13)
Manufacturing processes		
Blasting powder	Chronic, permanent	(8)
Coal tar fumes	Chronic, permanent	(8)
Perfumes (concentrated)	Chronic, permanent	(8)
Rubber vulcanization	Chronic, permanent	(26)
Tanning	Chronic, permanent	(8)

have been omitted from the tables for lack of space. Inconsequential variations on the original method are disregarded. The "recognition" methods are not credited to their original authors, even if different from the cited reference. The notation "Proetz" is used for any serial liquid-dilution method with sniffing from the vessels, even though the selection of test odorant(s) may be different from the original (16). Likewise, "Elsberg" identifies any blast injection method, irrespective of apparatus modifications and selection of odorant(s) differing from the prototype (38).

So far as could be determined from the published data, the incidence of hyposmia was evaluated under three headings: frequency, rating, and assessment. The frequency of occurrence in the worker population is expressed as a percentage where appropriate, but sometimes the observations relate to a single case history. The total number of workers examined is usually recorded in the original papers but is omitted here for simplicity. "Cohort" means either the entire group of exposed workers or a selected subgroup defined by the authors, e.g., "severe intoxication." The olfactory thresholds of affected workers were reported by many investigators, either as group averages or as tables or graphs, from which the reviewer derived the appropriate arithmetic or geometric mean. The authors nearly always provided, in the same or earlier papers, data on the thresholds of control groups of persons who had not been exposed to the subject chemical(s). For the sake of uniformity, the original data have been converted (single-case observation or group mean threshold) into an olfactory deficit, or sensitivity rating, according to the binary step scale proposed in Table 1. The larger the negative number, the more severe the hyposmia. In this way, the effects of different chemical exposures can be compared on a common scale so as to obtain a general idea of the resulting deficiencies. Nevertheless, the values, having been obtained by many different experimental methods, should not be compared too rigorously.

Also provided are verbal sensitivity-assessments of the degree of hyposmia, according to the classification in Table 1. Where possible, this is based on the numerical value of the sensitivity rating, but otherwise represents a best judgment drawn from the author's descriptions of the symptoms and/or odor chemicals used in the recognition tests. If the incidence of hyposmia as a number or percentage was not stated, this could generally be calculated from a graph or table by applying the principles illustrated in Fig. 1.

In the reference column, only the citation is given. Full authorship is provided in the references at the end of the chapter. For a given substance, it is not necessarily the only, or even the earliest citation, but it is usually the original article rather than a review.

Results from the Literature Survey

Acute Exposure Hyposmia has frequently been reported as an immediate symptom of acute exposure to a variety of chemicals. Eleven chemicals or mixtures are well documented in this respect (Table 3). Many of these are single-case observations, the consequences of accidents or other unusual circumstances. Exposure times ranged from a single inhalation up to a day's work. Although quantitative threshold measurements are lacking, it is clear from the descriptions that the patients suffered hyposmia or anosmia. A definite cause-and-effect relationship between the chemical injury and the hyposmia was apparent to the patient and the examining physician. The symptoms are grouped into three classes, with hyposmias that were temporary, recuperable, or permanent, respectively, in sections A, B, and C of Table 3. With different intensities of exposure, or with longer periods of observing the patient, the assessment of hyposmia and the possibility for recovery could change. Acute anosmias resulting from workplace chemical accidents should be regarded as traumatic injuries, in the opinion of Woelk (29).

Chronic Exposure: Recuperable Hyposmia Only one example, listed in section D of Table 3, has been found. This does not necessarily mean that recovery from chronic chemical hyposmia is rare. Persons who may have suffered an injury from a work exposure that has been discontinued are unlikely to consult a physician when their symptoms are spontaneously improving.

Chronic Exposure: Permanent Hyposmia It is much more difficult to prove hyposmia as a consequence of chronic chemical exposure because the symptom may not develop for years, and the worker may not have remained with the same chemical exposure during the whole of the latent period. Nevertheless, the industrial-hygienist authors listed in Tables 4-9 were convinced that hyposmia in a significant proportion of the sampled work force had been demonstrated and that it was caused by their exposure to a particular chemical, class of chemicals, or other industrial substance. The reviewer has grouped the 42 responsible chemicals and other materials into six tables, according to selected major divisions of the chemical industry: metallurgy, metallic compounds, dusts, nonmetallic inorganic compounds, organic compounds, and manufacturing processes involving complex mixtures. Although this is arbitrary, it serves to show which industries may be at risk, and it might help with discerning possible mechanisms by which the chemicals degrade the sense of smell.

Exposure times ranged from 1½ to 45 years. Olfactory sensitivity ratings were observed from −0.6 step, which is only slightly below the normal average, to −18 steps, which represents a profound anosmia, and even one case of complete anosmia. When evaluating the significance of the ratings, one should take into consideration the frequency (percent) occurrence for the group whose average rating is calculated. There are a few entries in Tables 4-9 where the frequency and rating of "hyposmias" is no different from the normal distribution illustrated in Fig. 1 and summarized in Table 1. Such ratings are enclosed in parentheses, to indicate their uncertain significance. Some of the other ratings, especially for cohorts, are so close to zero that it is doubtful if they would pass an appropriate test of significance (Student's *t*-test). They should not be altogether dismissed, however, because the conversion factors used by the reviewer to obtain the ratings in binary steps may have underestimated the degree of hyposmia shown in the original author's data.

Incidental Reports In Table 10 are gathered 67 additional reports of industrial substances, mostly chemicals, that are on record as having caused hyposmia in man but for which there was not enough information to qualify for listing in Tables 3-9. They were found, for the most part, in review articles, and probably represent observations of symptoms noted in the practical experience of industrial hygienists. It is doubtful whether the original articles, even if they could be located, contain any quantitative data, but the listings themselves constitute a clear warning that these substances can damage the sense of smell if handled without proper precautions. Enough information is provided in most cases for it to be possible to infer what type of hyposmia resulted (chronic, permanent, etc.).

In the opinion of F. Flury (quoted by Koelsch [8]), literally hundreds of volatile substances can lead to "smell poisoning." This is especially true of astringent or corrosive compounds that can cause long-lasting, even permanent loss of olfactory capability. Flury was writing in the early 1930s, when the practice of industrial hygiene was relatively primitive, but his warning should increase our respect today for the lesser-known toxic properties of chemicals.

Trigeminal Analgesia Most of the membranes of the nasal cavity are innervated by branches of the trigeminal nerve, which registers a burning, stinging, or "pungent" sensation when irritated by reactive chemicals, especially electrophilic compounds (50, 51). It is presumably the pain-sensitive fibers that are responding. The literature survey turned up a few examples of compounds that suppress the trigeminal sensitivity, i.e., cause a persistent analgesia (Table 11). Apart from brief mentions of carbon monoxide and smoke, it is low-molecular-weight chlorinated hydrocarbons that most often produce this effect.

Table 11 Industrial Chemicals Reported to Reduce the Sensitivity of the Trigeminal Nerve to Irritants

Substance	Exposure	Neuropathy	Reference
Carbon monoxide			(1)
Chloromethanes*			(114)
Dichloroethylene			(8)
Smoke and soot†			(9)
Trichloroethylene	1½ h	2 months	(52)‖
Trichloroethylene	6 weeks	> 1 year	(125)‖
Trichloroethylene‡	9 years	> 1 year	(117)
Trichloroethylene§			(53)‖

*CH_3Cl, CH_2Cl_2, $CHCl_3$, CCl_4.

†Locomotive drivers.

‡Intermittent abuse. Also caused anosmia.

§Of 188 chronically exposed degreasers, 17 percent suffered neuropathy.

‖Includes literature review.

Trichloroethylene neuropathy has an extensive literature because of its importance as a degreaser and as an anesthetic (52). The entire distribution of the trigeminal nerve can be anesthetized, and the glossopharyngeal nerve may also be affected. As little as 1½ hour of exposure can cause the neuropathy, which may, in severe cases, persist up to a year, with an "onion peel" pattern of recovery. The effect is probably due to demyelinization and axon degeneration. The neuropathy is especially marked with trichloroethylene that has been partially decomposed by alkali (soda lime, potassium tetroxide), which forms dichloroacetylene (53). Stabilizers such as triethylamine used in the commercial product (but not in the anesthetic grade) have also been implicated.

Nosebleeding, etc. Woelk (29) cited several examples of very strong odors causing reflex vasodilation and capillary bleeding in the olfactory region, and hence a temporary hyposmia. Many other autonomic nervous system reflexes initiated by industrial odors have been reported, and can lead to somatic complaints (headache, nausea, etc.) from persons living near a factory (54).

DISCUSSION

Significance of Hyposmia in the Chemical Industry

As remarked by Herberhold (1), the list of possible noxious agents for the sense of smell is astonishingly voluminous. Tables 3-10 include nearly 120 substances reported to exhibit this harmful property in varying severities. Reactive chemical vapors and gases, solvents, heavy metals, dusts, and a broad range of manufacturing processes have been implicated in this respect. Professionals responsible for occupational hygiene in almost all branches of the chemical industry should include the possibility of hyposmia among the factors they evaluate.

Comparison of Exposure and TLV Concentrations In a few studies, the average concentration, or range of concentrations, to which the affected workers were chronically exposed has been reported (Table 12). In every case, the exposure concentration was equal to or greater than the TLV for that substance currently recommended by the American Conference of Governmental Industrial Hygienists (4). For cadmium oxide and zinc chromate, the ratio of historical exposure to current TLV has been as high as 200-fold. Of course, some of these reports were from times or countries where less stringent standards, or no standards at all, were in effect. In the majority of studies here reviewed, no quantitative exposure data were reported. Adequate protection of the olfactory apparatus by adherence to the current TLVs is evidently marginal for some substances, and deserves more investigation for these and other materials.

Table 12 Average Chronic Exposure Concentrations Associated with Hyposmia, Compared with Threshold Limit Values (TLV, 8-h TWA) Recommended by ACGIH (4)

Substance	Table No.	Units	Concentration: Exposure	Concentration: TLV	Ratio exposure/TLV
Ammonia*	7	ppm	30	25	1.2
Benzine	8	ppm	400	300†	1.3
Cadmium compounds	5	mg/m^3	1.3	0.05	26
Cadmium oxide	5	mg/m^3	9	0.05	180
Cadmium oxide	5	mg/m^3	0.5	0.05	10
Carbon disulfide	7	ppm	62	10	6
Carbon monoxide	7	ppm	> 100	50	> 2
Nitrogen dioxide (NO_X)	7	ppm	3	3	1
Sulfur dioxide	7	ppm	90	2	45
Sulfur dioxide	7	ppm	155	2	77
Sulfur dioxide	7	ppm	80	2	40
Trichloroethylene	8	ppm	380	50	7
Zinc chromate	5	mg/m^3	10	0.05‡	200

*Not proved to cause hyposmia at this concentration. See footnote (†) of Table 7.
†TLV for gasoline.
‡Suspected carcinogenic potential for man.

Sense of Smell as a Safety Factor in the Workplace Volatile chemical hazards in the workplace are usually invisible in the air, and the only sensory awareness of their presence may arise from the sense of smell. For some substances, odor does provide an adequate warning of their presence well below the TLV, but for others the smell is too weak to afford any warning. This concept has recently been explored in depth elsewhere (2). Nevertheless, even if the average person can protect himself by attending to odor impressions, anybody with impaired olfactory function, and hence elevated personal detection threshold, is at a disadvantage and possibly even in danger. Clearly, every effort should be made to ensure that workplace chemical exposures do not add to the various causes of hyposmia that already exist.

Disability and Compensation for Hyposmia Accidental or chronic loss of the sense of smell not only is a personal deprivation, but may constitute an occupational disability. Sahli (13) cites the American Medical Association guideline that permanent bilateral anosmia should rate a 3 percent disability, and she remarks that some states include anosmia under workmen's compensation laws. West German authorities have suggested more liberal compensation, with a minimum of at least 10–20 percent disability even for plaintiffs who do not work, or appellants for whose work the sense of smell is irrelevant. The disability would rise to 20-40 percent for workers who benefit substantially from their olfactory sense on the job (pharmacist, chemist, fishmonger) and could become 100 percent for specialists such as head chef, tobacco blender, and perfumer, for whom a sensitive and cultivated nose is an indispensable qualification for their profession (1, 8, 9). Otolaryngologists are sometimes called on to evaluate olfactory disability claims as a basis for compensation awards: e.g., Pfander (55) on an acute, permanent hyposmia caused by sulfur dioxide, and Zenk (56) providing a series of referral opinions on workers chronically exposed to carbon disulfide.

Annual Olfactometric Testing for Workers? Herberhold (1) has suggested that, just as workers in very noisy occupations should have an annual hearing test, workers chronically exposed to chemical fumes should have an annual olfactometric examination. There would be several benefits to instituting such a program. It would educate workers to the general value of smell as a warning and could be adapted, by means of customized odor threshold tests, to guide the individual worker in the safe use of exhaust vents, respirators, etc., for specified chemicals. Any systematic loss of olfactory sensitivity, in a cohort of similarly exposed workers, could be an indicator of excessive exposure or of unsuspected toxicity, because the olfactory organ, owing to its location and constitution, may be among the most susceptible tissues in the body to chemical injury. Also, the extent of liability may be mitigated by the existence of a testing program that established a baseline sensitivity for workers who may later claim to have been injured by an industrial accident or environment, and that guards against hyposmic individuals being assigned to chemically hazardous work. Hyposmia can be a fatal handicap, as Nathanson (57) demonstrated, when he found degenerated olfactory mucosae at autopsy in two out of three cases of acute carbon monoxide poisoning by illuminating (coal) gas which, for most people, has a strong inherent warning odor.

Pathological Basis for Chemical Hyposmia

Although there seems to have been little research directed to the pathological mechanisms underlying the human hyposmias caused by chemical exposure, there have been some investigations, especially in experimental animals, that provide a partial understanding of the mechanisms involved.

Mechanisms for Hyposmia As described by earlier reviewers, chemically induced hyposmias and anosmias may be conveniently classified into three divisions: respiratory, essential, and central (8, 9, 11, 29). So-called respiratory or mechanical hyposmias are due to the indirect effect of various factors blocking the upper airways, and hence physically preventing access of the odoriferous molecules to the olfactory mucosa. Millers and cement-kiln workers can develop rhinoliths (8). Other substances can cause edema, polyps, or tumors that can block the narrow olfactory clefts. Essential hyposmia results from the toxic injury to the olfactory mucosa and nervous receptors—for example, by caustic chemicals such as zinc sulfate (58), metabolic inhibitors like hydrogen cyanide and hydrogen sulfide, and also repeated exposure to reactive chemicals or finely divided particles (1).

A distinction between respiratory and essential hyposmia is usually apparent by otolaryngological examination and by careful rhinomanometry (1). Central or intracranial hyposmias affecting the olfactory bulbs and brain are less well defined, and are invoked largely by elimination, when hyposmia is demonstrated but there is no sign of respiratory, and little or no indication of essential, hyposmia: for example, intoxications by carbon monoxide (59) or mercury (46).

Chemical Exposure and Olfactory Histology The olfactory receptor cells have a remarkable affinity for certain colloids, as demonstrated in mice by Rake (60) with Prussian blue, and in squirrel monkeys by De Lorenzo (61) with colloidal gold. The granules seem to be absorbed into the cytoplasm by formation of pinocytotic vacuoles, are rapidly transported within the neuron and axon, then cross the first-order synapse and enter the mitral cell dendrites. De Lorenzo (61) concludes that "the olfactory rod is busily engaged in 'drinking in' materials from the extracellular environment." The particles of poliomyelitis virus can probably be absorbed through the same pathway (62), and this route of infection in monkeys can be blocked by spraying the nose with 1 percent zinc sulfate solution, which also causes a recuperable hyposmia.

The cytological damage caused by zinc sulfate was described by Smith (63) in rats. All three principal types of cells in the olfactory mucosa were destroyed: receptor, supporting, and basal. Tissue damage in experimental conditions simulating possible industrial exposures were described by Meurman (64) for rats caged at very dusty locations in a cement factory, by Zenk (11) for rabbits exposed to 215 ppm carbon disulfide, and by Yamagishi et al. (65) for guinea pigs in 7 ppm nitrogen dioxide. Zenk (11) also measured changes in some enzymatic activities in the olfactory mucosa. As mentioned earlier, Buckley et al. (3) described their own and other recent studies, all demonstrating that the olfactory cells and nervous pathways are especially vulnerable to certain reactive airborne chemicals.

A variety of waterborne chemical agents was tested by Cancalon (66) in brief, 10-sec treatments on the olfactory cavity of the channel catfish. Among several heavy-metal salts, zinc chloride at 30 mM (about 0.4 percent) resulted in the maximum damaging effect (observed 4 days later), largely restricted to the receptor cells. Solutions below pH3 or above pH 9 caused total destruction of the whole area, including nonsensory tissues. Cancalon also tested the function of the receptor cells, by measuring the electroolfactogram, which is an oscillographic recording of the summated electrical potential from the olfactory mucosa. Rehn et al. (5) also demonstrated both olfactory epithelium degeneration and abolition of the electroolfactogram in mice exposed 0.5 sec to the saturated vapor of *N*-methylformimino-methylester. Getchell and Gesteland (67), using the electroolfactogram, investigated the complete abolition of receptor response in the frog by the sulfhydryl reagent *N*-ethylmaleimide. Criswell et al. (68) likewise showed that the World War I gas ethyl bromoacetate, also a sulfhydryl and alkylating agent, suppresses the olfactory response in the frog to all odorants tested, with the curious exception of aliphatic amines.

Regeneration and Turnover of Olfactory Receptors. The earlier research was reviewed by Takagi (69). The majority of investigators found that after degeneration of the olfactory epithelium was induced by section of the olfactory nerves or ablation of the bulb, or by treatment with zinc sulfate (63), there was no regeneration. Schultz (62), however, noted that the anosmia induced in humans by zinc sulfate, and the subsequent recovery in a few weeks, implied that the olfactory receptors were destroyed, but that the neurons may be capable of regeneration. Later workers reviewed by Takagi (69) indicated that a generation of entirely new olfactory cells or epithelium may be possible after the destruction of the tissues.

Even in the undamaged tissue, there is now ample evidence for a continuous renewal of olfactory cells, as reviewed by Moulton (70). In the mouse, the nuclei of the three main types of cells are stratified, with the supporting cell nuclei in the outermost layer, then a thick layer of receptor cell nuclei, and a lower, thin layer of basal cell nuclei. Moulton and Fink (71) injected mice with [^{3}H]thymidine, which is incorporated into dividing cells, and noted that the radioactively labeled nuclei in the first 4 days were largely confined to the basal layer. Between 4 and 20 days, 90 percent of the labeled cells had migrated into the receptor cell layer, and to a lesser extent into the supporting cells.

In a subsequent experiment with injection of colchicine, which blocks cell divisions at the metaphase, Moulton (72) was able to calculate the rates at which cells of each type were being replaced. The turnover rate of the entire cell population (basal, receptor, and supporting) was 28 ± 6 days. In all likelihood, the turnover rate of the receptor cells themselves was nearly the same. Evidently, cell divisions in the basal cell layer produce daughter cells, about half of which differentiate into new receptor cells and supporting cells. The receptor cells must in turn grow cilia and new axons, which reestablish the appropriate connections with the mitral cells in the olfactory bulb. Cancalon (66) described the recovery of structure and function (by electroolfactogram) in the olfactory mucosa of the catfish after various degrees of damage by chemical attack.

The renewal of neurons in the adult vertebrate is an extremely rare phenomenon but also extremely fortunate in the present context, because it suggests that chemical damage to the olfactory epithelium can be spontaneously repaired by regeneration of olfactory receptor cells. This can, of course, only be expected if enough basal cells survive to initiate the recovery. Cases of acute chemically induced hyposmia that are followed by recovery of olfaction in a few weeks or months may be explained by this regeneration of receptor cells. Nevertheless, unless the complete set of receptors is replaced, and their central nervous connections correctly renewed, there could be deficiencies such as partial anosmia, cacosmia, and heterosmia, as indeed sometimes follow olfactory injury.

Possible Treatments for Hyposmia As with most injuries, the less severe they are, the better are the prospects for recovery. Respiratory hyposmia can often be reversed by otolaryngological procedures such as removal of rhinoliths or surgery of polyps or tumor. Hyposmia due to inflammation or edema of the olfactory cleft frequently responds to antiinflammatory corticosteroid nose drops (37).

When the hyposmia is of the essential type, the best treatment is to discontinue, or at least decrease, the chemical exposure that caused the trouble. Yamagishi et al. (65) showed that changes induced in the olfactory epithelium of guinea pigs by 7 days' exposure to 7 ppm nitrogen dioxide were rapidly repaired within about 7 days after the exposure was stopped. Emmett (12) described a gradual recovery from the effects of 3 months of exposure to acetone, tetrahydrofuran, and cyclohexanone. Zenk (11) noted that even though hyposmia is one of the three cardinal signs of workplace cadmium poisoning, if exposure is discontinued, recovery of the sense of smell is possible. Even central olfactory deficiency due to chronic lead poisoning has been shown to improve after lead detoxification treatment (73).

Various drugs, vitamins, and minerals have been proposed from time to time as treatments for hyposmia. Osipova (74) treated workers having olfactory deficiency due to carbon disulfide exposure with injections of caffeine or eserine, which restored thresholds to near the normal average for several hours. Caffeine is an anti-cyclic AMPase, and might enhance the responsiveness of the intracellular transduction process. Eserine is an anticholinesterase, and could thereby prolong postsynaptic responsiveness. (See also Skouby and Zolstorff-Pedersen [75].) These seem overly drastic and nonselective drugs for the purpose.

Duncan and Briggs (76) had a high success rate with massive injections of vitamin A and oral dosage follow-up for patients with uncomplicated anosmia. This was most often of influenzal origin, but two of the markedly improved cases had unspecified toxic causes. Henkin et al. (77) reviewed earlier work of his group indicating that orally administered zinc sulfate (!) could correct a zinc deficiency in many hyposmic patients, and thereby restore normal olfaction. Unfortunately, in a randomized double-blind study on 106 patients, the zinc sulfate was effectively equivalent to placebo in the treatment of this disorder.

SUMMARY

There exists a substantial, though scattered, literature on the effects of industrial chemical exposure on the sense of smell of the workers. This is the first exhaustive and, so far as possible, quantitative review of the subject. In order to place the occupational health observations in perspective, it is necessary to consider the normal range of smell sensitivities in the population, as well as other factors affecting that sensitivity. Various olfactometric methods that have been used in industrial medicine are described, and an attempt is made to convert the data from each to a common numerical scale, based on binary steps of chemical stimulus concentration.

For purposes of systematizing the data, the observations were classified into (1) acute and chronic chemical exposures and (2) the resulting temporary, recuperable, or permanent hyposmias. The principal results of the literature survey are given in six tables that list the chronic, permanent hyposmias under the headings of metallurgy, metallic compounds, dusts, nonmetallic inorganic compounds, organic compounds, and manufacturing processes. The tables provide, wherever available, the average time and concentration of the chemical exposure, and the frequency, assessment, and quantitative rating of the chemical hyposmias in the workplace. Tables on acute olfactory injuries, incidental reports lacking in detail, and trigeminal nerve analgesia complete the survey.

This chapter concludes with a discussion of various fundamental and peripheral aspects of the problem, under the general headings of the significance of hyposmia in the chemical industry, and the pathological basis for chemically induced hyposmia.

REFERENCES

1 Herberhold C. Funktionsprüfungen und Störungen des Geruchssinnes. *Arch. Otorhinolaryngol.* 210:67–164 (1975).

2 Amoore JE, and E Hautala. Odor as an aid to chemical safety: Odor thresholds compared with threshold limit values and volatilities for 214 industrial chemicals in air and water dilution. *J. Appl. Toxicol.* 3:272–290 (1983).

3 Buckley LA, KT Morgan, JA Swenberg, RA James, TE Hamm, and CS Barrow. The toxicity of dimethylamine in F-344 rats and B6C3F1 mice following a 1-year exposure. *Fund. Appl. Toxicol.* 5:341–352 (1985).

4 ACGIH. *TLVs: Threshold Limit Values for Chemical Substances and Physical Agents in the Work Environment.* Cincinnati: American Conference of Governmental Industrial Hygienists (1984).

5 Rehn B, W Breipohl, C Schmidt, U Schmidt, and F Effenberger. Chemical blockade of olfactory perception by *N*-methylformimino-methylester in albino mice. II. Light microscopical investigations. *Chem. Senses* 6:317–328 (1981).

6 Naus A. *Olphactoric Properties of Industrial Matters.* Prague: Charles University (1975).

7 Doty RL. A review of olfactory dysfunctions in man. *Am. J. Otolaryngol.* 1:57–79 (1979).

8 Koelsch F. *Handbuch der Berufskrankheiten,* 2nd ed. Jena: VEB Gustav Fischer Verlag (1959).

9 Schwab W. Die Berufsschäden der oberen Luftwege und des oberen Speiseweges. *Arch. Ohren Nasen Kehlkopfheilk.* 185:243–378 (1965).

10 Lehnhardt E, and H Rollin. Berufsbedingte Riechstörungen. *HNO* 17:104–106 (1969).

11 Zenk H. Auswirkungen beruflicher Noxen auf das Geruchsvermögen. In *Aktuelle Themen der Oto-Rhino-Laryngologie,* edited by H Redetzky and H Thiele. Berlin:VEB Verlag Volk und Gesundheit, pp. 89–93 (1969).

12 Emmett EA. Parosmia and hyposmia induced by solvent exposure. *Br. J. Ind. Med.* 33:196–198 (1976).

13 Sahli BP. Anosmia: An occupational concern? *Occup. Health Nurs.* 30(2): 20–21 (1982).

14 Paschal, G. *Odors and the Sense of Smell: A Bibliography, 320 BC–1947.* New York: Airkem (1952).

15 Michels KM, DS Phillips, RH Wright, and J Pustek. Odor and olfaction: A bibliography, 1948–1960. *Percept. Motor Skills* 15:475–529 (1962).

16 Proetz AW. A system of exact olfactometry. *Ann. Otol. Rhinol. Laryngol.* 33:746–761 (1924).

17 Sherman AH, JE Amoore, and V Weigel. The pyridine scale for clinical measurement of olfactory threshold: A quantitative reevaluation. *Otolaryngol. Head Neck Surg.* 87:717–733 (1979).

18 Amoore JE, and BG Ollman. Practical test kits for quantitatively evaluating the sense of smell. *Rhinology* 21:49–54 (1983).

19 Amoore JE, D Venstrom, and AR Davis. Measurement of specific anosmia. *Percept. Motor Skills* 26:143–164 (1968).

20 Amoore JE, P Pelosi, and LJ Forrester. Specific anosmias to 5 α-androst-16-en-3-one and ω-pentadecalactone: The urinous and musky primary odors. *Chem. Senses Flavour* 2:401–425 (1977).

21 Amoore JE. Specific anosmia and the concept of primary odors. *Chem. Senses Flavour* 2:267–281 (1977).

22 Venstrom D, and JE Amoore. Olfactory threshold in relation to age, sex or smoking. *J. Food Sci.* 33:264–265 (1968).

23 Henkin RI. Complete anosmia: The absence of olfaction at primary and accessory olfactory areas. *Life Sci.* 5:1031–1040 (1966).

24 Henkin RI. The definition of primary and accessory areas of olfaction as the basis for a classification of decreased olfactory acuity. In *Olfaction and Taste II,* edited by T Hayashi. Oxford: Pergamon, pp. 235–252 (1967).

25 Alter M, and AP Seltzer. What do taste and smell disturbances tell you? *Patient Care* 8(21):76–88 (1974).

26 Van den Eeckhaut J. *L'Odorat Clinique.* Brussels: Office International de Libraire (1978).

27 Schiffman SS. Taste and smell in disease. *N. Engl. J. Med.* 308:1275–1279, 1337–1343 (1983).

28 Patterson PM, and BA Lauder. The incidence and probable inheritance of "smell blindness." *J. Hered.* 39:295–297 (1948).
29 Woelk HA. Die traumatische Anosmie und ihre Begutachtung. *Monatsschr. Unfallheilk.* 37:1–17 (1930).
30 Henkin RI. Disorders of taste and smell. *JAMA* 218:1946 (1971).
31 Mancioli G. Le turbe dell' odorato nei verniciatori. *Rass. Med. Ind.* 16:180–196 (1947).
32 Naus A. Alterations of the smell acuity caused by menthol. *J. Laryngol. Otol.* 82:1009–1011 (1968).
33 Cain WS, J Gent, FA Catalanotto, and RB Goodspeed. Clinical evaluation of olfaction. *Am. J. Otolaryngol.* 4:252–256 (1983).
34 Doty RL, P Shaman, and M Dann. Development of the University of Pennsylvania smell identification test: A standardized microencapsulated test of olfactory function. *Physiol. Behav.* 32:489–502 (1984).
35 Fordyce ID. Olfaction tests. *Br. J. Ind. Med.* 18:213–215 (1961).
36 Roseburg B, R Fikentscher, and H Spinar. Riechprüfungen mit Geruchsstreifen. *Monatsschr. Ohrenheilk. Laryngo-Rhinol.* 108:298–303 (1974).
37 Zusho H, H Asaka, and M Okamoto. Diagnosis of olfactory disturbance. *Auris Nasus Larynx* 8:19–26 (1981).
38 Elsberg CA, and I Levy. The sense of smell. I. A new and simple method of quantitative olfactometry. *Bull. Neurol. Inst. N.Y.* 4:5–19 (1935).
39 Elsberg CA, ED Brewer, and I Levy. The sense of smell. VI. The odorous substances to be used for tests of the olfactory sense. *Bull. Neurol. Inst. N.Y.* 4:286–293 (1935).
40 Elsberg CA, ED Brewer, and I Levy. The sense of smell. V. The relative importance of volume and pressure of the impulse for the sensation of smell and the nature of the olfactory process. *Bull. Neurol. Inst. N.Y.* 4:264–269 (1935).
41 Jerome EA. Olfactory thresholds measured in terms of stimulus pressure and volume. *Arch. Psychol.* 39(274):1–44 (1942).
42 Strauss EL. A study on olfactory acuity. *Ann. Otol. Rhinol. Laryngol.* 79:95–104 (1970).
43 Jones FN. A test of the validity of the Elsberg method of olfactometry. *Am. J. Psychol.* 66:81–85 (1953).
44 Fortunato V, and P Niccolini. Un pratico olfattometro basato sulla bottiglia di Elsberg moderni metodi di olfattometria. *Clin. Otorinolaryngoiatr.* 1:33–51 (1949).
45 Naus A, J Pihrt, and V Blaha. Olfactory disturbances in people working in dusty works (in Czech). *Cesk. Hyg.* 1:230–236 (1956).
46 Faleg G, R Lenzi, and F Marzi. Le alterazioni dell'olfatto nell' intossicazione cronica professionale da mercurio. *Folia Med. (Naples)* 42:1487–1493 (1959).
47 Okhnyanskaya LG, and DA Ginzburg. The olfactory humoral reflex in lead and mercury poisoning (in Russian). *Fiziol. Zh. SSSR im. I.M. Sechenova* 38:105–110 (1952).
48 Bushtueva KA. New studies on the effect of sulfur dioxide and of sulfuric acid aerosol on reflex activity of man. In *Limits of Allowable Concentra-*

tions of Atmospheric Pollutants, edited by VA Ryazanov, translated by BS Levine. Washington: U.S. Dept. of Commerce, Office of Technical Services, Vol. 5, pp. 86–92 (1962).

49 Malyarova LK. Biological action and hygienic significance of trichloroethylene as an atmospheric pollutant (in Russian). *Mater. Nauchno-Prakt. Konf. Molodykh Gig. Sanit. Vrachei.* 11:56–59 (1967). (Original not available, see *Chem. Abstr.* 1970, 72:24265c.)

50 Amoore JE. The stereochemical theory of olfaction. 1. Identification of the seven primary odours. *Proc. Sci. Sect. Toilet Goods Assoc.* No. 37, Special Suppl. 1–12 (1962).

51 Amoore JE. The stereochemical theory of olfaction. 2. Elucidation of the stereochemical properties of the olfactory receptor sites. *Proc. Sci. Sect. Toilet Goods Assoc.* No. 37, Special Suppl. 13–23 (1962)

52 Feldman RG, RM Mayer, and A Taub. Evidence for peripheral neurotoxic effect of trichloroethylene. *Neurology* 20:599–606 (1970).

53 Barret L, S Garrel, P Arsac, M Vincent, C Thony, JL Debru, and J Faure. Intérêt de l'étude des potentials évoqués du trijumeau dans l'intoxication chronique au trichloréthylène: Résultats préliminaires. *Toxicol. Eur. Res.* 4:159–162 (1982).

54 Winneke G, and J Kastka. Odor pollution and odor annoyance reactions in industrial areas of the Rhine-Ruhr region. In *Olfaction and Taste VI,* edited by J Le Magnen and P MacLeod. London: Information Retrieval, pp. 471–479 (1977).

55 Pfander F. Anosmie durch einmaliges Einatmen von Schwefeldioxyd. *HNO* 8:59–60 (1959).

56 Zenk H. Zum rhino-otologischen Bilde chronische Schwefelkohlenstoffeinwirkungen. *Z. Laryngol. Rhinol. Otol. Ihre Grenzgeb.* 50:170–175 (1971).

57 Nathanson, G. Des processus pathologiques occupant l'appareil olfactif chez les personnes ayant subi une intoxication aiguë, involuntaire, par l'oxyde de carbone. *Acta Otolaryngol.* 13:409–418 (1929).

58 Tisdall FF, A Brown, and RD Defries. Persistent anosmia following zinc sulfate nasal spraying. *J. Pediatr.* 13:60–62 (1938).

59 Zenk H. Die Auswirkungen berufsbedingter CO-Intoxikationen auf Geruchs-, Gehör-und Gleichgewichtsorgan. *Z. Laryngol. Rhinol. Otol. Ihre Grenzgeb.* 44:821–828 (1965).

60 Rake G. The rapid invasion of the body through the olfactory mucosa. *J. Exp. Med.* 65:303–315 (1937).

61 De Lorenzo AJD. The olfactory neuron and the blood-brain barrier. In *Taste and Smell in Vertebrates,* edited by GEW Wolstenholme and J Knight. London: Churchill, pp. 151–176 (1970).

62 Schultz EW. Future of chemoprophylaxis as a measure for the practical control of poliomyelitis. *J. Pediatr.* 13:38–59 (1938).

63 Smith CG. Changes in the olfactory mucosa and the olfactory nerves following intranasal treatment with one percent zinc sulfate. *Can. Med. Assoc. J.* 39:138–140 (1938).

64 Meurman OH. Experimental studies on the effect of pathological changes in the nasal mucous membrane on the olfactory bulb. *Acta Otolaryngol.* 38: 477–483 (1950).

65 Yamagishi M, K Konishi, Y Igarashi, and Y Nakano. Ultrastructural changes in olfactory epithelium in guinea pigs exposed to nitrogen dioxide gas (in Japanese). *Nippon Jibi Inkoka Gakkai Kaiho* 85:11–18 (1982).
66 Cancalon P. Degeneration and regeneration of olfactory cells induced by $ZnSO_4$ and other chemicals. *Tissue Cell* 14:717–733 (1982).
67 Getchell ML, RC Gesteland. The chemistry of olfactory reception: Stimulus-specific protection from sulfhydryl reagent inhibition. *Proc. Natl. Acad. Sci. U.S.A.* 69:1494–1498 (1972).
68 Criswell DW, FL McClure, R Schafer, and KR Brower. War gases as olfactory probes. *Science* 210:425–426 (1980).
69 Takagi SF. Degeneration and regeneration of the olfactory epithelium. In *Handbook of Sensory Physiology*, Vol. IV, *Chemical Senses*, Part 1, *Olfaction*, edited by LM Beidler. New York: Springer Verlag, pp. 75–94 (1971).
70 Moulton DG. Dynamics of cell populations in the olfactory epithelium. *Ann. N.Y. Acad. Sci.* 237:52–61 (1974).
71 Moulton DG, and RP Fink. Cell proliferation and migration in the olfactory epithelium. In *Olfaction and Taste IV*, edited by D Schneider. Stuttgart: Wissenschaftliche Verlagsgesellschaft MBH, pp. 20–26 (1972).
72 Moulton DG. Cell renewal in the olfactory epithelium. In *Olfaction and Taste V*, edited by DA Denton and JP Coghlan. New York: Academic Press, pp. 111–114 (1975).
73 Atchabarov BA, EA Kluchnikova and NV Gorbinova. The condition of the olfactory analyzer in lead intoxication (in Russian). *Mater. Gig. Tr. Prof. Patol.* 9:178–188 (1961).
74 Osipova VG. Alterations in the senses of smell and taste in chronic intoxications by carbon disulfide (in Russian). *Gig. Tr. Prof. Zabol.* 1:44–48 (1957).
75 Skouby AP, and K Zilstorff-Pedersen. The influence of acetylcholine-like substances, menthol and strychnine on olfactory receptors in man. *Acta Physiol. Scand.* 32:252–258 (1954).
76 Duncan RB, and M Briggs. Treatment of uncomplicated anosmia by vitamin A. *Arch. Otolaryngol.* 75:116–124 (1962).
77 Henkin RI, PJ Schechter, WT Friedewald, DL Demets, and M Raff. A double blind study of the effects of zinc sulfate on taste and smell dysfunction. *Am. J. Med. Sci.* 272:285–299 (1976).
78 Spealman CR. Odors, odorants and deodorants in aviation. *Ann. N.Y. Acad. Sci.* 58:40–43 (1954).
79 Meyer J. Wie riecht Blausäure? *Gasmaske* 7:112 (1935).
80 Buchan RF. Industrial selenosis. *Occup. Med.* 3:439–456 (1947).
81 NIOSH. *Occupational Exposure to Hydrogen Sulfide.* Washington: National Institute for Occupational Safety and Health, U.S. Govt. Printing Office (1977).
82 Symanski H. Ein Fall von Selenwasserstoffvergiftung. *Dtsch. Med. Wochenschr.* 75:1730 (1950).
83 Bredereck H. Verlust des Geruchsvermögens. *Nach. Chem. Tech.* 13(4):66 (1965).
84 Graves RJ. Loss of the sense of smelling. *Dublin J. Med. Chem. Sci.* 6:69 (1835).

85 MacIntyre I. Prolonged anosmia. *Br. Med. J.* 2:709 (1971).
86 Bedoni C, and L. Corbetta. Le alterazioni dell'olfatto in alcune malattie professionali. *Ann. Laringol. Otol. Rhinol. Faringol.* 57:641–650 (1958).
87 Mancioli G. Le turbe dell' odorato negli operai addetti al rivestimento elettrolitico dei metalli. *Rass. Med. Ind.* 18:25–34 (1949).
88 Osipova VG, and LG Okhnyanskaya. Stimulability of the olfactory analyzer in some professional diseases (in Russian). *Gig. Sanit.* 3:32–38 (1954).
89 Renninghoff F. Geruchsstörung durch Metallstaub. *HNO* 13:99–100 (1965).
90 Tatarskaya AA. Occupational diseases of the upper respiratory tract in persons engaged in departments of electrolytic refining of nickel (in Russian). *Gig. Tr. Prof. Zabol.* 4(6):35–38 (1960).
91 Modica V, M Rossi, and C Sfogliano. Danni olfattivi da inalazione di vapori e fumi metallici. *Clin. Otorinolaringoiatr.* 16:416–425 (1964).
92 Pyatayev GE. State of the olfactory function in zinc production workers (in Russian). *Zh. Ushn. Nos. Gorl. Bolezn.* 31(4):17–21 (1971).
93 Tarasenko NY, and RS Vorobieva. Hygienic problems connected with the use of cadmium (in Russian). *Vestn. Akad. Med. Nauk SSSR* 28(10):37–43 (1973).
94 Naus A. Cases of complete anosmia related to occupational etiology (in Czech). *Cesk. Hyg.* 24:501–504 (1979).
95 Friberg L. Health hazards in the manufacture of alkaline accumulators with special reference to chronic cadmium poisoning. *Acta. Med. Scand.,* Suppl. 138, No. 240 (124 pp.) (1950).
96 Adams RG, and N Crabtree. Anosmia in alkaline battery workers. *Br. J. Ind. Med.* 18:216–221 (1961).
97 Watanabe S, and Y Fukuchi. Occupational impairment of the olfactory sense of chromate producing workers (in Japanese). *Sangyo Igaku* 23:606–611 (1981).
98 Seeber H, R Fikentscher, and B Roseburg. Geruchs- und Geschmacksstörungen bei Chromfarbenarbeitern. *Z. Gesamte Hyg. Ihre Grenzgeb.* 22: 820–822 (1976).
99 Seeber H, and R. Fikentscher. Schäden der Nasenschleimhaut und Riechstörungen durch berufliche Chromstaubexposition. *Z. Gesamte Hyg. Ihre Grenzgeb.* 26:506–508 (1980).
100 Meurman OH. Does lime and cement dust damage the mucous membranes of the upper respiratory tract? (in Finnish). *Duodecim* 63:669–683 (1947).
101 Laciak J, and K Sipa. The importance of testing the olfaction of workers in some branches of the chemical industry (in Polish). *Med. Pr.* 9:85–90 (1958).
102 Rebattu JP, and B Boulud. La pathologie naso-sinusienne chez les travailleurs du bois en dehors du cancer. *J. Fr. Otorhinolaryngol.* 27:395–400 (1978).
103 Hansen D. Berufsbedingte Reichstörung infolge chronischer Kohlenoxydeinwirkung. *HNO* 18:140–142 (1970).
104 Rossberg G, H Schaupp, and W Schmidt. Geruchs- und Geschmacksvermögen bei Arbeitern der chemischen und metallverarbeitenden Industrie. *Z. Laryngol. Rhinol. Otol. Ihre Grenzgeb.* 45:571–589 (1966).

105 Laciak J, Z Modzelewski, A Kotkowska, and K Hajduk. Attempt at evaluation of the effect of small concentrations of nitrogen compounds upon the state of the upper respiratory tract (in Polish). *Med. Pr.* 28:427–432 (1977).

106 Kehoe RA, WF Machle, K Kitzmiller, and TJ Le Blanc. On the effects of prolonged exposure to sulphur dioxide. *J. Ind. Hyg.* 14:159–173 (1932).

107 D'Angelo E, V Modica, and C Sfogliano. Rilievi olfattometrici nei lavatori delle industrie dello zolfo. *Clin. Otorinolaringoiatr.* 16:426–435 (1964).

108 Harada N, M Fujii, H Dodo. Olfactory disorder in chemical plant workers exposed to SO_2 and/or NH_3. *J. Sci. Labour* Part 2, 59(3):17–23 (1983).

109 Rasskazova TV. Effect of occupational factors of superphosphate production on the mucous membrane of the upper respiratory tract (in Russian). *Zh. Ushn. Nos. Gorl. Bolezn.* 30(5):21–24 (1970).

110 Latkowski B, P Zalewski, K Najwer, K Zbrzezny, I Czyzewski, S Markucki, and Z Dzwonik. Evaluation of the taste and smell senses in petroleum chemistry workers, based on three years' observations (in Polish). *Med. Pr.* 32:51–57 (1981).

111 Ferrari C, and A Jemmi. Rilievi clinici sulle funzioni cocleovestibolare ed olfattiva nei lavatori del benzolo. *Acta Biomed. Ateneo Parmense* 37, Suppl. 2:207–220 (1966).

112 Kmita S. The influence of benzine vapors on the upper respiratory tract and on the organ of smell (in Polish). *Med. Pr.* 4:119–130 (1953).

113 Dragomiretsky VD, TV Rasskazova, and EY Berezner. Effect of low concentrations of solvents on the state of the mucous membrane of the upper respiratory tract of workers (in Russian). *Zh. Ushn. Nos. Gorl. Bolezn.* 30(5):16–18 (1970).

114 Fokina KV. The functional state of olfactory and vestibular analyzers in persons subjected to the action of chlorine products of methane (in Russian). *Gig. Sanit.* 32(2):22–26 (1967).

115 Despons J, and JLP Soulié. Anosmie d'origine externe probable paraissant due au pentachlorophénate de sodium. *Arch. Mal. Prof. Med. Trav. Secur. Soc.* 18:616–617 (1957).

116 Naus A, and J Pihrt. Disorders of smell caused by prolonged action of trichloroethylene vapors on the olfactory analyzer (in Czech). *Prac. Lek.* 12:14–17 (1960).

117 James WRL. Fatal addiction to trichloroethylene. *Br. J. Ind. Med.* 20:47–49 (1963).

118 Mancioli G. Le turbe dell' odorato negli operai addetti nelle industrie dei profumi. *Rass. Med. Ind.* 17:104–116 (1948).

119 Fiser D, S Radic, and F Kosicki. Testing of the olfactory and taste function with the workers of the factory for pepper processing "vitamin" in Horgos (in Serbo-Croatian). *Med. Pregl.* 30:21–23 (1977).

120 Dyumin OV, and TV Rasskazova. Alterations in the upper respiratory tract under effect of Pavinol in sewing factory workers (in Russian). *Zh. Ushn. Nos. Gorl. Bolezn.* 31(4):9–12 (1971).

121 Naus A, and J Pihrt. The influence of dust on the upper respiratory tract and smell analyzer in employees in the spice industry (in Czech). *Prac. Lek.* 9:404–407 (1957).

122 Fiser D, and S Radic. Testing of the olfactory and taste function in workers of the tobacco industry (in Serbo-Croatian). *Med. Pregl.* 30:125–127 (1977).
123 Szyfter W. Evaluation of the condition of the mucous membranes of the upper respiratory tract as well as smell and taste among workers exposed to the action of synthetic varnishes (in Polish). *Otolaryngol. Pol.* 32:122–123 (1978).
124 Kittel G. Diskussionsbemerkungen. *Z. Laryngol. Rhinol. Otol. Ihre Grenzgeb.* 45:589–590 (1966).
125 Mitchell ABS, and BG Parsons-Smith. Trichloroethylene neuropathy. *Br. Med. J.* 1:422–423 (1969).

Chapter 12

Absorption of Chemical Vapors by the Upper Respiratory Tract of Rats

W. T. Stott, J. C. Ramsey, and M. J. McKenna

INTRODUCTION

Many historical references may be found regarding the beneficial health effects of nasal breathing, usually expounding on the ability of the upper respiratory tract (URT) to filter, humidify, and warm inhaled air during its passage to the lungs (1). However, the URT has also been recognized for some time as a first line of defense of the lungs against several chemical irritants and toxicants. Experimental evidence of this was first provided by Jordon and Carlson in 1913 when they observed that pulmonary edema occurred more rapidly in tracheotomized rabbits and dogs than normal animals when exposed to ozone (2). Later Cameron et al. (3) related the pathological effects of several war gases to regional deposition in the URT, and Amdur (4) noted significant differences in the pulmonary responses of normal and tracheotomized guinea pigs exposed to ozone, sulfur dioxide, formaldehyde, or acetic acid.

The authors wish to express their appreciation to P. E. Kastl for excellent technical assistance and to Drs. R. R. Miller and R. J. Nolan for their support and insight into the conduct of these experiments.

Table 1 Examples of the Absorption of Gases and Chemical Vapors by the Upper Respiratory Tract of Animals

Compound	Animal	Percent absorbed	Reference
Sulfur dioxide	Human	85-99	(31)
	Dog	95-97	(5, 32)
Ozone	Rabbit, guinea pig	50	(33)
	Dog	30-70	(34)
Acrolein	Dog	80	(35)
Formaldehyde		99	(35)
Propionaldehyde		70-82	(35)
Hydrogen fluoride	Rat	99	(14)

As shown in Table 1, numerous gases and chemical vapors have been reported to be readily absorbed by the URT of a variety of species. Indeed, the URT of most animals is well suited for the absorption of vapors passing through it. Described by Brain (5) as analogous to an efficient "scrubbing tower," the URT of an animal may have a very large surface area and be covered with a mucosa rich in blood capillaries with fenestrated borders near the lumen surface (6, 7).

The epithelial lining of the URT of rodents has also been observed as a target tissue for some inhaled chemicals. Such compounds fall into two general categories: those causing a nonspecific degeneration of epithelium (e.g., ethylene dibromide), and those causing primarily lesions of the olfactory neuroepithelium (e.g., ethyl acrylate) (8–10).

The process by which inhaled vapors are absorbed by the URT has been discussed and described mathematically by Aharonson et al. (11), LaBelle et al. (12), and Morgan and Frank (13). These authors have depicted a model in which the partitioning of an inhaled chemical between the lumen and the mucus layer of the nasal cavity occurs while the vapor concentration steadily decreases as the inhaled air passes along the surface of the URT. Vapor uptake would thus be driven by the air/mucus partitioning of a vapor as described by its water solubility and related Henry's Law constant (air/water partition coefficient). Using Henry's Law constants, LaBelle et al. (12) were able to predict theoretical levels of uptake of numerous gases and vapors of varying water solubilities in URTs with several different extraction efficiencies. From a comparison of the URT absorption data obtained using ozone and sulfur dioxide, Morris and Smith (14) speculated that a high degree of chemical reactivity may also be required for the nearly complete absorption of a vapor by the URT. It was pointed out that the reactive ozone has a nearly 400-fold lower Henry's Law constant than the very water soluble and readily absorbed sulfur dioxide ($>$95 percent), yet approximately 50 percent of ozone is still absorbed by the URT of animals.

As reviewed by Aharonson et al. (11) and Morgan and Frank (13), the rate of vapor flow through the URT (i.e., the residence time of vapors in the URT) may also influence the level of chemical absorption that can occur. Utilizing data obtained in the URT of dogs for the uptake of ether, acetone, ozone, and sulfur dioxide at varying flow rates, Aharonson et al. (11) calculated that there was a greater total mass transfer of vapors across or into the mucosa at higher flow rates (i.e., shorter residence times) than at slower flow rates (longer residence times). Factors suggested as possible reasons for the increased transfer included (1) increases in URT surface area by recruitment of additional pathways in the nasal cavity, (2) increases in turbulence and thus contact of the air with the mucosa, (3) increases in URT blood flow in response to demand for water vapor and heat transfer to inhaled air, and (4) changes in the character and rate of production of mucus. However, as pointed out by Morgan and Frank (13), even while the mass transfer of vapors in the URT may increase with increasing flow rate, the percent of vapors entering the nasal cavity that are absorbed usually decreases and more of the inhaled vapors may still penetrate to the lungs.

While the absorption of a few gases and chemical vapors by the URT has been extensively studied, there is still relatively little information available on the URT absorption of chemicals of diverse physicochemical properties or of chemicals that affect different sites within the URT.

The work summarized here was undertaken to expand our understanding of this portion of the respiratory tract, its significance as both a portal of entry and a potential target organ in rodents, and to identify physicochemical and physiological parameters that may control absorption of chemicals by the upper respiratory tract of rodents.

MATERIALS AND METHODS

Chemicals

The chemicals used in these experiments were all of high purity (> 99 percent) and were chosen for their varying water solubilities and toxicological effects on the nasal mucosa of exposed rodents (Table 2). Styrene (STY), methylene chloride ($MeCl_2$), and propylene glycol monomethyl ether (PGME) do not cause lesions of the URT mucosa in exposed rodents. Ethyl acrylate (EA), nitroethane (NE), and propylene glycol monomethyl ether acetate (PGMEAc) primarily cause lesions of the olfactory neuroepithelium of exposed rodents. Ethylene dibromide (EDB) and epichlorohydrin (EPI) cause nonspecific lesions of the mucosa of exposed rodents. The water solubilities of the compounds within each of these groupings varied from relatively insoluble to moderately soluble or miscible.

Table 2 Physical and Biological Data for Chemicals Used in This Study

Chemical	Exposure concentration used (ppm)	Water solubility (ppm)	Reported lesions of the URT Mucosa of exposed rodents	Reference
Propylene glycol monomethyl ether	1000	Miscible	No visible lesions	(24)
Propylene glycol monomethyl ether acetate	1000	250,000	Degeneration of olfactory epithelium	(36)
Ethyl acrylate	225	20,000	Degeneration of olfactory epithelium	(8)
Nitroethane	1000	46,800	Degeneration of olfactory epithelium	(37)
Epichlorohydrin	100	76,500	Nonspecific degeneration of epithelium	(23)
Styrene	200	3,100	No visible lesions	(38)
Ethylene dibromide	75	4,300	Nonspecific degeneration of epithelium	(10, 39)
Methylene chloride	500	20,000	No visible lesions	(40)

Animal Model

The animal models used to obtain data on the uptake of vapors by the isolated URT, isolated LRT, and intact respiratory tract of rats have been described in detail by Stott and McKenna (15). Pentobarbital-anesthetized (60 mg/kg, i.p.) male Fischer 344 rats (200-260 g) were utilized in all experiments. These animals were reproducibly shown by plethysmography to have a respiratory minute volume of approximately 53 ± 3 ml/min.

The animal model used to measure absorption of vapors by the isolated URT and simultaneous excretion of vapors by the LRT is shown in Fig. 1. In this model, the tracheal connection of the URT and LRT was interrupted so that the URT could be exposed to vapors independently of the LRT by which the rat spontaneously breathed from a stream of room air (150 ml/min flow). The test atmospheres were drawn through the URT at approximately 0.055 liter/min or 0.105 liter/min from a Saran bag connected to the animal's snout (mouth sealed) through the URT and out of the cephalad endotracheal tube and to a gas chromatograph (GC). Effluent concentrations of each vapor were quantitated by GC analysis after reaching an apparently steady level, usually within 10-20 min. Simultaneous excretion of a chemical present in the blood via the LRT was determined by GC analysis of the caudate endotracheal tube effluent (as shown). Absorption of vapors by the LRT and simultaneous excretion of vapors by the URT could be determined by switching the gas bag to the inlet for the

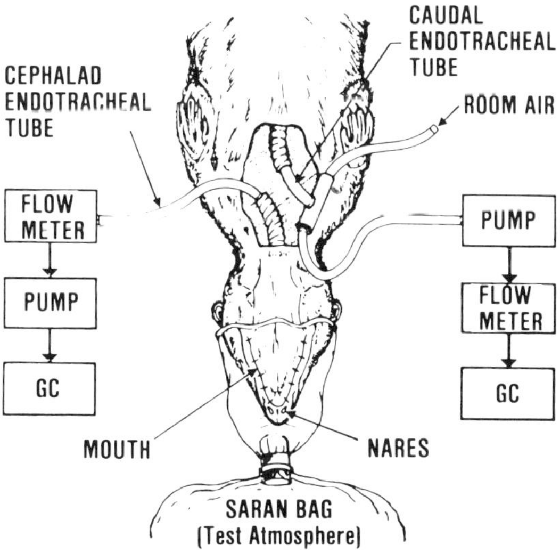

Figure 1 Ventral view of animal model used to determine absorption of chemical vapors by the URT and simultaneous excretion of absorbed compounds by the LRT. [*Reprinted with permission from Stott, W. T., and M. J. McKenna (15).*]

pulmonary air stream, reversing the flow through the URT, and attaching the GC to the effluent from the URT.

Measurements of vapor uptake by the intact respiratory tract of anesthetized rats were made using a small, nose-only exposure chamber. Test atmospheres were supplied to the chamber at a flow rate of approximately 150 ml/min and subsequently to a GC for quantitation of effluent vapor concentrations.

Rates of absorption and simultaneous excretion of an inhalant were determined when effluent concentrations reached a constant level using equations 1 and 2, respectively. Results were expressed as the percentage absorption of vapors passing into the isolated URT or LRT, or the intact animal (i.e., a = o and c = respiratory minute volume in Eq. 1).

$$\text{mole/min absorbed} = \frac{(b\text{-}a)(c)}{d} \qquad (1)$$

$$\text{mole/min excreted} = \frac{(a)(c)}{d} \qquad (2)$$

(Abbreviations: a = mole chemical/mole effluent gas; b = mole chemical/mole test atmosphere; c = liter/min flow rate; d = 24.45 liter/mole.)

Using the concentration data obtained, the rates of chemical absorption that would be expected to occur in an intact exposed animal via the URT and LRT were calculated using equations 3 and 4. The total dose received by the entire respiratory tract is simply the sum of equations 3 and 4 multiplied by the time of exposure. The rate of absorption by intact, nose-only-exposed animals was also calculated (Eq. 5).

$$\text{mole/min absorbed by URT (U)} = (\text{mol})(f_{urt}) \qquad (3)$$

$$\text{mole/min absorbed by LRT} = (\text{mol-U})(f_{lrt}) \qquad (4)$$

$$\text{mole/min absorbed by intact respiratory system (intact animal exposure)} = (\text{mol})(f) \qquad (5)$$

(Abbreviations: U = mole/min absorbed by URT; mol = mole/min passing into the rat; f = fraction absorbed.)

Pharmacokinetic Modeling

In an attempt to better understand the factors controlling URT absorption of vapors, as well as the interrelationship of the isolated URT and LRT absorption within the intact respiration tract, several kinetic models were constructed to simulate the absorption and excretion data obtained in these experiments (Figs. 2, 3). These models are simply a modification of a generalized physiological model described by Anderson (16), Anderson et al. (17), and Ramsey and Anderson (18), which was used by these authors to describe the absorption of inhaled STY by exposed animals. These and other published works (19) provide a very detailed review of the uses of physiological pharmacokinetic modeling, and therefore only the modifications that were made to the generalized model will be described.

The model describing the uptake and simultaneous excretion of chemical vapors by the URT and LRT is shown in Fig. 2. Two tissue compartments were used to represent the two portions of the respiratory tract, each receiving a defined percent of the cardiac output (QC) and being ventilated at a defined airflow rate (Q) with a known concentration of vapors (CI or CIP). The rest of the body (e.g., muscle, fat, liver) was considered as a single compartment equivalent to the known volume of distribution for each chemical in the rat. Nonrespiratory elimination of absorbed chemicals was assumed to be equivalent to their central compartment elimination rate constants observed in rats. Physiological constants included (1) a total cardiac output in pentobarbital-anesthetized rats of 14.8 liter/h•kg (20), of which 1.5-3.0 percent was estimated

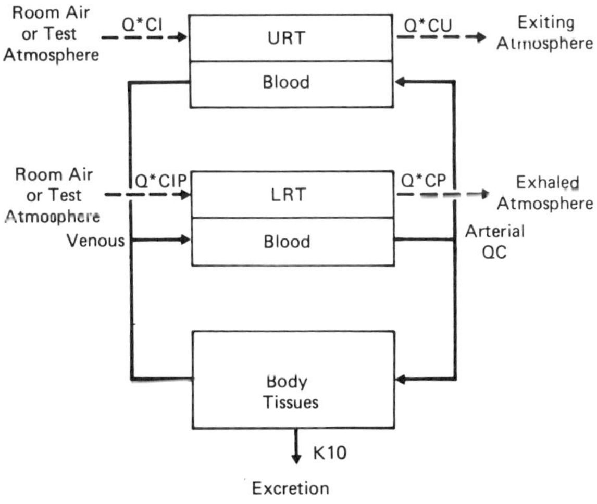

Figure 2 Schematic of physiological model of upper and lower respiratory tract absorption and excretion of chemical vapors. Abbreviations: Q, airflow; QC, total cardiac output; CI and CIP, vapor concentrations going to URT and LRT, respectively; CU and CP, vapor concentrations exiting URT and LRT, respectively; K10, central compartment excretion constant. The URT and LRT compartments are depicted as being independently ventilated with the desired atmospheres while being perfused with arterial and venous blood, respectively. For URT absorption and LRT excretion of vapors, CI = test atmosphere and CIP = room air. The reverse was true for LRT absorption and URT excretion of vapors.

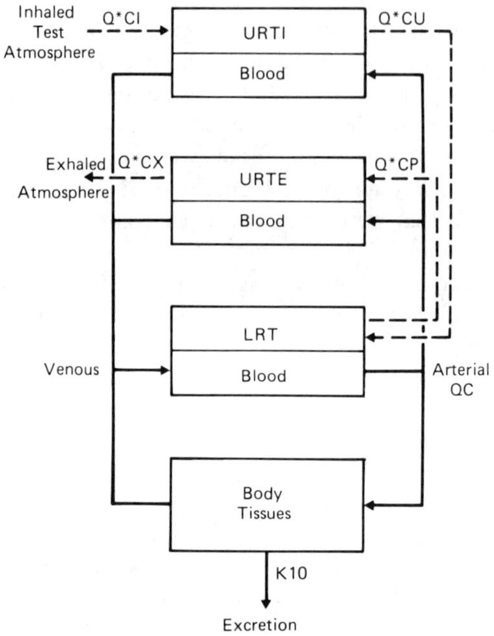

Figure 3 Schematic of physiological model of the absorption of chemical vapors by the intact respiratory tract (nose-only-exposed rat). Abbreviations are as in Fig. 2 plus: CX, vapor concentration exiting URTE. The desired atmosphere is depicted as flowing through the URT compartment during inhalation, passing to the LRT compartment, and then passing out through the URT compartment again during exhalation. All compartments are also perfused with a certain amount of the cardiac output.

to perfuse the URT and 97-98.5 percent the rest of the body tissues; (2) a URT capillary blood volume of 0.052 ml (10 percent of a measured total URT blood volume in rat); (3) an estimated 0.34 ml of capillary blood in pulmonary tissues (21); and (4) ventilation of the respiratory tract at 53.2 ml/min.

The uptake of vapor and rate of change in the amount of chemical within each compartment of the model were quantitated by a set of differential equations. Note that no Michaelis-Menten expression describing saturable metabolism was included in the model as no known metabolically saturating levels of any vapor were used, with the possible exception of $MeCl_2$. In the case of URT absorption of vapors, the rate of change in the amount of a chemical within the blood of the URT compartment was related to the net amount being absorbed as inhalant plus that returning to and leaving the URT compartment via the blood flow. This is shown in equation 6.

$$\text{RABU} = \text{Q*(CI-CVU/PB)} + \text{QU*(CA-CVU)} \quad (6)$$

(Abbreviations not defined above: RABU = rate of change in chemical content of the URT compartment; CVU = concentration of chemical in venous blood leaving the URT; PB = blood/air partition coefficient; QU = blood flow through URT: CA = concentration of chemical in arterial blood.)

The concentration of vapors leaving the URT (CU) measured experimentally were equivalent to CVU/PB, and the concentration of a chemical in the venous blood leaving the URT was equivalent to ABU/CVU. By using an appropriate set of constants for each compound (Table 3), a defined concentration of vapors, and integrating equation 6 simultaneously with other equations describing the rates of change of chemicals in other tissue compartments, an estimation of the rate of vapor uptake by the isolated URT and LRT was possible.

In the intact system, a net absorption of an inhaled chemical by the URT may take place during inhalation, and a slight net absorption or excretion of vapors may occur during exhalation; thus the model depicting the intact animal (Fig. 3) contained a "nasal cavity" for each situation (URTI and URTE). Inhaled atmospheres were passed through the URTI first, then through the lungs, and then they exited through the URTE. The equations used to quantitate the

Table 3 Physical and Biological Data Used for Physiological Modeling Portion of the Study

Compound	Partition coefficient* (blood or water/air)	Central compartment excretion constant† (h^{-1})	Volume of distribution† (liter/kg)
PGME	403 (B)	0.23	0.91
PGMEAc	141 (W)	4.9	1.01
EA	2.3 (W)	15.8	0.36
NE	21 (B)	1.7	0.16
EPI	11 (W)	0.16‡	0.35‡
STY	39 (B)§	2.7§	1.15§
EDB	3.9 (B)	1.8‖	0.23‖
$MeCl_2$	9.7 (B)#	10.6**	0.30**

*Determined experimentally at 37°C in a 100 ml sealed vial containing 5 ml heparinized whole blood or distilled water unless noted otherwise. B = blood; W = water.

†Determined experimentally upon i.v. administration to rats (blood concentration curve analysis) unless noted otherwise.

‡Smith (personal communication).

§Ramsey and Anderson (18). The rate constant is based on the rapid (α) distributive phase.

‖Watanabe and Fox (personal communication).

#Sato and Nakajima (41).

**McKenna (42).

concentration of a given chemical and its rate of change in the two URT tissue compartments were basically the same as those described previously.

RESULTS AND DISCUSSION

Animal Model

The results of the present study support the previous findings of others that the URT of rats may absorb relatively high levels of some inhaled chemical vapors. At a flow rate equivalent to the respiratory minute volume of the rats used, greater than 90 percent of PGME and PGMEAc and 50–70 percent of EA, NE, EPI, STY, and EDB vapors passing through the isolated URT of rats were absorbed (Table 4). $MeCl_2$ was only poorly absorbed by the URT (13 percent). With the exception of STY and $MeCl_2$, the percent absorption of vapors by the URT approximated that observed in the isolated LRT and nose-only-exposed

Table 4 Absorption and Excretion of Chemical Vapors by the Isolated URT and LRT and by the Intact Respiratory Tract of Rats*

	Percent absorption†			Percent excretion‡	
Compound	URT	LRT	Intact	URT	LRT
PGME	96.3	106	87	0.2	0.5
	3.1	7.3	6.8	0.1	0.6
PGMEAc	93.9	99	85	3.8	2.8
	4.1	38	12	3.6	0.2
EA	66.4	61	65	1.7	1.8
	5.9	8.6	7.3	0.2	0.8
NE	64.8	71	58	2.8	2.0
	5.9	5.0	12	2.0	0.4
EPI	60.8	73	51	ND	ND
	9.8	8.6	7.7		
STY	57.4	94	92	4.5	0.9
	7.8	3.6	9.5	5.0	0.4
EDB	48.9	51	58	ND	ND
	2.5	17	9.1		
$MeCl_2$	13.2	37	44	4.8	11.7
	3.6	4.1	10	3.8	2.9

[*From Stott and McKenna (15).*]

*Average ± standard deviations of 4–9 animals.

†Absorption expressed as a percent of chemical available for absorption at a ventilation rate of 53 ml/min.

‡Excretion expressed as a percent excretion of absorbed chemical. ND, none detected.

rat. Constant rates of absorption were achieved within 10--20 min of the start of exposure and remained quite constant for up to 2 h, an observation similar to one made by Aharonson et al. (11) regarding the uptake of acetone vapors in tracheostomized dogs. They are also representative of those observed at lower vapor concentrations.

The data suggest that a simple correlation of water solubility and vapor absorption by the URT does not exist. The relatively water-insoluble STY and EDB were absorbed nearly as well as the moderately soluble EA, NE, and EPI whereas two compounds of similar solubility, STY and $MeCl_2$, were absorbed to a very different degree (57 and 13 percent, respectively).

In addition to the absorption of chemical vapors, the URT was also noted to excrete compounds present in the bloodstream, although only a small percent of the vapors simultaneously absorbed by the LRT ($<$ 5 percent). However, this excretion, when coupled with any slight solute back-pressure which may build up in mucus during the inhalation of vapors, will limit the absorption of any low concentration of vapors returning through the URT during exhalation. As with the URT, few of the compounds absorbed by the URT were simultaneously excreted by the LRT with the exception of $MeCl_2$ (12 percent). As occurred in the absorption of chemical vapors, the rate of excretion of vapors by the URT was observed to reach a nearly constant level relatively quickly, usually within 20 min. This occurred even with those compounds that had not yet reached steady-state blood levels (e.g., PGME), presumably because of the inability to detect small absolute changes in chemical vapor concentrations of effluents.

It is important to note, however, the potential effects that the necessary surgical manipulation of the respiratory tract in the animal model used might have on the absorption and excretion of vapors by the URT. These include (1) the interruption of the normal bidirectional, alternating ventilation of the URT and thus potential desorption of dissolved vapors during exhalation; (2) interruption of the removal of dissolved vapors by mucociliary clearance to the gut; (3) alterations in the bloodflow to the URT by drying; and (4) the lack of trigeminal-mediated changes in the ventilation of the URT. While the unidirectional, constant flow of vapors in the animal model may have prevented some loss of vapors dissolved in the mucus which would occur during exhalation in the normal animal, significant solute back-pressures would be expected to occur only at vapor concentrations much higher than those used (11, 13).

While the normal clearance of mucus from the URT to the gut was interrupted in the animal model, the placement of the cephalad cannula also resulted in the removal of mucus from the URT, much as would normally occur upon swallowing the mucus. Degasing of the mucus in the water trap used between the cannula and GC would have resulted in a slight lowering of the calculated percent absorption of vapors.

Alterations in the URT blood flow, most likely as a result of drying of the mucosa, were noted to occur in the animal model. As shown in Table 5, the

Table 5 Blood Perfusion of the Upper Respiratory Tract of Rats*

	Exposure	Percent cardiac output
Intact respiratory tract	Air	0.49 ± 0.15
	200 ppm ethyl acrylate vapors	1.11 ± 0.44
Surgically isolated upper respiratory tract†	Air	1.04 ± 0.82
	200 ppm ethyl acrylate vapors	1.26 ± 0.78

*Data were obtained in pentobarbital-anesthetized rats (60 mg/kg, i.p.) using radiolabeled microsphere methodology (43).

†Animal model described in the text.

URT blood flow of cannulated rats was double that of normal animals. However, blood flows between the two groups of rats were observed to be similar (1.1-1.3 percent QC) when exposed to EA vapors, suggesting that similar blood perfusion levels could have occurred in the other exposed rats.

Finally, normally occurring trigeminal-mediated decreases in respiratory rates were not observed to occur in these pentobarbital-anesthetized rats. Such a reflex action in exposed rats can significantly reduce the intake of vapors and thus the amount of vapor absorbed by the URT (22). Overall, with some obvious limitations, the animal model appeared to generally reflect the functioning of the URT as a part of the normal respiratory tract.

Effects of Flow Rate

The percent absorption of most vapors by the isolated URT of rats was noted to decrease as the rate of flow through the URT increased (Fig. 4). Doubling of the average flow rate from 53 ml/min to 105 ml/min resulted in a decrease in the residence time of vapors in the URT from 18.9 min/liter to 9.5 min/liter. With the exception of the very water-soluble PGME and PGMEAc vapors, the decreased residence time resulted in up to a 27 percent decrease in the actual percentage absorption of vapors.

In an attempt to determine if flow-induced changes in the efficiency of the URT in absorbing vapors occurred similar to those reported by Aharonson et al. (11), an uptake coefficient value (R) was calculated for each vapor at each flow rate. Defined by Aharonson et al. (11) as the rate of flux of a gas through the nasal mucosa on a unit area basis, this value has been used as a measure of the efficiency of URT vapor absorption relative to the URT residence time of the vapors. As shown in Table 6, R values remained steady or increased with decreasing residence times for nearly all of the chemicals tested. The absorption efficiencies of PGME, PGMEAc, EPI, and NE were particularly increased with

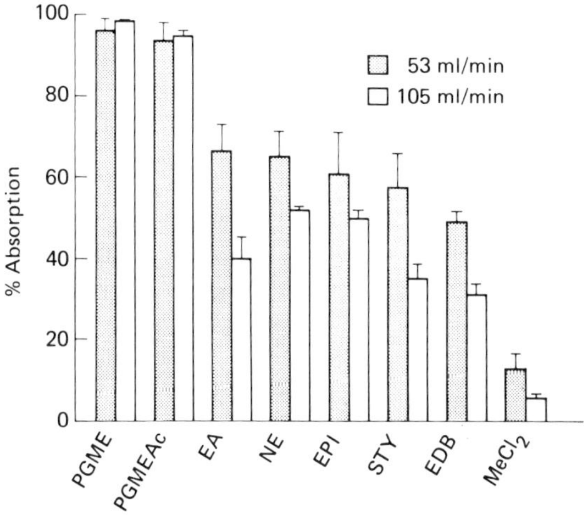

Figure 4 Comparison of the absorption of chemical vapors by the URT ventilated at 1 and 2 times the respiratory minute volume of the pentobarbital-anesthetized rats used (53 and 105 ml/min, respectively). Data represent the average of 3-9 rats with S.D. [*Reprinted with permission from Stott, W. T., and M. J. McKenna (15).*]

Table 6 Relative Efficiency (Uptake Coefficient) of the Upper Respiratory Tract of Rats to Absorb Chemical Vapors Having Different Residence Times (min/liter of inhalant) in the Nasal Cavity*

	Uptake coefficient (× 10^6 liter/min/mm Hg)	
Compound	**18.9† min/liter**	**9.5‡ min/liter**
PGME	407	775
PGMEAc	3160	4640
EA	77	72
NE	86	104
EPI	55	98
STY	53	55
EDB	47	52
$MeCl_2$	7.6	8.1

*The "efficiency" of uptake is defined as the rate of flux (i.e., mass transfer) of vapors across the nasal mucosa/unit area (11, 13): Uptake coefficient = (flow rate/barometric pressure) ln (partial pressure vapor into/out of the URT). An increase in the uptake coefficient = increased efficiency of absorption.

†Average flow rate of 0.053 liter/min in the animal model.

‡Average flow rate of 0.105 liter/min in the animal model.

increased flow rates. As noted above, several factors such as altered blood flow, mucus flow, URT surface area, and resistance may be responsible for these results.

URT "Dose" Calculation

Considering the potential for the isolated URT to absorb large percentages of certain chemical vapors passing through it, we thought it useful to quantitatively define the URT as a portal of entry of inhaled compounds into the systemic circulation and to compare this role with that of the lung in the normal, intact, functioning respiratory tract of an animal. To accomplish this, the rate of uptake of vapors by the URT and LRT as part of an intact respiratory tract was calculated using equations 3 and 4 and percent absorption values determined in the animal model at a flow rate of 105 ml/min. The sum of these calculated uptake rates was then compared to rates calculated for the intact respiratory tract using experimentally derived percent absorption values obtained with nose-only-exposed animals. The results, normalized to a 100 ppm exposure of each chemical vapor, are presented in Fig. 5.

In most cases, there was reasonable agreement in the rates of absorption between the composite and intact respiratory tracts, suggesting that the animal

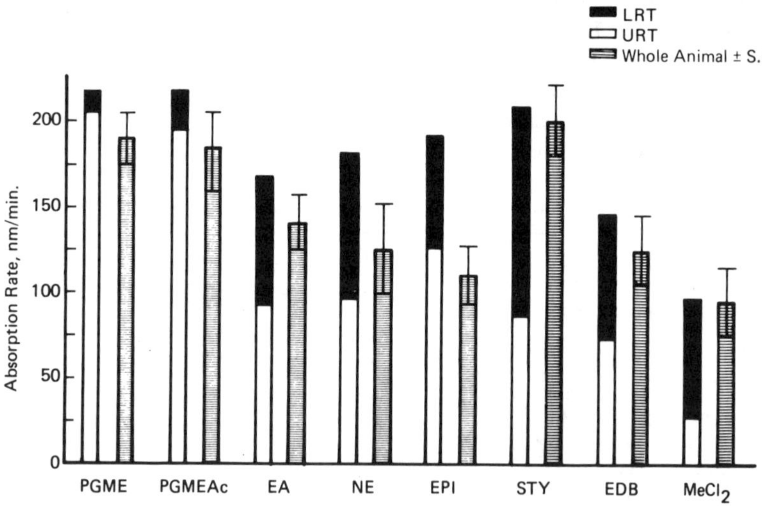

Figure 5 Comparison of calculated rates of absorption of chemicals received via the isolated URT plus LRT during a normal breathing cycle and that observed in the intact respiratory system (data from Table 2). All data were normalized to a 100-ppm exposure level of each chemical which, using equation 1, is equivalent to a 218 nmole/min total intake of vapor. Values were calculated usings equations 3 to 5 (see text). [*Reprinted with permission from Stott, W. T., and M. J. McKenna (15).*]

model used to obtain data on URT and LRT absorption of vapors did approximate the functioning of these parts of the respiratory tract in the normal animal. The apparent slight overpredictions of absorption of most of the compounds tested may have been due in part to (1) some unavoidable rebreathing of exhaled air by nose-only-exposed rats, (2) the presence of an effective "dead space" in the URT in nose-only-exposed rats, and (3) the lack of fluctuating airflows, with their fluctuating percent absorption rates, in the animal model which can occur in the URT during normal breathing cycles.

The large differences noted for EPI and NE may relate to a more serious problem in the measurement of URT absorption of these two compounds. In accordance with these calculations, over 90 percent of inhaled PGME and PGMEAc vapors and 41-65 percent of EA, EPI, STY, NE, and EDB vapors were removed from inhaled air prior to reaching the lungs of nose-only-exposed rats under the conditions of the study.

The above calculations suggest that the "dose" of a chemical received by the nasal mucosa of an animal on a unit surface area basis may be as much as several thousand times that received by the lungs, even for compounds of low or intermediate solubility. Thus, it is not surprising that EPI and EDB vapors have been observed to cause lesions of the URT mucosa of rats at much lower exposure levels than those causing lesions of the LRT, even though they were absorbed to a similar degree by the isolated URT and LRT (Table 2) (10, 23).

A high rate of chemical vapor absorption itself, however, does not correlate with the production of morphologic lesions of the URT mucosa. PGME was readily absorbed by the isolated URT yet does not cause these lesions in exposed rats (24). Likewise, the potential site of activity within the URT mucosa of exposed rats does not appear to be related to their URT absorption. Compounds primarily causing lesions of the olfactory epithelium (NE, EA, PGMEAc) were absorbed by the isolated URT at rates greater than or equivalent to those compounds that primarily cause lesions of the respiratory epithelium (EPI, EDB) (Table 1).

Physiological Modeling

The physiological pharmacokinetic models utilized in the present study to predict vapor absorption by the isolated URT, isolated LRT, and nose-only-exposed rats were designed to be very simplistic in their characterization of the body and capable of using readily obtainable constants. These models (1) considered the URT as a rapidly mixed chamber unlike the more physiologically appropriate, open-ended tube model described by Aharonson et al. (11) and Morgan and Frank (13); (2) essentially disregarded the mucus as a significant absorptive bed; and (3) utilized the blood/air partitioning coefficients of vapors rather than Henry's Law constants as the driving force behind absorption of vapors by the URT.

As shown in Table 7, the models could accurately predict the experimentally observed levels of vapor absorption by the isolated LRT and nose-only-exposed animal models. The overestimation of $MeCl_2$ uptake was attributed to the nearly metabolically saturating exposure level used in the study (500 ppm). Prediction of the absorption of vapors by the URT proved to be more complex. Not surprisingly, URT blood flow and blood/air partition coefficients were identified as the parameters having the greatest impact on vapor absorption. When 1.5 percent of the cardiac output and the in vitro measured blood/air partition coefficients (Table 3) were used, the model predictions were considerably lower than the observed absorption rates (Fig. 6). However, when 3.0 percent of the cardiac output coupled with a 25 percent increase in the blood/air partition coefficients was used, the differences in predicted versus observed values for most compounds were relatively small. These values for QU and PB are not unrealistic. Several URT blood flows measured in rats exposed to EA vapors were observed to be in excess of 2.5 percent, and it has been reported by Anggard (25) that nearly 60 percent of the blood flow through the nasal mucosa of cats occurs via arteriovenous anastomers, a source of blood flow that would have been missed by the microsphere method used in these experiments. In addition, measurements of PB in vitro can only approximate in vivo situations, and in some cases were not obtainable owing to chemical reactivity and/or blood metabolic activity (PGMEAc, EA, and EPI).

The large underestimations of URT absorption, EA, EPI, and EDB made by the model were not unexpected. EA has been observed to be readily hydrolyzed

Table 7 Agreement of Physiological Model Predicted versus Experimentally Observed Values for Chemical Absorption in the Isolated Lower Respiratory Tract (LRT) of Rats and Nose-Only-Exposed Rats

	Percent of experimental value	
Compound	LRT	Intact respiratory tract
PGME	94	115
PGMEAc	100	116
EA	113	106
EPI	80	111
STY	104	105
NE	104	123
EDB	81	66
$MeCl_2$	240	198

*Values are presented as a percent of experimental values = (predicted X 100)/(observed) (i.e., 100 percent = perfect agreement).

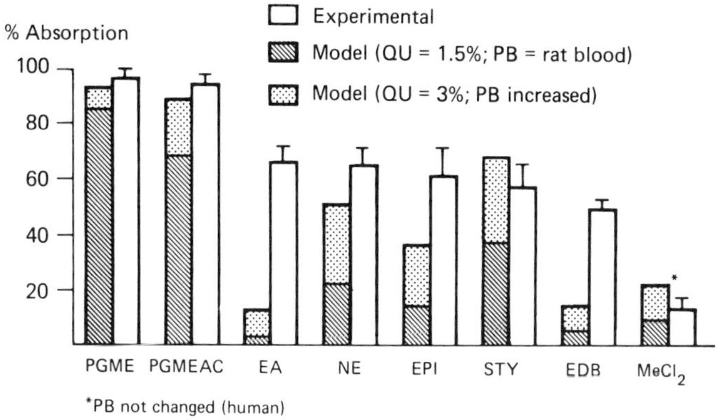

Figure 6 Comparison of predicted versus experimentally observed absorption of chemical vapors by the upper respiratory tract of rats using the physiological and animal models, respectively. QU equals the percent cardiac output perfusing the URT and PB is the in vitro measured blood/air partition coefficient of the chemicals (PB increased = 25 percent increase in PB).

by nasal cavity area esterases in vitro (26), and considerable amounts may be hydrolyzed in the mucosa prior to entering the bloodstream. The reactive compounds EPI and EDB are known to undergo metabolism and to bind with tissue macromolecules (27, 28). Indeed, the nasal mucosa is well supplied with xenobiotic-metabolizing enzyme systems (29, 30). Thus, these three chemicals may be absorbed by the URT at a rate faster than predicted based solely on physical blood/air partitioning. It was concluded that the blood/air partitioning of chemicals can account for absorption of chemicals by the URT, but only if several other metabolic (systemic as well as localized) and physiological parameters are also considered.

SUMMARY

The upper respiratory tract (URT) of animals has been noted to absorb large amounts of several inhaled vapors, some of which have caused lesions of the nasal mucosa. This absorption has usually been related to the water solubility of chemicals and, in some cases, has been noted to be dependent on the rate of airflow through the URT. In the work reported here, the absorption of propylene glycol monomethyl ether (PGME), PGME acetate (PGMEAc), ethyl acrylate (EA), epichlorohydrin (EPI), styrene (STY), nitroethane (NE), ethylene dibromide (EDB), and methylene chloride ($MeCl_2$) vapors, by the surgically isolated URT of rats, was determined and compared to that by isolated lungs and nose-only-exposed rats. Nearly all PGME and PGMEAc, and 30-70 percent of EA, EPI, STY, NE, and EDB were absorbed by the URT. In most cases this absorption was found to be airflow-dependent and did not relate directly to the water solubility of a compound or to its ability to cause lesions of the URT mucosa. It was estimated that the nose-only-exposed rats received > 90 percent of absorbed PGME and PGMEAc and between 41-65 percent of absorbed EA, EPI, STY, NE, and EDB via their URT. Several predictive pharmacokinetic models were also developed to help identify significant physicochemical and physiological factors that may control URT absorption of chemical vapors.

REFERENCES

1 Proctor DF. Historical background. In *The Nose,* edited by DF Proctor, I Andersen. Amsterdam: Elsevier (1982).

2 Jordan EA, and AJ Carlson. Ozone: Its bactericidal, physiologic and deodorizing action. *JAMA* 61:1007–1012 (1913).

3 Cameron GR, JH Gaddum, and RHD Short. The absorption of war gases by the nose. *J. Pathol.* 58:449–456 (1946).

4 Amdur MD. The physiological response of guinea pigs to atmospheric pollutants. *Int. J. Air Poll.* 1:170–183 (1959).

5 Brain JD. The uptake of inhaled gases by the nose. *Ann. Otol. Rhinol. Laryngol.* 79:529–539 (1970).

6 Swindle PF. The architecture of the blood vascular networks in the erectile and secretory lining of the nasal passages. *Ann. Otol. Rhinol. Laryngol.* 44: 913–932 (1935).

7 Proctor DF, and DL Swift. Temperature and water vapor adjustment. In *Respiratory Defense Mechanism,* edited by JD Brain, DF Proctor and LM Reid. New York: Marcel Dekker, pp. 95–124 (1977).

8 Miller RR, JA Ayres, LW Rampy, JM Smith, CS Weil, JJ Clary, and GC Jersey. Ethyl acrylate vapor inhalation study: 3 month sacrifice of rats and 6 month sacrifice of rats and mice. Presented at the *19th Ann. Meeting Soc. Toxicol.,* Washington, DC., March 9–13, Abst. 159 (1980).

9 Miller RR, JA Ayres, GC Jersey, and MJ McKenna. Inhalation toxicity of acrylic acid. *Fund. Appl. Toxicol.* 1:271–277 (1981).

10 Nitschke KD, RJ Kociba, DG Keyes, and MJ McKenna. A thirteen week repeated inhalation study of ethylene dibromide in rats. *Fund. Appl. Toxicol.* 1:437–442 (1981).

11 Aharonson, EF, H Menkes, G Gurtner, DL Swift, and DF Proctor. Effect of respiratory airflow rate on removal of soluble vapors by the nose. *J. Appl. Physiol.* 37:654–657 (1974).

12 LaBelle CW, JE Long, and EE Christofano. Synergistic effects of aerosols. *Arch. Ind. Health* 11:297–304 (1955).

13 Morgan MS, and R Frank. Uptake of pollutant gases by the respiratory system. In *Respiratory Defense Mechanism,* edited by JD Brain, DF Proctor, LM Reid. New York: Marçel Dekker, pp. 157–189 (1977).

14 Morris JB, and FA Smith. Regional deposition and absorption of inhaled hydrogen fluoride in the rat. *Toxicol. Appl. Pharmacol.* 62:81–89 (1982).

15 Stott WT, and MJ McKenna. The comparative absorption and excretion of chemical vapors by the upper, lower, and intact respiratory tract of rats. *Fund. Appl. Toxicol.* 4:594–602 (1984).

16 Andersen ME. Physiological pharmacokinetic models for the inhalation of gases and vapors. *Proc. Twelfth Conf. Environ. Toxicol.* 299–320 (1982).

17 Andersen ME, ML Gargas, and JC Ramsey. Inhalation pharmacokinetics: Evaluating systemic extraction, total in vivo metabolism, and the time course of enzyme induction for inhaled styrene in rats based on steady-state blood:air concentration ratios. *Toxicol. Appl. Pharmacol.* 73:176–187 (1984).

18 Ramsey JC, and ME Anderson. A physiologically based description of the inhalation pharmacokinetics of styrene in rats and humans. *Toxicol. Appl. Pharmacol.* 73:159–175 (1984).

19 Fiserova-Bergerova V. *Modeling of Inhalation Exposure to Vapors: Uptake, Distribution, and Elimination,* Vols. I and II. Boca Raton, FL: CRC Press, (1983).

20 Blood FR, DL Smith, and FE D'Amour. Cardiac output in the rat at normal and at high altitudes and its relationship to gas embolism. *Am. J. Physiol.* 163:268–271 (1950).

21 Weibel ER. *Morphometry of the Human Lung.* New York: Academic Press (1963).

22 Alarie Y. Sensory irritation of the upper airways by airborne chemicals. *Toxicol. Appl. Pharmacol.* 24:279–297 (1973).

23 Quast JF, JW Henck, and MJ McKenna. A 90-day inhalation toxicity study of epichlorohydrin in laboratory animals. Presented at *18th Ann. Meeting Soc. Toxicol.*, New Orleans, LA, March 11–15, Abstr. 85 (1979).

24 Miller RR, JA Ayres, LL Calhoun, JT Young, and MJ McKenna. Comparative short-term inhalation toxicity of ethylene glycol monomethyl ether and propylene glycol monomethyl ether in rats and mice. *Toxicol. Appl. Pharmacol.* 51:368–377 (1981).

25 Anggard A. Capillary and shunt blood flow in the nasal mucosa of the cat. *Acta Otolaryngol.* 78:418–422 (1974).

26 Stott WT, and MJ McKenna. Hydrolysis of several glycol ether acetates and acrylate esters by nasal mucosal carboxylesterase *in vitro. Fund. Appl. Toxicol. 5,* 399–404 (1985).

27 Fishbein L. Industrial mutagens and potential mutagens. I. Halogenated aliphatic derivatives. *Mutat. Res.* 32:267–308 (1976).

28 Jones AR, P Davies, K Edward, and H Jackson. Antifertility effects and metabolism of alpha and beta epichlorohydrins in the rat. *Nature* 83:224 (1969).

29 Dahl AR, WM Hadley, FF Hahn, JM Benson, and RO McClellan. Cytochrome P-450-dependent monooxygenases in olfactory epithelium of dogs: Possible role in tumorigenicity. *Science* 216:57–59 (1982).

30 Brittebo EB, and H Tjaelve. Tissue-specificity of n-nitrosodibutylamine metabolism in Sprague-Dawley rats. *Chem.-Biol. Interact.* 38:231–242 (1982).

31 Spiezer FE, and NR Frank. The uptake and release of SO_2 by the human nose. *Arch. Environ. Health* 12:725–728 (1966).

32 Frank NR, RE Yoder, JD Brain, and E Yokoyama. SO_2 (^{35}S labeled) absorption by the nose and mouth under conditions of varying concentration and flow. *Arch. Environ. Health* 18:315–322 (1969).

33 Miller FJ, CA McNeal, JM Kirtz, DE Gardner, DL Coffin, and DB Menzel. Nasopharyngeal removal of ozone in rabbits and guinea pigs. *Toxicology* 14:273–281 (1979).

34 Yokoyama E, and R Frank. Respiratory uptake of ozone in dogs. *Arch. Environ. Health* 25:132–138 (1972).

35 Egle JL. Retention of inhaled formaldehyde, propionaldehyde, and acrolein in the dog. *Arch. Environ. Health* 25:119–124 (1972).

36 Miller RR, EA Hermann, JT Young, LL Calhoun, and PE Kastl. Propylene glycol monomethyl ether acetate: Metabolism, disposition and short-term vapor inhalation toxicity studies. *Toxicol. Appl. Pharmacol. 74,* 521–530 (1984).

37 Gushow TS, TJ Bell, JD Burek, WJ Potts, and MJ McKenna. Nitroethane: A 13-week inhalation toxicity study in rats and mice. *Toxicologist* 2, Abstr. 561 (1982).

38 Jersey GC, MF Balmer, JF Quast, CN Park, DJ Schuetz, JE Beyer, KJ Olson, SB McCollister, and LW Rampy. Two-year chronic inhalation toxicity and carcinogenicity study on monomeric styrene in rats. Toxicology Research Laboratory Report, Dow Chemical U.S.A., Midland, MI. (1978).

39 Reznik G, SF Stinson, and JM Ward. Respiratory pathology in rats and mice after inhalation of 1,2-dibromo-3-chloropropane or 1,2-dibromoethane for 13 weeks. *Arch. Toxicol.* 46:233–240 (1980).

40 Burek JD, KD Nitschke, TJ Bell, DL Wackerle, RC Childs, JE Beyer, DA Dittenber, LW Rampy, and MJ McKenna. Methylene chloride: A two-year inhalation toxicity and oncogenicity study in rats and hamsters. *Fund. Appl. Toxicol.* 4:30–47 (1984).

41 Sato A, and T Nakajima. A structure-activity relationship of some chlorinated hydrocarbons. *Arch. Environ. Health* 34:69–75 (1979).

42 McKenna MJ. The pharmacokinetics of inhaled methylene chloride in rats. *Proc. Ninth Ann. Conf. Environ. Toxicol.,* Dayton, OH, AMRL-TR-79-68, pp. 184–209 (1979).

43 Stott WT, MD Dryzga, and JC Ramsey. Blood flow distribution in the mouse as compared to the rat. *J. Appl. Toxicol.* 3:310–312 (1983).

Chapter 13

Metabolism of Xenobiotics and Steroid Hormones in the Nasal Mucosa

E. B. Brittebo, A. Castonguay, J. J. Rafter, B. Kowalski, M. Åhlman, and Ingvar Brandt

INTRODUCTION

Via the inhaled air, the mucosa of the respiratory tract is exposed to particles and volatile environmental chemicals. While the pulmonary enzymatic system that metabolizes the absorbed chemicals has been known for many years, the drug-metabolizing enzyme activity in the nasal mucosa has been demonstrated only recently. In these studies it was shown that the mucosa of the respiratory tract, particularly the nasal mucosa, has a marked ability to metabolize some carcinogenic N-nitrosamines (1-4). Subsequent investigations showed that the nasal mucosa possesses a considerable amount of cytochrome P-450-dependent monooxygenase activity and that many other types of chemicals are metabolized in this tissue (5-9).

The present work was supported in part by a research fellowship to E.B.B. from the Swedish Medical Research Council. Parts of the investigations were supported by grants from the Swedish Medical Research Council (E.B.B.), the Swedish Council for Planning and Coordination of Research (E.B.B., I.B.), the National Cancer Institute (A.C.), the Swedish Cancer Society (J.J.R.), the European Science Foundation (B.K.), and the Research Committee of the National Swedish Environment Protection Board (M.Å.).

The drug-metabolizing system of the nasal mucosa has the ability to transform xenobiotics into nontoxic excretable products. In some cases, however, relatively inert foreign compounds may be metabolically activated to chemically reactive intermediates, which become covalently bound to tissue macromolecules. The formation of such reactive electrophilic intermediates is generally considered to be of importance in the pathogenesis of various tissue lesions induced by chemicals. Since the drug-metabolizing activity of the nasal mucosa is considerable, the nasal mucosa would be a likely target for the deleterious effects of certain chemicals that are bioactivated in the tissue. Because of the complicated structure of the nasal cavity of rodents, the presence of lesions in this region has not always been carefully examined. However, more recently, lesions in the mucosa of the nasal cavity of rodents have been demonstrated to occur after exposure to various compounds (10). These lesions, including tumors in the nasal region, have been induced not only by inhalation of volatile xenobiotics but also by peroral and subcutaneous administration of nonvolatile chemicals.

In considering the nasal mucosa as a site of drug metabolism, this chapter will focus on some volatile and nonvolatile xenobiotics that have previously been shown to induce tumors in the nasal region of rodents. In addition, studies are included demonstrating that the nasal mucosa is also a site of steroid hormone metabolism. The distribution of the chemicals and their metabolites in the respiratory tract has been studied by whole-body autoradiography and microautoradiography. Various analytical methods such as high-performance liquid chromatography (HPLC), gas chromatography, and mass spectrometry have been used to identify the metabolites produced during incubation of some of the studied compounds with the nasal mucosa in vitro.

MATERIALS AND METHODS

In Vivo Studies

Whole-body Autoradiography Originally developed by Ullberg (11), the technique was used to study the distribution of various compounds in the respiratory tract as well as in other tissues of rodents. In these experiments, groups of mice or young rats were injected into the tail vein with about 5μCi of ^{14}C-labeled compounds. The animals were killed by exposure to gaseous carbon dioxide at various predetermined time intervals after administration, embedded in an aqueous gel of carboxymethyl-cellulose, and frozen by immersion in hexane cooled with solid carbon dioxide ($-78°$C). Sagittal whole-body sections (20 μm) were cut by a microtome at $-20°$C and the tape-fastened sections were freeze-dried. When performing autoradiography of volatile compounds it is possible to distinguish between the volatile parent compound and its nonvolatile metabolites by the use of heated tissue sections. In the case of 1,2-dibromoethane, selected sections were heated at +50°C for 12-16 h to ensure a complete evaporation of the volatile radioactivity in the tissues before exposure to X-ray film. To study the distribution of firmly bound radioactivity after injection of various ^{14}C-labeled compounds, selected sections were extracted stepwise with a series of organic solvents of different polarity. This procedure makes it possible to remove the unbound radioactivity in the tissues. Tissue sections (20 μm thick) were extracted stepwise with 5 percent trichloroacetic acid, absolute ethanol, n-heptane, absolute ethanol, and 50 percent ethanol for 1 min, respectively. After washing for 5 min in running water, the sections were dried at room temperature and, together with adjacent, nonextracted sections, pressed against X-ray film (Structurix; Agfa Gevaert, Belgium). After 1-6 months of exposure at − 20°C, the autoradiograms were developed.

Microautoradiography This technique utilizes paraffin-embedded sections to study the distribution of firmly bound metabolites within the nasal region of rodents. The animals were injected intravenously with ^{14}C-labeled compounds and killed as described above. The nasal region was dissected and fixed in 4 percent formaldehyde in phosphate buffer (pH 7). After fixation, the tissue was decalcified in 44 percent formic acid:70 percent ethanol (1:1) for about 1 week. The tissue was dehydrated in an ethanol series, transferred to xylene, and embedded in paraffin. Sections 5 μm thick were cut and mounted on glass slides. After deparaffinization of the sections in xylene and hydration in series of ethanol, the slides were dipped in NTB-2 (Eastman Kodak) liquid film emulsion, and stored for 1-10 weeks at 4°C in the dark. After exposure, the film was developed and the sections stained with hematoxylin-eosin. In some cases, sections were stained with periodic acid Schiff (PAS) before being dipped in the film emulsion. Since the sections are extracted with organic solvents, these microautoradiograms will show only the radioactivity that is firmly bound to the tissues. Because of the high energy of ^{14}C radiation, the resolution of the autoradiograms do not allow determination of the radioactivity in individual cells.

In Vitro Studies

Short-term Culture of Rat Nasal Septa Procedures to culture the rat nasal septa were employed (up to 24 h) in the study of the metabolism of $(2'\text{-}^{14}C)N'$-nitrosonornicotine, as described by Brittebo et al. (12). The nasal septa from F-344 rats were placed on a dry Metricel filter, and Williams supplemented medium E was added to the dish. The dishes were rocked at 37°C in an atmosphere of 95 percent oxygen and 5 percent carbon dioxide. After incubation, the media were collected and stored at − 20°C until analyzed by HPLC as described by Hecht et al. (13). The identification and quantitation of ^{14}C-labeled N′-nitrosonornicotine and its metabolites were performed by HPLC using a Waters Associates model ALC/GPC-204 high-speed liquid chromatograph equipped with two μBondapak-C_{18} columns in series as described earlier (12). The elution program consisted of an acetate buffer of pH 4.5 for 10 min, followed by a linear gradient up to 60 percent of aqueous methanol (50 percent). The radioactivity present in the fractions was determined by liquid scintillation. Mixtures of synthetic reference compounds were coinjected and used as UV markers. The radioactive metabolites were identified by coelution with the UV markers.

Incubation of Excised Rat Nasal Mucosa Rat nasal mucosa was incubated (up to 3 h) in the study of the metabolism of ^{14}C-labeled phenacetin, testosterone, and progesterone. The nasal mucosa from both the respiratory and olfactory regions of Sprague-Dawley rats was removed from the nasal cavity walls, septum, and turbinates. The tissue slices were incubated in a Krebs-Ringer phosphate buffer at 37°C in an atmosphere of oxygen.

During incubation with ([1-^{14}C]-ethyl)phenacetin, the ^{14}C-labeled CO_2 formed was trapped on filter papers soaked with aqueous KOH and placed in the center well of Warburg vials. The radioactivity on the filter papers was determined by liquid scintillation as described previously (14).

The incubates of (4-^{14}C)-progesterone or (4-^{14}C)-testosterone were extracted with chloroform:methanol (2:1), and the organic phase was collected and chromatographed on a thin-layer of silica gel as described previously (15). Following autoradiography of the thin-layer plates, the labeled areas were collected and the radioactive products were eluted with acetone. The radioactive extracts were evaporated and silylated. Gas chromatographic-mass spectrometric analyses were carried out as described previously using 3 percent SE-30 as the stationary phase (16).

RESULTS AND DISCUSSION

N-nitrosamines

N-nitrosamines are a class of potent carcinogens which display remarkable organ specificity in their carcinogenic action. In rodents, one of the frequent target organs for N-nitrosamines is the nasal cavity. Spontaneous tumors at this site are rare, and in fact before recognizing N-nitrosamines as chemical carcinogens, little was known about the induction of tumors in this region. In the middle of the 1960s a number of studies reported the induction of tumors in the nasal mucosa of mice, rats, and hamsters by various N-nitrosamines (17-20). These studies showed that nasal tumors were induced irrespective of the route of administration of the N-nitrosamines–intravenous or subcutaneous injections, skin painting, or inhalation.

Because of the powerful biological actions of the N-nitrosamines, including acute cellular injury, carcinogenesis, and mutagenesis, extensive studies on the mechanisms of their toxicity have been conducted during the past two decades (21, 22). These studies have showed that N-nitrosamines are metabolized to reactive electrophiles that alkylate cellular macromolecules (23). Initially, most of these studies were conducted with various liver preparations, although it is well known that the N-nitrosamines induce tumors in many extrahepatic tissues, e.g., in the nasal mucosa.

In a series of whole-body autoradiographic studies of various N-nitroso compounds in mice, it appeared that N-nitrosamine metabolites are firmly bound to and retained in specific extrahepatic tissues, including the mucosa of the entire respiratory tract (24, 25). Since the accumulation of metabolites at this site appeared shortly (1 min) after an intravenous injection of the N-nitrosamines, a local metabolism of the N-nitrosamines was proposed. Further studies in vitro showed that the metabolism of N-nitrosamines indeed takes place in some extrahepatic tissues and that the nasal mucosa is a site with a pronounced ability to metabolize various N-nitrosamines. The studies on the metabolism of a number of N-nitrosamines including N-nitrosodiethylamine, N-nitrosopyrrolidine, N-nitrosodibutylamine, N-nitrosopiperidine, NN′-dinitrosopiperazine, and N′-nitrosonornicotine in the nasal mucosa of rodents have been discussed in a recent review (26).

The metabolism of one of these N-nitrosamines, N′-nitrosonornicotine, in the rat nasal mucosa has since been studied in more detail. When administered in high doses, N′-nitrosonornicotine has been described as inducing necrosis in the nasal mucosa of rats (27). After repeated subcutaneous injections, benign and malignant tumors including neuroepitheliomas of the olfactory region have been observed in rats and hamsters (28, 29). Whole-body autoradiography showed that after an intravenous injection of ^{14}C-labeled N′-nitrosonornicotine (NNN), a specific localization of tissue-bound metabolites occurred in the mucosa of the ethmoturbinates of rats (3). Microautoradiography showed that the highest amount of tissue-bound radioactivity was present in the subepithelial (Bowman's) glands of the olfactory region. There was also a low labeling of the olfactory and respiratory epithelium and in the epithelium of the maxillary sinus and nasolacrimal duct, as well as in some acinous glands and excretory ducts in the mucosa. In contrast, the epithelium of the vomeronasal organ was not labeled (30).

When in vitro studies were performed, it was found that the rat nasal mucosa has a high capacity to metabolize NNN to reactive products which become firmly bound to the tissue (3). Microautoradiography performed on nasal septa incubated with NNN showed that the radioactive products were bound to the subepithelial glands and to the olfactory and respiratory epithelia of the mucosa (Fig. 1) (12). In this study, it was also demonstrated that the nasal mucosa has a high capacity to metabolize N′-nitrosonornicotine to metabolites that are released into the culture medium. Separation of NNN and

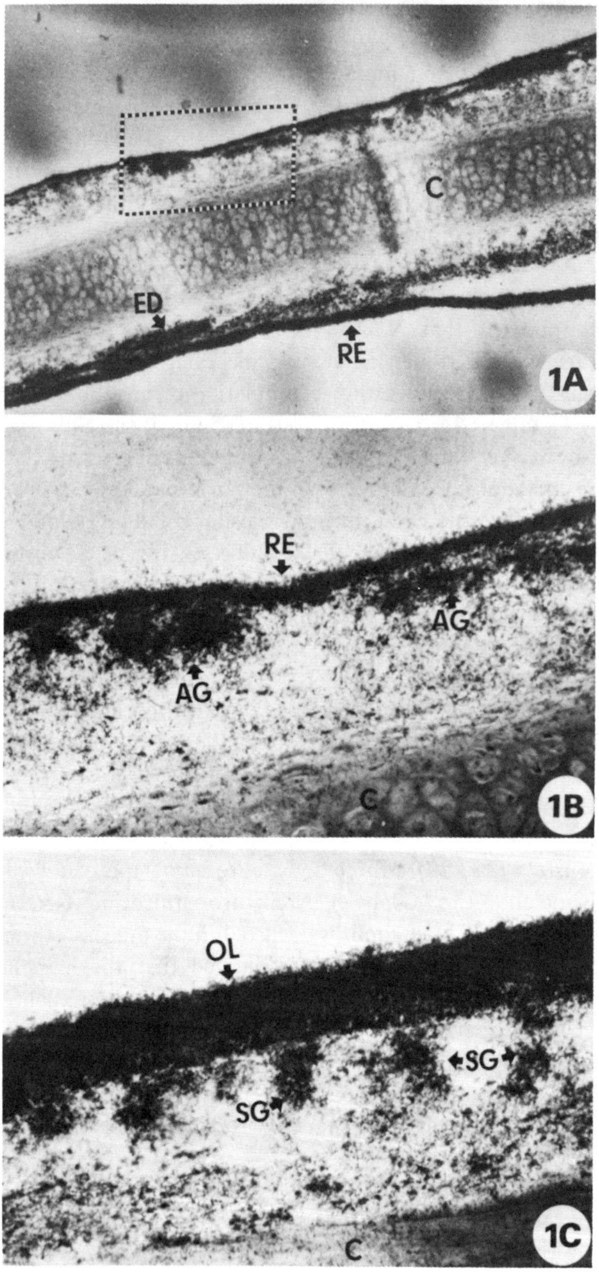

Figure 1 Microautoradiograms of rat nasal septa that were incubated with [2′-^{14}C] N′-nitrosonornicotine (37 μm) for 24 h. (*A*) Nasal septum with heavily labeled respiratory epithelium (RE), acinous glands (AG), and excretory ducts (ED). The labeling of the other parts of the nasal mucosa and cartilage (C) is low. (Magnification ×72). (*B*) Enlargement of a part from *A* as indicated. (Magnification ×240). (*C*) Part of the nasal septum showed marked labeling of the olfactory epithelium (OL) and subepithelial glands (SG). The labeling of the other parts of the nasal mucosa and cartilage (C) is low. (Magnification ×240). Black silver grains correspond to radioactivity present in the H&E-stained section. [*From Brittebo et al. (12).*]]

its metabolites by reverse-phase HPLC showed that within 2 h of incubation more than one-half of the initial amount of NNN had been metabolized (Fig. 2). After 24 h of culture, unchanged NNN could not be detected in the medium. The observed metabolic transformations of NNN and its metabolites are illustrated in Fig. 3.

The high rates of formation and release of the keto acid metabolite 8 (Fig. 3) and the hydroxy acid metabolite 10 (Fig. 3) into the media during the incubations of NNN indicated that the nasal mucosa possesses a marked α-carbon hydroxylating ability. There is substantial evidence suggesting that α-carbon hydroxylation is the initial and crucial step in the activation of most nitrosamines to ultimate carcinogenic species. The α-hydroxynitrosamines formed have very short lifetimes under physiological conditions, and they rearrange to respective diazohydroxides (31). As indicated in Fig. 3, reactive electrophilic intermediates such as diazohydroxides can be formed during the metabolism of NNN. These intermediates probably react immediately with water or with cellular macromolecules in the vicinity of their site of formation. In situ formation and binding of reactive intermediates probably play an important role in the etiology of neuroepitheliomas induced by NNN in the nasal mucosa in rats.

The α-carbon hydroxylation of NNN can take place on the sterically hindered 2′-carbon or on the more accessible 5′-carbon. When comparing the levels of products from 2′-carbon and 5′-carbon hydroxylation by rat nasal mucosa, a clear preference for 2′-carbon hydroxylation was seen, although the ratio decreased with the time of culture. In this context it is interesting to note

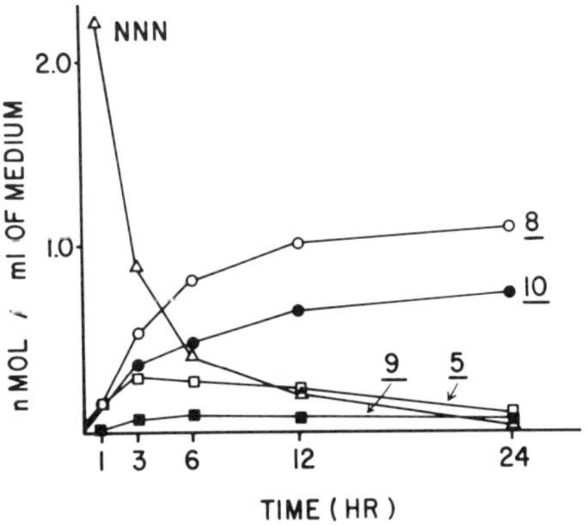

Figure 2 Levels of N′-nitrosonornicotine (NNN) and NNN-metabolites as a function of time of culture of rat nasal septa with [2′-^{14}C] N-nitrosonornicotine (3.8 μM). Each point represents a single determination. Symbols: Δ, N′-nitrosonornicotine; ○, keto acid 8; ●, hydroxy acid 10; □, keto alcohol 5; ■, diol 9. Numbers refer to Fig. 3. [*From Brittebo et al. (12).*]

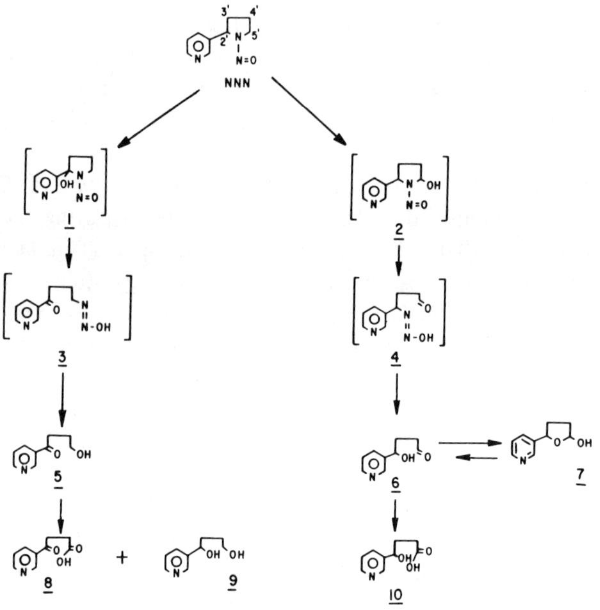

Figure 3 Metabolic transformations of N′-nitrosonornicotine in cultured rat nasal septa. Structures in brackets are hypothetical intermediates. [*From Brittebo et al. (12).*]

that a preference for 2′-carbonhydroxylation of NNN has been observed also in rat esophagus, whereas no preference for 2′-carbonhydroxylation of NNN was observed in the rat liver (32). After peroral administration of NNN in rats, tumors were observed in the esophagus whereas the rat liver does not seem to be a significant target tissue for the carcinogenic effects of NNN (27). Addition of metyrapone to the culture medium of the rat nasal septa produced a differential effect in that metyrapone inhibited the 5′-carbon hydroxylation of NNN more strongly than the 2′-carbon hydroxylation (Table 1). Since the action of metyrapone on drug metabolism is associated with an ability of the compound to interact with cytochrome P-450 (33), an involvement of this monooxygenase system also in the metabolism of NNN by the nasal mucosa seems probable. The observed differential effect of metyrapone on the 2′- and 5′-carbon hydroxylation of NNN in the nasal mucosa indicates, however, that there may be differences between the properties of the enzymatic systems that hydroxylate the 2′- and 5′-positions of NNN in this tissue.

Phenacetin

Epidemiological studies have shown a positive association between chronic abuse of phenacetin-containing analgesics and occurrence of tumors in the urinary tract in man (34). In animal experiments, long-term peroral administration of phenacetin has been reported to induce tumors in the nasal region as well as in the urinary tract (35, 36). The tumors in the rat nasal cavity are described as adenocarcinomas arising from serous and mucous glands, squamous cell carcinomas, and transitional cell carcinomas (35).

The toxic effects of phenacetin have been suggested to be mediated by reactive metabolites that bind to tissue constituents (37, 38). The realization that the nasal mucosa can metabolize N-nitrosamines stimulated our interest in the possibility that in situ metabolic activation might likewise be involved in the pathogenesis of the phenacetin-induced lesions in this tissue. Therefore studies on the distribution and metabolism of phenacetin in the rat and rabbit respiratory tract were recently initiated and (1-^{14}C-ethyl)phenacetin was synthesized for this purpose (14).

Whole-body autoradiography showed that 5 min after an intravenous injection of (^{14}C-ethyl)phenacetin in the rat, a high level of radioactivity was present in the mucosa of the ethmoid region of the nasal cavity, in the lateral nasal gland, and in the tracheobronchial mucosa (Fig. 4). In the other tissues, including the urinary tract, there was a low, homogeneously distributed radioactivity which did not exceed that of the blood. By extraction of tissue sections with organic solvents and water, it was possible to remove the homogeneously distributed radioactivity present in the tissues whereas the radioactivity in the mucosa of the respiratory tract could not be extracted.

Microautoradiography showed that after intravenous injection of (^{14}C-ethyl)phenacetin, most of the radioactivity was bound to the PAS-positive subepithelial glands (Bowman's glands) in the olfactory region of the rat nose (Fig. 5). The olfactory epithelium was also labeled, although to a lower extent

Table 1 Effect of Metyrapone on the Metabolism of N′-nitrosonornicotine by Rat Nasal Mucosa

	Metabolites (μM)/3 h/nasal septa*				
Treatment	5	8	9	10	NNN
Metyrapone (50 μM)	0.19 ± 0.04	0.25 ± 0.07	0.05 ± 0.02	0.09 ± 0.03†	2.94‡ ± 0.90
Control	0.20 ± 0.04	0.40 ± 0.14	0.08 ± 0.03	0.35 ± 0.09	1.45 ± 0.30

*Mean ± SD ($n = 3$). Numbers refer to Fig. 3.

†Significantly different from control value ($p < 0.01$; Student's t-test).

‡Significantly different from control value ($p < 0.1$; Student's t-test).

Note: Nasal septa from adult female F-344 rats were cultured in Williams medium E or Williams medium E (one septum per 5 ml) containing metyrapone. After 30 min, the media were replaced by either Williams medium E containing [2′-^{14}C] NNN (3.8 μM) or Williams medium E containing [2′-^{14}C] NNN (3.8 μM) and metyrapone. Media were harvested after 3 h and metabolites analyzed by HPLC as described in Materials and Methods. [*From Brittebo et al. (12)*].

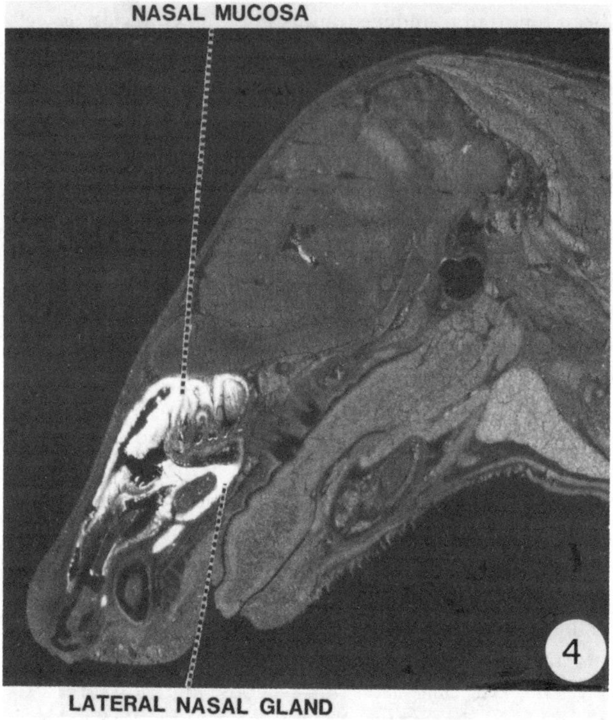

Figure 4 Autoradiogram showing the distribution of radioactivity 5 min after an i.v. injection of (^{14}C-ethyl)-phenacetin in a Sprague-Dawley rat. There is a high uptake of radioactivity in the mucosa of the ethmoid region and in the lateral nasal gland. [*From Brittebo and Åhlman (14).*]

than the subepithelial glands (Fig. 5). The respiratory epithelium covering the nasolacrimal duct, the maxillary sinus, and parts of the septum was not labeled. There was a high level of radioactivity in the lateral nasal gland and in a few small glands and excretory ducts situated beneath the respiratory epithelium of the septum, whereas there was no labeling of the epithelia of the vomeronasal organ. In the trachea and large bronchi, radioactivity was bound to the epithelium whereas the labeling of the terminal bronchioles was low.

Previous studies in the rat have demonstrated that the major metabolic pathway of phenacetin is oxidative deethylation, yielding acetaminophen, and acetaldehyde, which is further metabolized to CO_2. As shown in Table 2 and Fig. 6, the rat and rabbit nasal mucosa had a marked ability to produce $^{14}CO_2$ from (^{14}C-ethyl)phenacetin in vitro, as compared to the liver, lung, and kidney.

Addition of the cytochrome P-450 inhibitors metyrapone and SKF 525A decreased the formation of $^{14}CO_2$ from (^{14}C-ethyl)phenacetin by the rat nasal mucosa, liver, and lung. Autoradiography of pieces of rat and rabbit nasal

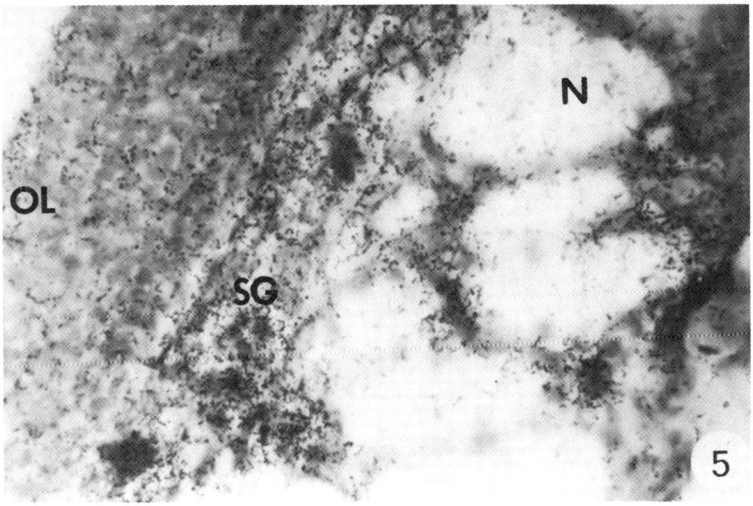

Figure 5 Microautoradiogram from the nose of a Sprague-Dawley rat killed 4 h after an i.v. injection of (^{14}C-ethyl)-phenacetin. Radioactivity (black silver grains) is preferentially present in the PAS-positive subepithelial glands (SG) underneath the olfactory epithelium (OL). The radioactivity in the nerve bundles (N) is low. (PAS-hematoxylin-stained sections, X883.) [*From Brittebo and Åhlman (14).*]

Table 2 Production of $^{14}CO_2$ from (^{14}C-ethyl)-phenacetin In Vitro by Various Tissues from Rat and Rabbit*

Tissue	Rat†	Rabbit†
Nasal mucosa	10.76 ± 1.03	3.37 ± 0.85
Liver	1.59 ± 0.13	0.51 ± 0.08
Lung	0.45 ± 0.06	0.39 ± 0.06
Kidney	0.08 ± 0.02	–
Kidney cortex	–	0.09 ± 0.01
Kidney medulla	–	0.02 ± 0.01

*Tissue slices were incubated with (^{14}C-ethyl)-phenacetin (0.9 μM) for 60 min, and the $^{14}CO_2$ formed was trapped and determined.

†Values represent pmole $^{14}CO_2$ per mg wet weight tissue (mean ± SE; n = 3-4). [*From Brittebo and Åhlman (14).*]

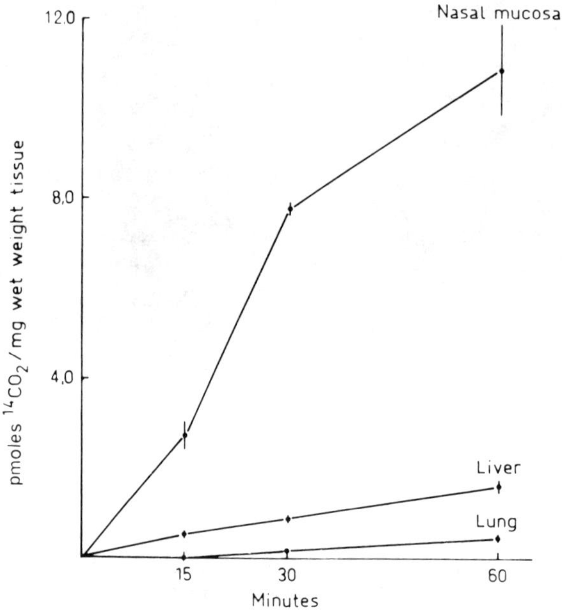

Figure 6 Formation of $^{14}CO_2$ from (^{14}C-ethyl)-phenacetin at incubation of slices of the nasal mucosa, lung, and liver at various time intervals. Each point represents the mean ±SE; $n = 3$–4. [*From Brittebo and Åhlman (14).*]

regions and trachea incubated with (^{14}C-ethyl)phenacetin showed that a binding of radioactivity also occurred in the nasal and tracheal mucosa in vitro.

The obtained results thus indicate that metabolism of (^{14}C-ethyl)phenacetin takes place in situ in the rat nasal mucosa; i.e., in a target tissue for phenacetin carcinogenesis. The metabolism of (^{14}C-ethyl)phenacetin to $^{14}CO_2$ occurred at a much higher rate in the nasal mucosa than in the liver, indicating that considerable amounts of ^{14}C-acetaldehyde are formed in the nasal mucosa. The ^{14}C-labeled acetaldehyde released intracellularly may become bound via cross-links or some other mechanism to the cellular constituents in the nasal mucosa. In addition the ^{14}C-labeled acetaldehyde is utilized in the general cell metabolism, finally resulting in the formation of $^{14}CO_2$ and metabolic incorporation of radioactivity into cellular constituents. Thus, the radioactivity bound to the mucosa of the upper respiratory tract may be due to a reactive intermediate containing the ^{14}C-labeled ethyl group as well as to a binding of ^{14}C-acetaldehyde or an incorporation of ^{14}C-acetaldehyde metabolites via the general biosynthetic pathways in the tissue. Since the chemical nature of the radioactive compound bound to the nasal mucosa has not been determined in the present study, the actual extent of these three types of binding cannot be assessed. Chemically reactive metabolites of phenacetin can be formed by several pathways involving cytochrome P-450, or via a prostaglandin synthetase-mediated reaction (37–39). Since recent studies by Woutersen et al. (40) have shown that inhalation of acetaldehyde induces degenerative lesions and tumors in the olfactory region of rats, it seems possible that the carcinogenic effect of phenacetin in the nasal mucosa is due to a high local formation of acetaldehyde, in addition to formation of other reactive intermediates. A similar mechanism has been proposed for the nasal carcinogen hexamethylphosforamide, which is rapidly demethylated to formaldehyde in the nasal mucosa (8).

1,2-Dibromoethane

1,2-Dibromoethane (EDB) is widely used as a grain fumigant, and the occurrence of residues of this compound in various agricultural products has recently caused great public concern. EDB is also used as a lead scavenger in gasoline (41). Studies on the toxic effect of EDB have shown that several lesions can be induced including liver necrosis, testicular atrophy, and tumors in the stomach, lung, and nasal cavity. EDB-induced tumors in the nasal cavity of mice are reported to occur following long-term inhalation and are described as being adenocarcinomas and squamous cell carcinomas located in the turbinates of the nasal cavity (42). Inhalation of relatively high levels of EDB induces atrophy and necrosis of the olfactory epithelium in mice and rats (43).

Because EDB is a volatile compound, it is possible to study the distribution of the nonvolatile metabolites in the body by the use of autoradiography with heated tissue sections in which the volatile radioactivity has been evaporated. By means of this procedure, a high level of nonvolatile metabolites was registered in the mucosae of the entire respiratory system and of the upper alimentary tract, and in the liver of mice killed 1 min to 4 days after an intravenous injection of ^{14}C-labeled EDB (Fig. 7). Autoradiograms prepared with tissue sections that had been extensively washed with organic solvents showed that a considerable amount of the radioactivity in the mucosae could not be extracted but remained firmly bound to the tissues. Microautoradiography of the nasal region again showed that the highest amount of tissue-bound radioactivity was present in the subepithelial (Bowman's) glands located beneath the olfactory epithelium of the ethmoturbinates. In the epithelium of the trachea, bronchi, bronchioli, palate, esophagus, and forestomach there was also a selective binding of radioactive material.

The rapid localization of nonvolatile metabolites in the mucosae of the respiratory tract and upper gastrointestinal tract suggests that local metabolism of EDB takes place in these tissues and that reactive EDB metabolites formed may play a role in the pathogenesis of EDB-induced tumors at these sites.

2,3,7,8-Tetrachlorodibenzo-*p*-dioxin

Chlorinated dibenzo-*p*-dioxins are formed as contaminants during the synthesis of several commercially important chemicals. 2,3,7,8-Tetrachlorodibenzo-*p*-

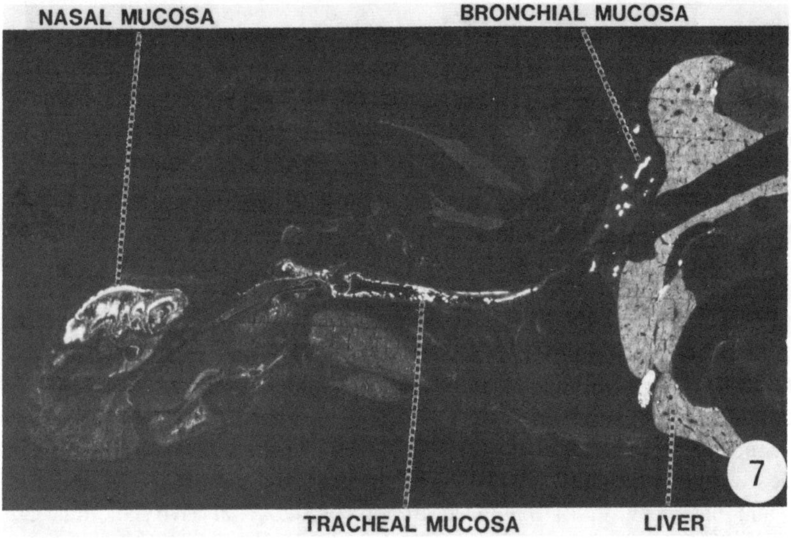

Figure 7 Autoradiogram showing the distribution of nonvolatile metabolites 1 min after an i.v. injection of 1,2-dibromo(^{14}C)-ethane in a C57B1 mouse. There is a high level of metabolites in the nasal and tracheobronchial mucosa and in the liver.

dioxin (TCDD) is an often studied representative of this group of chemicals. Investigations of the toxicity of TCDD have demonstrated that this compound causes a wide variety of biological effects in experimental animals. Lesions such as hepatic necrosis, thymic atrophy, fetal malformations, and malignant tumors have been observed following administration of TCDD (44). In a long-term study of TCDD in rats by Kociba et al. (45), an increased incidence of hepatocellular carcinomas was registered as well as tumors in the nasal turbinates, hard palate, and lung.

Several reports have been presented showing a significant uptake and accumulation of TCDD in the liver of rodents (46). In the liver, TCDD is slowly metabolized to more polar products which subsequently are excreted via the bile and urine or bound to hepatic macromolecules, although in very minute amounts (46). The autoradiographic study on the distribution of ^{14}C-labeled TCDD intravenously injected in C57B1, NMRI, and CBA mice showed that a high uptake of radioactivity had occurred in the liver, as previously described by others. In addition to the hepatic accumulation, there was a selective localization of radioactivity in the nasal mucosa (47). Within the nasal region, the radioactivity was preferentially observed in the mucosa of the ethmoturbinates, but marked labeling also occurred in the mucosa of the septum and lateral nasal cavity walls (Fig. 8). The radioactivity in these sites appeared at 4 h after injection, but became increasingly accentuated at 24 h and later. The other sites of the respiratory system (the tracheobronchial mucosa and lung) consistently showed low amounts of radioactivity in all animals. In pregnant mice of late gestation, a distinct localization of radioactivity was also observed in the fetal nasal mucosa.

The chemical structure of the radioactive material taken up in the nasal mucosa is not known at present, nor is the reason for the selective accumulation in the mucosa. In the liver and other tissues, TCDD has been shown to be a potent inducer of cytochrome P-450-dependent monooxygenases, e.g., aryl hydrocarbon hydroxylase (AHH) (48, 49). A twofold increase of AHH activity was recently observed in the nasal mucosa following administration of TCDD in rats (50).

Steroid Hormones

It is well established that the lung is a site of steroid hormone metabolism, although because of the heterogeneous cellular composition of the lung, little is known about the cellular localization of the metabolism in this organ. Previous studies by Appelgren (51-54) have shown, however, that a distinct localization of radioactivity appears in the nasal and bronchial mucosa of mice intravenously injected with various ^{14}C-labeled steroids—e.g., testosterone, 5α-dihydrotestosterone, 4-androstene-3,17-dione, pregnenolone, and progesterone.

The selective uptake of radioactivity in the mucosa of the respiratory tract indicated that the mucosa may have an ability to metabolize those steroid hormones into products that are reversibly bound and retained in this tissue.

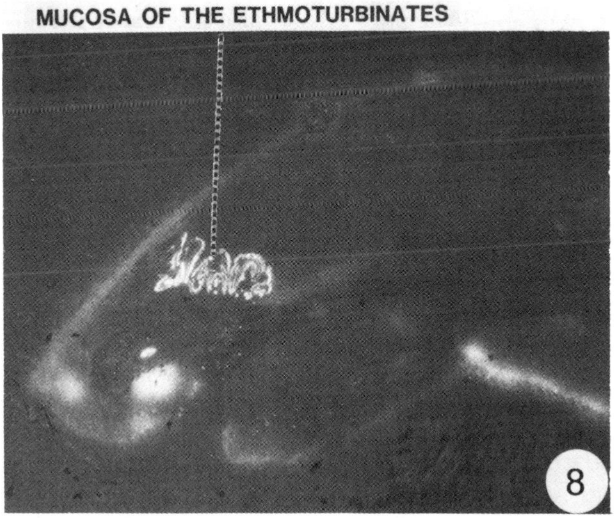

Figure 8 Autoradiogram showing the distribution of radioactivity 24 h after an i.v. injection of ^{14}C-labeled 2,3,7,8-tetrachlorodibenzo-*p*-dioxin in a CBA mouse. There is a high level of radioactivity in the mucosa of the ethmoturbinates.

Initial experiments showed that the nasal mucosa of mice and rats can metabolize progesterone, and a selective uptake of radioactivity in the bronchial mucosa was demonstrated to occur also at in vitro conditions (6). For further studies, progesterone and testosterone were chosen as representatives of C_{21} and C_{19} steroids. The metabolites formed during incubation of these steroid hormones with excised rat nasal mucosa were isolated and identified (15). The pattern of metabolites demonstrated that both progesterone and testosterone are reduced as well as hydroxylated at multiple positions on the steroid skeleton (Tables 3, 4). The major testosterone metabolites formed were identified as 4-androstene-3,17-dione, 5α-dihydrotestosterone, 3α-hydroxy-5α-androstane-17-one, and 5α-androstane-3α,17β-diol, indicating the presence of 5α-reductase, 3α-, and 17β-hydroxysteroid oxidoreductase activities in the nasal mucosa. These enzyme activities were also indicated by the formation of 5α-pregnane-3,20-dione and 3α-hydroxy-5α-pregnane-20-one from progesterone. In addition, minor amounts of 3β-hydroxy-5α-pregnane-20-one, 20α-, and 20β-hydroxy-pregn-4-en-3-one were formed from progesterone, indicating the presence of low levels of 3β-, 20α-, and 20β-hydroxysteroid oxidoreductase in the mucosa. Several hydroxylated products of progesterone and testosterone were also identified as minor metabolites. The isolation of 1β-, 2α-, 6β-, 15β-, and 16α-hydroxylated testosterone metabolites and 2α-, 6α-, 6β-, 15α-, and 16α-hydroxylated progesterone metabolites shows the presence of steroid hydroxylases in rat nasal mucosa.

The physiological significance of the metabolic transformations of steroid hormones in the nasal mucosa is not known. The porcine nasal mucosa has been demonstrated, however, to be a steroid-sensitive tissue since odoriferous steroids, e.g., 5α-androst-16-en-3-one, have been identified as acting pheromones and are used in spray formulations to ascertain estrus in sows (55). Previous studies on the metabolism of 5α-androst-16-en-3-one by porcine nasal mucosa have demonstrated the presence of 3α- and 3β-hydroxysteroid oxidoreductase (55), whereas other steroid-metabolizing enzyme activities have not previously been recorded in this tissue. Although the chemical nature of rat pheromones is not known, it might be speculated that the occurrence of a considerable steroid-metabolizing capacity in the rat nasal mucosa may be due to a need for activation and/or inactivation of inhaled pheromonal steroids also in this species.

In other mammalian tissues, hydroxylation of progesterone in position 17 yields an intermediate in the synthesis of androgens. In the nasal mucosa experiments, there was no indication of 17-hydroxylase activity, nor were any androgens formed from progesterone. Likewise, in incubations with testosterone, no aromatization of the substrate to estrogens could be observed. These observations suggest that the nasal mucosa is not involved in the biosynthesis of physiologically active steroid hormones but more likely in the inactivation of steroids. It should be pointed out, however, that the rat nasal mucosa can form biologically active reduced androgens, i.e., 5α-dihydrotesto-

Table 3 Gas-liquid-chromatographic and Mass-spectrometric Characteristics of Isolated Metabolites Produced from Progesterone at Incubation with Rat Nasal Mucosa

t.l.c. zone	Radioactivity recovered (%)	t_r	Characteristic mass-spectrometric peaks (m/e)	Compounds identified
1	16.3	0.70	316(M^+, base peak), 298, 258, 246, 231	5α-pregnane-3, 20-dione
2	57.9	0.84	314(M^+, base peak), 272, 229, 124	progesterone
3	15.1	0.64	390(M^+), 375, 300(M^+ − 90, base peak), 285, 215	3α-hydroxy-5α-pregnane-20-one
4	2.8	0.81	390(M^+), 375(base peak), 300(M^+ − 90), 285, 215	3β-hydroxy-5α-pregnane-20-one
5	1.4	1.20	388(M^+), 344, 329, 272, 117(base peak)	20α-hydroxypregn-4-en-3-one
6	0.6	0.90	388(M^+), 117(base peak)	20β-hydroxypregn-4-en-3-one
7	1.4	—	—	—
8	0.9	1.07	402(M^+), 387, 346(base peak)	6β-hydroxyprogesterone
9	0.9	1.47	402(M^+), 387, 346(base peak)	6α-hydroxyprogesterone
10	0.6	1.08	478(M^+), 463(base peak), 299, 143, 142, 129	2α,3α-dihydroxy-5α-pregnane-20-one
11	0.4	1.40	402(M^+), 387, 312(M^+ − 90), 303, 231, 172(base peak)	15α-hydroxyprogesterone
12	0.7	—	—	—
13	0.3	0.97	478(M^+), 388(M^+ − 90), 345, 298(M^+ − 2 × 90), 255, 172(base peak), 159, 157, 109	3α,16α-dihydroxy-5α-pregnane-20-one
14	0.8	—	—	—

Note: t.l.c., thin-layer chromatography, t_r, relative retention time (5α-cholestane = 1.00); M^+, molecular ion. [*From Brittebo and Rafter (15).*]

Table 4 Gas-liquid-chromatographic and Mass-spectrometric Characteristics of Isolated Metabolites Produced from Testosterone at Incubation with Rat Nasal Mucosa

t.l.c. zone	Radioactivity recovered (%)	t_r	Characteristic mass-spectrometric peaks (m/e)	Compounds identified
1	4.4	–	–	–
2	7.8	0.52	286(M^+, base peak), 244, 124	4-androstene-3, 17-dione
3	14.1	0.53	362(M^+), 347, 272(M^+ – 90), 257, 129(base peak)	5α-dihydrotestosterone
4	8.3	0.38	362(M^+), 347, 272(M^+ – 90, base peak), 271, 257	3α-hydroxy-5α-androstane-17-one
5	40.4	0.67	360(M^+), 345, 270(M^+ – 90), 129(base peak)	testosterone
6	7.4	0.49	436(M^+), 421, 346(M^+ – 90), 331, 256(M^+ – 2 × 90), 241, 217, 215, 129 (base peak)	5α-androstane-3α,17-diol
7	0.9	–	–	–
8	1.6	–	–	–
9	2.8	1.36	448(M^+, base peak), 358(M^+ – 90), 269, 268(M^+ – 2 × 90), 191, 129	16α-hydroxytestosterone
		0.96	448(M^+), 433(base peak), 332, 317, 201, 129	2α-hydroxytestosterone
10	2.9	0.69	450(M^+), 435(base peak), 360(M^+ – 90), 347, 271, 147, 143	2α-hydroxy-5α-dihydrotestosterone
11	2.7	0.80	448(M^+, base peak), 433, 392, 358(M^+ – 90), 268(M^+ – 2 × 90), 129	6β-hydroxytestosterone
12	1.5	0.93	448(M^+), 433, 358(M^+ – 90), 332(base peak), 217, 191	1β-hydroxytestosterone
13	2.3	1.06	448(M^+), 433, 358(M^+ – 90), 304, 268(M^+ – 2 × 90), 217(base peak), 191	15β-hydroxytestosterone
		0.82	524(M^+), 509(base peak), 434(M^+ – 90), 419, 255, 143, 142, 129	5α-androstane-2α, 3α, 17β-triol
14	3.0	–	–	–

Note: t.l.c., thin-layer chromatography, t_r, relative retention time (5α-cholestane = 1.00); M^+, molecular ion. [*From Brittebo and Rafter (15).*]

sterone and 5α-androstane-3α, 17β-diol, from testosterone. It is generally held that 5α-dihydrotestosterone formed in situ from testosterone is a mediator of androgen action in some tissues. The possibility that the nasal mucosa might be a target for the biologically active reduced metabolites of testosterone therefore needs to be further considered.

Concluding Remarks

A common finding in the present autoradiographic studies of various radio-labeled nasal carcinogens intravenously injected in mice and rats was the rapid and selective uptake of radioactivity in the olfactory mucosa of the nasal cavity. In some cases the selective uptake of radioactivity in this region seemed to be due to an in situ metabolism of the carcinogens to products that are bound to and retained in the mucosa. The chemical structure of the metabolites that bind to the mucosa is unknown, but it seems probable that they represent reactive electrophilic intermediates that are formed at the metabolism in the nasal mucosa. In the case of N′-nitrosonornicotine, the metabolites released into the culture media at in vitro incubation with nasal septa were identified. This study indicated that unstable α-hydroxynitrosamines are formed and converted into electrophilic intermediates, diazohydroxides, which react with the tissue constituents in the nasal mucosa. In other extrahepatic sites of metabolism, e.g., the lung, the xenobiotic metabolizing activities are often restricted to a few cell types or tissue structures. The mucosa of the nasal cavity is also a complex tissue composed of different structural components with several types of cells. The squamous, respiratory, and olfactory epithelia cover a connective tissue containing glands, blood vessels, and nerve bundles. Because of the heterogeneous nature of the nasal mucosa, it is difficult to determine the capacity of the various cell types to metabolize xenobiotics. However, microautoradiographic study of nasal septa incubated with N′-nitrosonornicotine showed a preferential binding of radioactivity in the respiratory and olfactory epithelia and in sub-epithelial (Bowman's) glands in the mucosa. Since the intermediates diazo-hydroxides, postulated to be formed during the metabolism of N′-nitrosonor-nicotine, are highly reactive, they will probably bind to tissue constituents at their site of formation. It therefore seems reasonable to believe that the metabolism of N′-nitrosonornicotine and probably also of other xenobiotics is confined to specific areas in the mucosa, most likely to the epithelia and glands of Bowman.

A considerable level of cytochrome P-450-dependent monooxygenase activity has recently been recorded in the nasal mucosa, especially in the olfactory region of the nasal cavity (5, 8, 9). In recent years it has been established that cytochrome P-450 is a family of isozymes with differing substrate specificities. At the incubation of rat nasal mucosa with progesterone and testosterone, metabolites hydroxylated at several different positions were identified, indicating the presence of various steroid hydroxylases in this tissue. Since different forms of cytochrome P-450 are considered to be involved in the hydroxylation at different sites of the steroid molecule, the identification of several hydroxylated steroid metabolites in the nasal mucosa suggests that several forms of cytochrome P-450 are also present in the nasal mucosa.

It is interesting to note that the uptake and binding of the studied nasal carcinogens and steroid hormones was highest in the olfactory region. That the highest level of cytochrome P-450–dependent monooxygenase activities has been registered in the olfactory region may indicate that the metabolic activity of the nasal mucosa is related to the process of olfaction.

SUMMARY

The distribution and metabolism of the ^{14}C-labeled nasal carcinogens N′-nitrosonornicotine, phenacetin, 1,2,-dibromoethane, and 2,3,7,8-tetrachlorodibenzo-*p*-dioxin and the steroid hormones progesterone and testosterone were studied in mice and rats. As shown by whole-body autoradiography, there was a selective uptake of radioactivity in the mucosa of the ethmoturbinates shortly after intravenous injections of these ^{14}C-labeled carcinogens and steroids. Microautoradiography showed that tissue-bound metabolites were present preferentially in the subepithelial glands of the olfactory nasal mucosa after intravenous injections of N′-nitrosonornicotine, phenacetin, and 1,2-dibromoethane. In vitro experiments demonstrated that rat nasal mucosa has a marked ability to metabolize N′-nitrosonornicotine to various hydroxylated products, indicating an initial α-carbon hydroxylation giving rise to electrophilic intermediates–i.e., diazohydroxides. These intermediates probably react with tissue constituents in the vicinity of their site of formation, suggesting that the metabolism is confined to specific areas in the mucosa, i.e., the epithelia and subepithelial glands. Identification of products formed during incubation of progesterone and testosterone with rat nasal mucosa showed that there is a preferential formation of reduced metabolites, indicating the presence of 5α-reductase and 3α-, 3β-, 17β-, 20α-, and 20β-hydroxysteroid oxidoreductase activities in the mucosa. Progesterone metabolites hydroxylated at positions 2α, 6α, 6β, 15α, and 16α and testosterone metabolites hydroxylated at positions 1β, 2α, 6β, 15β, and 16α were also identified, indicating the presence of several steroid hydroxylases in the nasal mucosa. Since different forms of cytochrome P-450 are considered to be involved in the hydroxylation at different sites of the steroid molecule, the obtained results suggest that several forms of cytochrome P-450 are present also in the rat nasal mucosa.

REFERENCES

1 Brittebo, EB, B Löfberg, and H Tjälve. Sites of metabolism of N-nitrosodiethylamine in mice. *Chem. Biol. Interact.* 34:209–221 (1981).

2 Brittebo, EB, B Löfberg, and H Tjälve. Extrahepatic sites of metabolism of N-nitrosopyrrolidine in mice and rats. *Xenobiotica* 11:619–625 (1981).

3 Brittebo, EB, and H Tjälve. Formation of tissue-bound N'-nitrosonornicotine metabolites by the target tissues of Sprague-Dawley and Fisher rats. *Carcinogenesis* 2:959–963 (1981).

4 Brittebo, EB, and H Tjälve. Tissue specificity of N-nitrosodibutylamine metabolism in Sprague-Dawley rats. *Chem. Biol. Interact.* 38:231–242 (1982).

5 Brittebo, E. N-Demethylation of aminopyrine by the nasal mucosa in mice and rats. *Acta Pharmacol. Toxicol.* 51:227–232 (1982).

6 Brittebo, E. Metabolism of progesterone by the nasal mucosa in mice and rats. *Acta Pharmacol. Toxicol.* 51:441–445 (1982).

7 Brittebo, EB, and I Brandt. Metabolism of chlorobenzene in the mucosa of the murine respiratory tract. *Lung* 162:79–88 (1984).

8 Dahl, AR, WM Hadley, FF Hahn, JM Benson, and RO McClellan. Cytochrome P-450–dependent monooxygenases in olfactory epithelium of dogs. Possible role in tumorigenicity. *Science* 216:57–59 (1982).

9 Hadley, WM, and AR Dahl. Cytochrome P-450–dependent monooxygenase activity in rat nasal epithelial membranes. *Toxicol. Lett.* 10:417–422 (1982).

10 Reznik, G, and SF Stinson. *Nasal Tumours in Animals and Man,* Vol. III, *Experimental Nasal Carcinogenesis.* Boca Raton, FL: CRC Press, pp. 1–253 (1983).

11 Ullberg, S. Studies on the distribution and fate of ^{35}S-labelled benzylpenicillin in the body. *Acta Radiol.* Suppl. 118:1–110 (1954).

12 Brittebo, EB, A Castonguay, K Furuya, and SS Hecht. Metabolism of tobacco-specific nitrosamines by cultured rat nasal mucosa. *Cancer Res.* 43: 4343–4348 (1983).

13 Hecht, SS, D Lin and CB Chen. Comprehensive analysis of urinary metabolites of N'-nitrosonornicotine. *Carcinogenesis* 2:833–838 (1981).

14 Brittebo, EB, and M Åhlman. Metabolism of a nasal carcinogen–phenacetin–in the mucosa of the upper respiratory tract. *Chem. Biol. Interact.* 50:233–246 (1984).

15 Brittebo, EB, and JJ Rafter. Steroid metabolism by rat nasal mucosa: Studies on progesterone and testosterone. *J. Steroid Biochem.* 20:1147–1151 (1984).

16 Gustafsson, JÅ. Steroid hydroxylations. In *Methods in Enzymology,* edited by S Fleischner and L Packer. New York: Academic Press, Vol. LII, pp. 377–388 (1978).

17 Herrold, K. Induction of olfactory neuroepithelial tumours in Syrian hamsters by diethylnitrosamine. *Cancer* 17:114–121 (1964).

18 Hoffman, F, and A Graffi. Nasenhöhlentumoren bei Mäusen nach perkutaner Diäthylnitrosaminapplikation. *Arch. Geschulstforsch.* 23:274–288 (1964).

19 Druckrey, H, S Ivankovic, HD Mennel, and R Preussmann. Selektive Erzeugung von Carcinomen der Nasenhöhle bei Ratten durch N,N'-Di-Nitrosopiperazin, Nitrosopiperidin, Nitrosomorpholin, Methyl-allyl-, Dimethyl- und Methyl-vinyl-nitrosamin. *Z. Krebsforch.* 66:138–150 (1964).

20 Thomas, C. Zur Morphologie der Nasenhöhlen Tumoren bei der Ratte. *Z. Krebsforsch.* 67:1–10 (1965).

21 Olajos, EJ. Biological interactions of N-nitroso compounds: A review. *Ecotoxicol. Environment. Safety* 1:175–196 (1977).

22 Olajos, EJ, and F Coulston. Comparative toxicology of N-nitroso compounds and their carcinogenic potential to man. *Ecotoxicol. Environment. Safety* 2:317–367 (1978).

23 Michejda, CJ, MB Kroeger-Koepke, SR Koepke, and DH Sieh. Activation of nitrosamines to biological alkylating agents. In *N-Nitroso Compounds,* edited by RA Scanlan and SR Tannenbaum. ACS Symposium Series No. 174. Washington, DC: American Chemical Society, pp. 3–20 (1981).

24 Johansson-Brittebo, E, and H Tjälve. Studies on the distribution and metabolism of N-(^{14}C)-nitrosopyrrolidine in mice. *Chem. Biol. Interact.* 25:243–253 (1979).

25 Brittebo, EB, and H Tjälve. Autoradiographic observations on the distribution and metabolism of N′-(^{14}C)-nitrosonornicotine in mice. *J. Cancer Res. Clin. Oncol.* 98:233–242 (1980).

26 Brittebo, EB, and H Tjälve. Metabolism of N-nitrosamines by the nasal mucosa. In *Nasal Tumours in Animals and Man,* Vol. III, *Experimental Nasal Carcinogenesis,* edited by G Reznik and SF Stinson. Boca Raton, FL: CRC Press, pp. 233–250 (1983).

27 Hoffman, D, R Raineri, SS Hecht, R Maronpot, and EL Wynder. A study of tobacco carcinogenesis. XIV. Effects of N′-nitrosonornicotine and N′-nitrosoanabasine in rats. *JNCI* 55:977–981 (1975).

28 Singer, GM, and HW Taylor. Carcinogenicity of N′-nitrosonornicotine in Sprague-Dawley rats. *JNCI* 57:1275–1276 (1976).

29 Hecht, SS, CB Chen, T Ohmori, and D Hoffman. Comparative carcinogenicity in F-344 rats of the tobacco specific nitrosamines, N′-nitrosonornicotine and 4-(N-methyl-N-nitrosamino)-1-(3-pyridyl)-1-butanone. *Cancer Res.* 40: 298–302 (1980).

30 Löfberg, B, EB Brittebo, and H Tjälve. Localization and binding of N′-nitrosonornicotine metabolites in the nasal region and in some other tissues of Sprague-Dawley rats. *Cancer Res.* 42:2877–2883 (1982).

31 Mochizuki, M, T Anjo, K Takeda, E Suzuki, N Sekiguchi, GF Huang, and M Okada. Chemistry and mutagenicity of α-hydroxynitrosamines. In *N-Nitroso Compounds: Occurrence and Biological Effects,* edited by H Bartsch, IK O'Neill, M Castegnaro, and M Okada. IARC Scientific Publication No. 41. Lyon: International Agency for Research on Cancer, pp. 553–559 (1982).

32 Hecht, SS, B Reiss, D Lin and GM Williams. Metabolism of N′-nitrosonornicotine by cultured rat esophagus. *Carcinogenesis* 3:453–456 (1982).

33 Netter, KJ, GF Kahl, and MP Magnusson. Kinetic experiments on the binding of metyrapone to liver microsomes. *Naunyn-Schmiedebergs Arch. Pharmakol.* 265:205–215 (1969).

34 IARC Monographs on the Evaluation of the Carcinogenic Risk of Chemicals to Humans, Vol. 24. *Some Pharmaceutical Drugs.* Lyon: International Agency for Research on Cancer, pp. 135–159 (1980).

35 Isaka, H, H Yoshii, A Otsuji, M Koike, Y Nagai, M Koura, K Sugiyasu, and T Kanabayashi. Tumours of Sprague-Dawley rats induced by long-term feeding of phenacetin. *Gan* 70:29–36 (1979).
36 Johansson, SL. Carcinogenicity of analgesics: Long-term treatment of Sprague-Dawley rats with phenacetin, phenazone, caffeine and paracetamol (acetaminophen). *Int. J. Cancer* 27:521–529 (1981).
37 Hinson, JA. Reactive metabolites of phenacetin and acetaminophen: A review. *Environ. Health Perspect.* 49:71–79 (1983).
38 Gilette, JR, SD Nelson, GJ Mulder, DJ Jollow, JR Mitchell, LR Pohl, and JA Hinson. Formation of chemically reactive metabolites of phenacetin and acetaminophen. *Adv. Exp. Med. Biol.* 136:931–950 (1981).
39 Andersson, B, M Nordenskjöld, A Rahimtula, and P Moldeus. Prostaglandin synthetase–catalyzed activation of phenacetin metabolites to genotoxic products. *Mol. Pharmacol.* 22:479–485 (1982).
40 Woutersen, RA, LM Appelman, VJ Feron, and CA van der Heijden. Inhalation toxicity of acetaldehyde in rats. II. Carcinogenicity study: Interim results after 15 months. *Toxicology* 31:123–133 (1984).
41 IARC Monographs on the Evaluation of the Carcinogenic Risk of Chemicals to Humans, Vol. 15. *Some Fumigants, the Herbicides 2,4-D and 2,4,5-T, Chlorinated Dibenzo-dioxins and Miscellaneous Industrial Chemicals.* Lyon: International Agency for Research on Cancer, pp. 195–209 (1977).
42 Stinson, SF, G Reznik, and JM Ward. Characteristics of proliferative lesions in the nasal cavities of mice following chronic inhalation of 1,2-dibromoethane. *Cancer Lett.* 12:121–129 (1981).
43 Reznik, G, SF Stinson, and JM Ward. Respiratory pathology in rats and mice after inhalation of 1,2-dibromo-3-chloropropane or 1,2-dibromoethane for 13 weeks. *Arch. Toxicol.* 46:233–240 (1980).
44 Poland, A, and JC Knutson. 2,3,7,8-Tetrachlorodibenzo-*p*-dioxin and related halogenated aromatic hydrocarbons: Examination of the mechanism of toxicity. *Annu. Rev. Pharmacol. Toxicol.* 22:517–554 (1982).
45 Kociba, RJ, DG Keyes, JE Beyer, RM Carreon, CE Wade, DA Dittenberg, RP Kalnins, LE Frauson, CN Park, SD Barnard, RA Hummel, and CG Humiston. Results of a two-year chronic toxicity and oncogenicity study of 2,3,7,8-tetrachlorodibenzo-*p*-dioxin in rats. *Toxicol. Appl. Pharmacol.* 46: 279–303 (1978).
46 Gasiewicz, TA, JR Olson, LH Geiger, and RA Neal. Absorption, distribution and metabolism of 2,3,7,8-tetrachloro-dibenzodioxin (TCDD) in experimental animals. In *Human and Environmental Risks of Chlorinated Dioxins and Related Compounds,* edited by RE Rucker, AL Young, and AP Gray. New York: Plenum, pp. 495–525 (1983).
47 Appelgren, LE, I Brandt, EB Brittebo, M Gillner, and JÅ Gustafsson. Autoradiography of 2,3,7,8-tetrachloro-(^{14}C)-dibenzo-*p*-dioxin (TCDD): Accumulation in the nasal mucosa. *Chemosphere* 12:545–548 (1983).
48 Hook, GER, JK Haseman, and GW Lucier. Induction and suppression of hepatic and extrahepatic microsomal foreign compound metabolizing enzyme systems by 2,3,7,8-tetrachlorodibenzo-*p*-dioxin. *Chem. Biol. Interact.* 10:199–214 (1975).

49 Haaparanta, T, H Glaumann, and JÅ Gustafsson. Induction of cytochrome P-450 dependent reactions in the rat ventral prostate by β-napthoflavone and 2,3,7,8-tetrachlorodibenzo-*p*-dioxin. *Toxicology* 29:61–75 (1983).

50 Bond, JA. Some biotransformation enzymes responsible for polycyclic aromatic hydrocarbon metabolism in rat nasal turbinates: Effects on enzyme activities of in vitro modifiers and intraperitoneal and inhalation exposure of rats to inducing agents. *Cancer Res.* 43:4805–4811 (1983).

51 Appelgren, LE. Sites of steroid hormone formation. Autoradiographic studies using labelled precursors. *Acta Physiol. Scand.* Suppl. 301:1–108 (1967).

52 Appelgren, LE. The distribution of labelled testosterone in mice. *Acta Endocrinol.* 62:505–512 (1969).

53 Appelgren, LE. The distribution of labelled androstendione in mice. *Steroidologia* 2:87–99 (1971).

54 Appelgren, LE. Autoradiographic studies on labelled 5α-dihydrotestosterone in mice. *Steroids Lipids Res.* 3:286–298 (1972).

55 Gower, DB, MR Hancock, and LH Bannister. Biochemical studies on the boar pheromones, 5α-androst-16-en-3-one and 5α-androst-16-en-3α-ol, and their metabolism by olfactory tissue. In *Biochemistry of Taste and Olfaction,* edited by RH Cagan and MR Kare. New York: Academic Press, pp. 7–31 (1981).

Chapter 14

Mechanisms of Nasal Toxicity Induced by Formaldehyde and Acrolein

Henry d'A. Heck, Mercedes Casanova,
Michael J. McNulty, and Chiu-wing Lam

INTRODUCTION

Formaldehyde and acrolein are important commercial aldehydes, currently manufactured in volumes of 5.4×10^9 and 0.5×10^9 lb/yr, respectively (1, 2). Nearly 90 percent of commercial acrolein is converted directly to acrylic acid, so the potential for human exposure is low (2). Commercial formaldehyde is mainly used for the synthesis of resins, which are employed in the manufacture of building products. Formaldehyde is also used in the textiles, paper, and leather-goods industries, and as a disinfectant and preservative. Exposure to formaldehyde from these sources is recognized to be widespread.

Formaldehyde and acrolein are also generated in large amounts from non-commercial sources. Both aldehydes are components of the exhaust from internal combustion engines (3), and formaldehyde and other aldehydes are contributors to photochemical smog (4). The amounts of formaldehyde and acrolein in the smoke of a single cigarette range from approximately 50 to 150 μg (5, 6). Inasmuch as humans are exposed to low to moderate concentrations of both aldehydes, studies have been undertaken to investigate the mechanisms of their toxic effects in rodents.

COVALENT BINDING OF FORMALDEHYDE TO RESPIRATORY MUCOSAL DNA

Formaldehyde has been shown to react with DNA in cultured mammalian cells, forming DNA-protein crosslinks (7, 8). These findings demonstrated that formaldehyde has the ability to damage DNA, and they are consistent with the known mutagenic (9) and carcinogenic (10) activity of formaldehyde. Until recently, however, no evidence existed that formaldehyde can crosslink DNA to proteins in vivo. In addition, there was no direct evidence that formaldehyde was itself the agent responsible for DNA-protein crosslinking.

The initial evidence that inhalation exposure to formaldehyde can cause DNA-protein crosslinking in vivo was the observation that exposure of rats to formaldehyde at concentrations equal to or greater than 6 ppm decreased the extractability of DNA from proteins in homogenates of the respiratory mucosa (11). Extractions of DNA were carried out using a strongly denaturing aqueous-immiscible organic solvent mixture. When the tissue was extracted in this manner, the DNA was separated into two fractions. The aqueous (AQ) phase contained DNA that by all spectrophotometric and chromatographic criteria appeared to be pure, double-stranded DNA. The interfacial (IF) layer also contained DNA, but this DNA appeared to be crosslinked to proteins, since the DNA could not be recovered without proteolytic digestion of the interface. Importantly, the amount of IF DNA depended on the airborne concentration of formaldehyde to which the rats had been exposed, increasing with increasing concentrations. It was tentatively concluded, therefore, that formaldehyde can react with respiratory mucosal DNA in vivo.

However, it was recognized that the inability to separate DNA from proteins does not constitute proof of the formation of DNA-protein crosslinks by formaldehyde. Therefore, further studies were undertaken using [^{14}C]- and [^{3}H]formaldehyde to investigate the mechanisms of labeling of macromolecules (DNA, RNA, and proteins) in the nasal mucosa. The use of two isotopes allowed the two mechanisms of labeling; (1) metabolic incorporation and (2) covalent binding, to be differentiated. The results of these experiments are described in detail elsewhere (12). A brief summary of the main findings, focusing on the DNA from the respiratory mucosa, is presented here.

The labeling of macromolecules in the respiratory mucosa was studied in rats that had been preexposed for 6 h to unlabeled formaldehyde on the day preceding the exposure to the labeled compound. Preexposure was undertaken to stimulate cell turnover in the respiratory mucosa, a physiological response to toxic injury that occurs after exposure to certain concentrations of formaldehyde (13) and that increases the fraction of single-stranded DNA. Regions of DNA that are single-stranded are known to be susceptible to the formation of adducts with formaldehyde, whereas double-stranded DNA does not appear to form such adducts (14). The pre-exposure to unlabeled formaldehyde and the exposure to [^{14}C]- and [^{3}H]formaldehyde were both carried out at the same airborne concentration.

Measurements of the ^{14}C specific activity of IF and AQ DNA from the respiratory mucosa following exposure to 0.3, 2, 6, 10, or 15 ppm of [^{14}C]- and [^{3}H]formaldehyde are shown in Table 1. The specific activity of DNA was maximal at 6 ppm and decreased at higher concentrations. In addition, the ^{14}C specific activity of the AQ DNA was significantly greater than that of the IF DNA at 6 ppm, but no significant difference between the specific activities of the two DNA fractions was found at other concentrations.

Based on several arguments that are advanced in the paper by Casanova-Schmitz et al. (12), it can be concluded that the major route of labeling of DNA in the respiratory mucosa was metabolic incorporation. The maximum in the specific activity of the DNA at 6 ppm therefore implies that the incorporation of [^{14}C]formaldehyde into respiratory mucosal DNA was maximal at this concentration. This result is consistent with the observation that the incorporation of [^{3}H]thymidine into respiratory mucosal DNA after exposure to formaldehyde at 6 ppm was greater than after exposure to 15 ppm (13). The decreased incorporation of ^{14}C into DNA that occurred at 10 and 15 ppm relative to that at 6 ppm was probably due to cytotoxic effects of formaldehyde at high concentrations.

The observation that the ^{14}C specific activity of the AQ DNA from the respiratory mucosa was significantly higher than that of the IF DNA at 6 ppm is important. This result implies that the AQ DNA had incorporated a significantly larger amount of ^{14}C than had the IF DNA at 6 ppm. In addition, it demonstrates that the two DNA fractions must have differed structurally, for otherwise they could not have been separated by solvent extraction into portions with differing specific activities. However, no difference between the specific activities of AQ and IF DNA was found at either 0.3 or 2 ppm, demonstrating that the structural difference noted above is not an inherent property of respiratory mucosal DNA and must have been induced in the DNA by

Table 1 ^{14}C Specific Activities of Respiratory Mucosal DNA (nmole Equiv [^{14}C] Formaldehyde/mg) in Rats Exposed to [^{14}C]- and [^{3}H] Formaldehyde*

	Airborne formaldehyde concentration (ppm)				
DNA fraction	**0.3**	**2**	**6**	**10**	**15**
Aqueous	0.54 ± 0.13	1.78 ± 0.61	6.56 ± 1.07	4.31 ± 1.45	3.91 ± 0.89
Interfacial	0.45 ± 0.14	1.51 ± 0.41	3.55 ± 0.24	3.12 ± 0.23	2.80 ± 0.22

*Rats were exposed for 6 h to [^{14}C]- and [^{3}H]formaldehyde 1 day after a single pre-exposure (6 h) to the same concentration of unlabeled formaldehyde. DNA was isolated as described by Casanova-Schmitz et al. (12). Values shown are mean ± SD, $n = 3$ groups of rats at each concentration (4 animals per group).

exposure to formaldehyde at 6 ppm. A plausible explanation to account for this structural difference is that formaldehyde exposure at 6 ppm resulted in the formation of DNA-protein crosslinks in the IF DNA fraction.

Quantitative evidence for the formation of DNA-protein crosslinks by formaldehyde was obtained by measuring the $^3H/^{14}C$ ratios of the two DNA fractions (12). The $^3H/^{14}C$ ratio of the IF DNA increased with increasing formaldehyde concentrations, whereas no increase in the $^3H/^{14}C$ ratio of the AQ DNA was detected (Fig. 1). This finding suggests that the labeling of IF DNA by [^{14}C]- and [^3H]formaldehyde was due to both metabolic incorporation and covalent binding, but that the labeling of AQ DNA was due primarily or exclusively to metabolism.

The difference between the $^3H/^{14}C$ ratios of IF and AQ DNA was statistically significant at concentrations equal to or greater than 2 ppm. In addition, the isotope ratio difference was highly correlated with the percentage of IF DNA obtained in each experiment (Fig. 2). This result indicates that the difference between the $^3H/^{14}C$ ratios is due to DNA-protein crosslinking in the interfacial DNA, and that the crosslinks are composed of exogenous formaldehyde.

It can be shown that the $^3H/^{14}C$ ratio of a macromolecule following

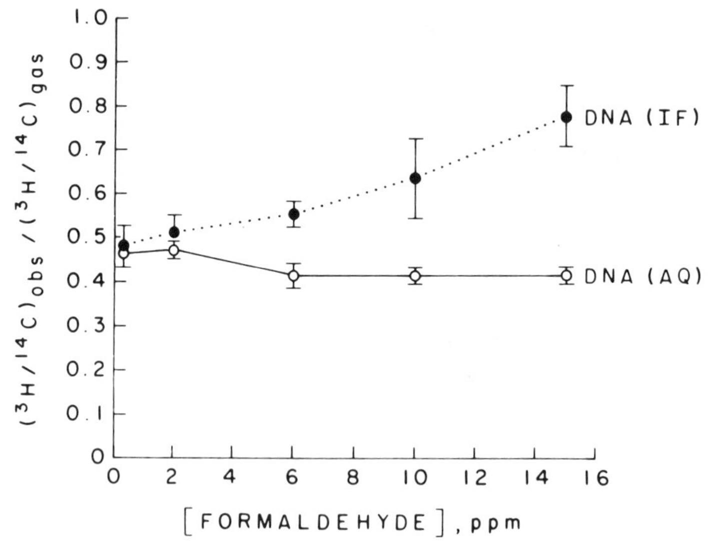

Figure 1 Normalized $^3H/^{14}C$ ratios (observed ratio divided by $^3H/^{14}C$ ratio of inhaled [^{14}C]- and [^3H]formaldehyde) of AQ DNA and IF DNA from the respiratory mucosa of rats exposed for 6 h to 0.3, 2, 6, 10, or 15 ppm of [^{14}C]- and [^3H]formaldehyde, 1 day after a single preexposure (6 h) to the same concentration of unlabeled formaldehyde. Values are mean ± SD; $n = 3$ groups of rats at each concentration (4 animals per group). [*From Casanova et al. (12).*]

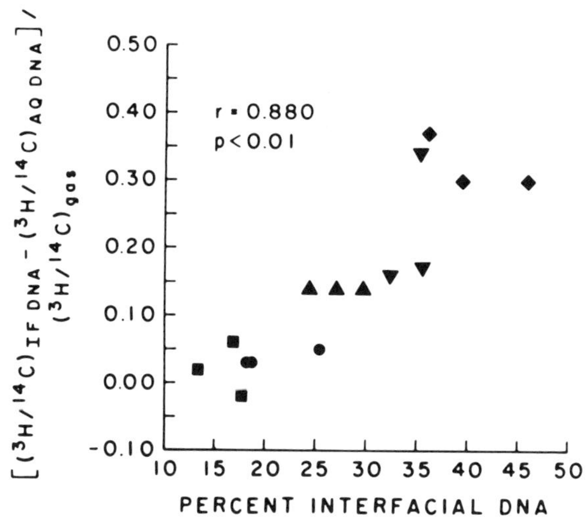

Figure 2 Plot of the difference between the normalized $^3H/^{14}C$ ratio of IF DNA and that of AQ DNA from the respiratory mucosa vs. the percent IF DNA. Formaldehyde concentrations are 0.3 (■), 2 (●), 6 (▲), 10 (▼), and 15 (◆) ppm. [*From Casanova et al. (12).*]

exposure to a toxicant labeled with both isotopes is quantitatively related to the fraction of the total ^{14}C that is due to covalent binding, f_b (12).

$$f_b = \frac{(^3H/^{14}C)_o - (^3H/^{14}C)_m}{(^3H/^{14}C)_b - (^3H/^{14}C)_m} \tag{1}$$

The definitions of the terms in this equation are: $(^3H/^{14}C)_o$ = observed $^3H/^{14}C$ ratio of macromolecule; $(^3H/^{14}C)_m$ = $^3H/^{14}C$ ratio characteristic of metabolic incorporation of ^3H and ^{14}C (derived from [^3H]- and [^{14}C]formaldehyde) into the macromolecule; $(^3H/^{14}C)_b$ = $^3H/^{14}C$ ratio characteristic of covalent binding of [^3H]- and [^{14}C]formaldehyde to the macromolecule under the reaction conditions. The values of these isotope ratios can be measured, and the fraction of covalently bound [^{14}C]formaldehyde can be calculated (12). Knowledge of the total ^{14}C content permits the concentration of covalently bound formaldehyde to be determined (column 2 of Table 2).

The concentration–response profile for covalent binding of [^{14}C]formaldehyde to DNA exhibits a linear portion above 6 ppm but is nonlinear below this concentration (Fig. 3). The nonlinearity of the binding curve is demonstrated by the data shown in the third column of Table 2, which summarizes the concentration of formaldehyde covalently bound to DNA divided by the airborne concentration of formaldehyde. Analysis of these data using Newman-Keuls' multiple-range test shows that the ratios at 0.3 and 2 ppm are not significantly different from each other, nor are the ratios at 6, 10, and 15 ppm

Table 2 Absolute Concentrations of Covalently Bound [^{14}C] Formaldehyde in Respiratory Mucosal DNA and Concentrations of Covalently Bound Formaldehyde Relative to the Inhaled Formaldehyde Concentration

Airborne formaldehyde concentration (ppm)	Absolute concentration of covalently bound [^{14}C] formaldehyde* (nmole/mg of DNA)	Concentration of covalently bound [^{14}C] formaldehyde per ppm inhaled formaldehyde*
0.3	0.002 ± 0.003	0.007 ± 0.009
2	0.022 ± 0.006	0.011 ± 0.003
6	0.233 ± 0.023	0.039 ± 0.004
10	0.406 ± 0.099	0.041 ± 0.010
15	0.631 ± 0.064	0.042 ± 0.004

*Covalently bound formaldehyde was calculated using the equations given in Appendix 2 of Casanova-Schmitz et al. (12). Values shown are mean ± SE; $n = 3$ groups of rats at each concentration, 4 animals per group.

significantly different from one another. However, the ratios at 0.3 and 2 ppm are significantly lower than those at 6, 10, and 15 ppm. Inasmuch as the linear hypothesis requires that all such normalized ratios have the same value, these data provide strong evidence that covalent binding of formaldehyde to DNA is not a linear function of the airborne concentration at low formaldehyde concentrations.

The explanation for low-dose nonlinearity in the binding of formaldehyde to DNA is not entirely clear at this time. However, at least two mechanisms could explain such nonlinear behavior. First, physiological and biochemical defense mechanisms, such as mucociliary clearance, metabolism, and repair, could be inactivated or may become less efficient with increasing formaldehyde concentrations, resulting in a disproportionate increase in the concentration of DNA-protein crosslinks. Second, the marked increase in cell turnover caused by formaldehyde exposure at 6 ppm relative to that at 2 ppm (13) could increase the availability of sites in the DNA for reaction with formaldehyde. As noted earlier, formaldehyde binds to single-stranded regions of DNA, but not to regions that are double-stranded.

EFFECTS OF GLUTATHIONE (GSH) DEPLETION BY PHORONE ON DNA-PROTEIN CROSSLINKING BY FORMALDEHYDE

Formaldehyde dehydrogenase (FDH), an important enzyme in the metabolism of endogenous formaldehyde, is present in the respiratory and olfactory mucosa of the rat (15). The activity of FDH in homogenates of respiratory and olfactory tissue is similar to its activity in liver homogenates. Uotila and Koivusalo (16) have shown that FDH does not directly catalyze the oxidation of formaldehyde, but catalyzes the oxidation of the hemithioacetal adduct of formaldehyde with GSH (S-hydroxymethylglutathione) to S-formylglutathione. Glutathione is also an essential (probably allosteric) activator of FDH (17). Inasmuch as glutathione is necessary for the activity of FDH, it might be expected that depletion of GSH would diminish the capacity of nasal mucosal tissues to oxidize formaldehyde and, therefore, could result in an enhancement of toxicity, as evidenced by DNA-protein crosslinking.

Formaldehyde exposure (15 ppm, 6 h/day, 9 days) did not result in measurable depletions of GSH in the respiratory mucosa (15). Therefore, the capability of other compounds, all known depletors of GSH in the liver, to lower the concentration of nonprotein sulfhydryls (NPSH) in the respiratory mucosa was determined. The compounds (diethyl maleate, buthionine sulfoximine, and phorone [diisopropylidene acetone]) were injected intraperitoneally to rats, and the concentrations of NPSH in the respiratory mucosa and liver were determined 2 h after injection. The results of these experiments showed that all three compounds depleted respiratory mucosal NPSH to varying degrees but that the most complete depletions occurred by administration of phorone.

At a dose of 300 mg/kg i.p., phorone lowered respiratory mucosal NPSH by

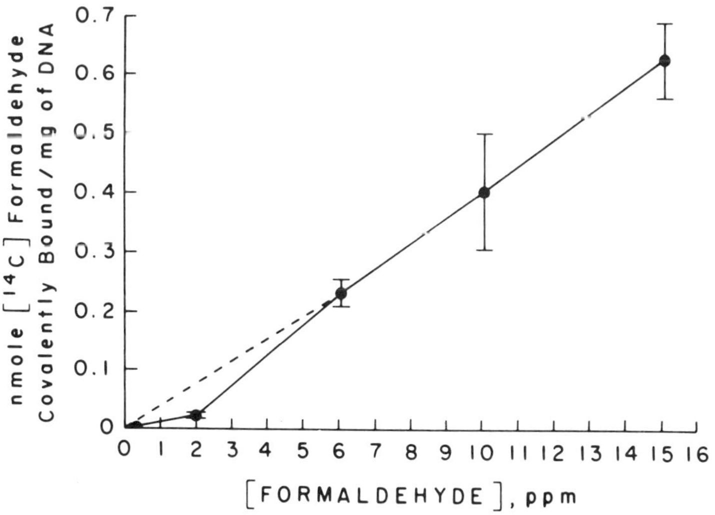

Figure 3 Concentration of covalently bound [^{14}C]formaldehyde in the DNA from the respiratory mucosa of rats exposed for 6 h to 0.3, 2, 6, 10, or 15 ppm of [^{14}C]- and [^{3}H]-formaldehyde, 1 day after a single preexposure (6 h) to the same concentration of unlabeled formaldehyde. Values shown are mean ± SE; $n = 3$ groups of rats at each concentration (4 animals per group). [*From Casanova et al. (12).*]

approximately 90 percent (from approximately 3.04 to 0.30 μmole/g of tissue). Concentrations of NPSH in the livers of the same rats were decreased from approximately 7.2 to 0.68 μmole/g. The concentration of NPSH in nasal tissue remained low for approximately 5 h before beginning to rebound. Maximum depletions were achieved at a dose of 250–300 mg/kg, with administration of higher doses causing no further depletion of NPSH.

To investigate the effect of GSH depletion on DNA-protein crosslinking by formaldehyde, the percent IF DNA from the respiratory and olfactory mucosa of rats injected with phorone was compared with that of rats not injected with phorone. The results of these studies are summarized in Table 3. In rats injected with vehicle, there was a small increase in the percent IF DNA from the respiratory mucosa (Δ% = 4.96) as a result of exposure to 6 ppm of formaldehyde for 3 h. (This increase was expected, since earlier studies had shown that formaldehyde exposure at concentrations of 6 ppm and above increases the percent IF DNA from the respiratory mucosa of rats [11]). There was no detectable increase in the percent IF DNA from the olfactory mucosa as a result of exposure to 6 ppm of formaldehyde, consistent with the earlier studies.

Table 3 also shows that, in rats injected with phorone followed by exposure to 6 ppm of formaldehyde, there was a substantial increase in the percent IF DNA from the respiratory mucosa (Δ% = 15.05). Thus, the increase in the yield of interfacial DNA resulting from formaldehyde exposure was approximately threefold larger in rats injected with phorone than in control rats injected with vehicle. However, no significant increase in the percent IF

Table 3 Percent Interfacial DNA from Respiratory and Olfactory Mucosa of Rats (unexposed or exposed to formaldehyde [6 ppm, 3 h/day, 2 days]) Injected Either with Vehicle or with Phorone (250 mg/kg)*

		Formaldehyde concentration		
Nasal mucosa	**Treatment**	**0 ppm**	**6 ppm**	**Δ%**
Respiratory	Corn oil	15.08 ± 1.67	20.04 ± 2.10	4.96 ± 2.68
	Phorone	12.14 ± 1.36	27.19 ± 0.97	15.05 ± 1.67
Olfactory	Corn oil	10.94 ± 1.06	10.61 ± 0.58	−0.33 ± 1.21
	Phorone	9.95 ± 2.25	10.95 ± 0.99	1.00 ± 2.46

*Rats were injected i.p. either with phorone dissolved in corn oil or with corn oil 1 h prior to the second exposure to formaldehyde, and they were sacrificed immediately after the exposure. Percent interfacial DNA was determined as described previously (11). Values are mean ± SD; n = 3 groups of rats in each treatment group (3 rats per animal group), except for the 0 ppm-phorone treatment group, where n = 7 animal groups.

DNA from the olfactory mucosa was noted. Importantly, phorone alone, i.e., without simultaneous formaldehyde exposure, caused no detectable increase in the percent IF DNA from either the respiratory or the olfactory mucosa. Thus, depletion of GSH diminished the capacity of the respiratoy mucosa to protect itself against DNA-protein crosslinking by exogenous formaldehyde, but depletion itself did not result in detectable DNA-protein crosslinking by endogenous formaldehyde. These results indicate, first, that oxidation of formaldehyde by FDH is an important defense mechanism, and second, that depletion of GSH does not itself cause DNA-protein crosslinking; simultaneous exposure to exogenous formaldehyde is necessary for this reaction to occur.

DEPLETION OF SULFHYDRYL GROUPS IN THE NASAL MUCOSA BY INHALATION OF ACROLEIN

The reaction of acrolein with sulfhydryl compounds is rapid and essentially irreversible, resulting in the formation of a thiol ether (18). In the case of glutathione, this reaction is complete within seconds at millimolar concentrations of the thiol (pH 7.4, 20°C) (19) Acrolein has been shown to deplete glutathione in isolated rat hepatocytes (20), and sulfhydryl compounds (such as N-acetylcysteine) protect against the toxicity of acrolein in vitro (21). In addition, acrolein can react with sulfhydryl groups in the active sites of enzymes, causing a loss of enzyme activity (22-24). Hence, it would be expected that inhalation exposure to acrolein might decrease the concentrations of nonprotein and protein sulfhydryl groups in nasal mucosal tissue.

The concentrations of NPSH, total sulfhydryls, and protein sulfhydryls (PSH) in the respiratory and olfactory mucosa were determined in rats exposed to selected concentrations of acrolein for 3 h (Table 4). At concentrations above 0.1 ppm, acrolein significantly depleted the NPSH concentration of the respiratory mucosa. In contrast, the concentration of PSH was lowered only slightly, if at all. A small decrease in the concentration of NPSH but no decrease in the concentration of PSH was observed in the olfactory mucosa.

The greater depletion of NPSH than of PSH indicates that nonprotein sulfhydryls in the nasal mucosa react more readily than protein sulfhydryls with inhaled acrolein. This result suggests that most of the PSH in the nasal mucosa are inaccessible owing to protein folding. It is also possible that the greater reactivity of acrolein with NPSH was due, in part, to a glutathione transferase-mediated reaction between GSH and glycidaldehyde, the latter having been identified as a metabolite of acrolein in vitro (25). Glycidaldehyde is a substrate for hepatic glutathione-S-epoxide transferase (26, 27). However, no direct evidence has been presented that acrolein is metabolized to glycidaldehyde in vivo.

Table 4 Sulfhydryl Concentrations in the Respiratory and Olfactory Mucosa of Acrolein-exposed Rats*

Acrolein (ppm)	Nonprotein SH (μmole/g tissue)	Total SH (μmole/g tissue)	Protein SH (μmole/g tissue)
Respiratory mucosa			
0.0	2.58 ± 0.21 (100%)	12.30 ± 0.09 (100%)	9.72 ± 0.23 (100%)
0.1	2.09 ± 0.21 (81%)	12.01 ± 0.10 (98%)	9.92 ± 0.23 (102%)
0.5	1.66 ± 0.04† (64%)	10.59 ± 0.11† (86%)	8.93 ± 0.12 (92%)
1.0	1.38 ± 0.19† (53%)	9.90 ± 0.22† (81%)	8.52 ± 0.29 (88%)
2.4	0.98 ± 0.03† (38%)	10.16 ± 0.46† (83%)	9.18 ± 0.46 (94%)
Olfactory mucosa			
0.0	2.71 ± 0.11 (100%)	13.29 ± 0.22 (100%)	10.58 ± 0.25 (100%)
0.1	2.95 ± 0.13 (109%)	12.71 ± 0.38 (96%)	9.76 ± 0.40 (92%)
0.5	2.85 ± 0.24 (105%)	12.73 ± 0.11 (96%)	9.48 ± 0.26 (90%)
1.0	2.09 ± 0.16† (77%)	12.72 ± 0.30 (96%)	10.63 ± 0.34 (100%)
2.4	1.97 ± 0.09† (73%)	11.81 ± 0.48 (89%)	9.84 ± 0.49 (93%)

*Rats were exposed to selected concentrations of acrolein for 3 h and were sacrificed immediately after exposure. NPSH concentrations were determined by a modification of the method described by Casanova-Schmitz et al. (15). Total SH concentrations were determined by the method of Sedlak and Lindsay (29). Values are mean ± SE; $n = 4$ rats, analyzed individually.

†Denotes significant differences ($p < 0.05$) from 0 ppm exposure group, following treatment of the data by ANOVA and Scheffé's test (30).

POSSIBLE POTENTIATION OF FORMALDEHYDE TOXICITY BY ACROLEIN

The data summarized in this paper and elsewhere (12) demonstrate that inhalation exposure to formaldehyde at concentrations equal to or greater than 2 ppm results in the formation of DNA-protein crosslinks in the respiratory mucosa of the rat, and that crosslinking of DNA to proteins by formaldehyde depends nonlinearly on the formaldehyde concentration at low concentrations of the aldehyde. In addition, evidence has been presented that DNA-protein crosslinking by formaldehyde is enhanced by depletion of GSH, implying an important role for glutathione and FDH in defense against toxic injury by inhaled formaldehyde.

Acrolein exposure at concentrations equal to or greater than 0.5 ppm significantly lowered the concentration of respiratory mucosal NPSH. In contrast, no depletions of NPSH were detected when rats were exposed repeatedly to 15 ppm of formaldehyde (15). The differing effects of acrolein and formaldehyde on respiratory mucosal NPSH concentrations are consistent with the stabilities of the adducts formed between GSH and the two aldehydes.

Environmental exposure to formaldehyde and acrolein frequently involves a simultaneous exposure to both compounds. For example, the concentration of both aldehydes in cigarette smoke is approximately the same (5, 6). The present studies suggest that the toxicologic effects of formaldehyde may be enhanced by a concurrent exposure to low concentrations of acrolein. In addition to being competitive agonists for receptors associated with the trigeminal nerve (28), acrolein and formaldehyde can also compete for glutathione in the respiratory mucosa. Depletion of GSH by acrolein could increase the concentration of DNA-protein crosslinks produced by formaldehyde in comparison to that which would result from exposure to formaldehyde alone. (In principle, acrolein can also react with cellular DNA, but conclusive evidence that this reaction occurs either in vivo or in cell culture is currently lacking [2].) Investigations of the possible potentiating effects of acrolein on DNA-protein crosslinking by formaldehyde would elucidate the toxicologic significance of exposures to mixtures of both compounds.

SUMMARY

Formaldehyde and acrolein are very potent upper respiratory tract irritants. Both compounds react rapidly with thiols to form either a reversible hemithioacetal adduct (formaldehyde) or a stable thiol ether (acrolein). The hemithioacetal adduct of formaldehyde with glutathione (GSH) is the substrate for the enzyme formaldehyde dehydrogenase (FDH), and the activity of FDH is relatively high in homogenates of the rat nasal respiratory mucosa. Inhalation of formaldehyde at concentrations equal to or greater than 2 ppm caused DNA-protein crosslinking to occur in the rat nasal respiratory mucosa, the target tissue in the chronic bioassay of formaldehyde. The yield of DNA-protein crosslinks was higher in rats depleted of GSH (by i.p. injection with phorone) and exposed to 6 ppm of formaldehyde than in rats injected with vehicle and exposed to formaldehyde. When rats were exposed to acrolein at concentrations above 0.1 ppm, there was a significant depletion of nonprotein sulfhydryls (NPSH) in the nasal respiratory mucosa. Detectable depletions of NPSH in the olfactory mucosa occurred only at acrolein concentrations equal to or greater than 1 ppm. In neither tissue was there a measurable change in the concentration of protein sulfhydryls as a result of acrolein exposure. Unlike acrolein, formaldehyde did not deplete nasal respiratory NPSH, even at concentrations as high as 15 ppm. These results indicate that oxidation of formaldehyde catalyzed by FDH is an important defense mechanism against formaldehyde-induced DNA-protein crosslinking, and they suggest that simultaneous exposure to acrolein could potentiate the toxicity of formaldehyde by depleting GSH in the target tissue.

REFERENCES

1 Webber, D. Basic chemical output returns to growth. *Chem. Eng. News* 62(19):8–10 (1984).

2 Beauchamp, RO Jr., KT Morgan, AD Kligerman, DA Andjelkovich, and Hd'A Heck. A critical review of the literature on acrolein toxicity. *CRC Crit. Rev. Toxicol.* 14:309-380 (1985).
3 Lipari, F, and SJ Swarin. Determination of formaldehyde and other aldehydes in automobile exhaust with an improved 2,4-dinitrophenylhydrazine method. *J. Chromatogr.* 247:297-306 (1982).
4 Bailey, RA, HM Clark, JP Ferris, S Krause, and RL Strong. *Chemistry of the Environment.* New York: Academic Press, p. 268 (1978).
5 Mansfield, CT, BT Hodge, RB Hege Jr, and WC Hamlin. Analysis of formaldehyde in tobacco smoke by high performance liquid chromatography. *J. Chromatogr. Sci.* 15:301-302 (1977).
6 Horton, AD, and MR Guerin. Determination of acetaldehydes and acrolein in the gas phase of cigarette smoke using cryothermal gas chromatography. *Tobacco Sci.* 18:19-22 (1974).
7 Ross, WE, and N Shipley. Relationship between DNA damage and survival in formaldehyde-treated mouse cells. *Mutat. Res.* 79:277-283 (1980).
8 Grafstrom, RC, AJ Fornace, H Autrup, JF Lechner, and CC Harris. Formaldehyde damage to DNA and inhibition of DNA repair in human bronchial cells. *Science* 220:216-218 (1983).
9 Goldmacher, VS, and WG Thilly. Formaldehyde is mutagenic for cultured human cells. *Mutat. Res.* 116:417-422 (1983).
10 Kerns, WD, KL Pavkov, DJ Donofrio, MM Connell, RI Mitchell, EJ Gralla, and JA Swenberg. Carcinogenicity of formaldehyde in rats and mice after long-term inhalation exposure. *Cancer Res.* 43:4382-4392 (1983).
11 Casanova, M, and Hd'A Heck. Effects of formaldehyde exposure on the extractability of DNA from proteins in the rat nasal mucosa. *Toxicol. Appl. Pharmacol.* 70:121-132 (1983).
12 Casanova, M, TB Starr, and Hd'A Heck. Differentiation between metabolic incorporation and covalent binding in the labeling of macromolecules in the rat nasal mucosa and bone marrow by inhaled [^{14}C]- and [^{3}H]formaldehyde. *Toxicol. Appl. Pharmacol.* 76:26-44 (1984).
13 Swenberg, JA, EA Gross, HW Randall, and CS Barrow. The effect of formaldehyde exposure on cytotoxicity and cell proliferation. In *Formaldehyde: Toxicology, Epidemiology and Mechanisms,* edited by JJ Clary, JE Gibson, and RS Waritz. New York: Dekker, pp. 225-236 (1983).
14 Von Hippel, PH, and K-Y Wong. Dynamic aspects of native DNA structure: Kinetics of the formaldehyde reaction with calf thymus DNA. *J. Mol. Biol.* 61:587-613 (1971).
15 Casanova, M, RM David, and Hd'A Heck. Oxidation of formaldehyde and acetaldehyde by NAD^+-dependent dehydrogenases in rat nasal mucosal homogenates. *Biochem. Pharmacol.* 33:1137-1142 (1984).
16 Uotila, L, and M Koivusalo. Formaldehyde dehydrogenase from human liver. Purification, properties, and evidence for the formation of glutathione thiol esters by the enzyme. *J. Biol. Chem.* 249:7653-7663 (1974).
17 Uotila, L, and B Mannervik. A steady-state-kinetic model for formaldehyde dehydrogenase from human liver. A mechanism involving NAD^+ and the hemimercaptal adduct of glutathione and formaldehyde as substrates and

free glutathione as an allosteric activator of the enzyme. *Biochem. J.* 177: 869–878 (1979).

18 Smith, CW. *Acrolein.* New York: Wiley, (1962).

19 Esterbauer, H, H Zollner, and N Scholz. Reaction of glutathione with conjugated carbonyls. *Z. Naturforsch.* C30:466–473 (1975).

20 Zitting, A, and T Heinonen. Decrease of reduced glutathione in isolated rat hepatocytes caused by acrolein, acrylonitrile, and the thermal degradation products of styrene copolymers. *Toxicology* 17:333–341 (1980).

21 Dawson, JR, K Norbeck, I Anundi, and P Moldéus. The effectiveness of N-acetylcysteine in isolated hepatocytes, against the toxicity of paracetamol, acrolein, and paraquat. *Arch. Toxicol.* 55:11–15 (1984).

22 Rando, RR. Allyl alcohol-induced irreversible inhibition of yeast alcohol dehydrogenase. *Biochem. Pharmacol.* 23:2328–2331 (1974).

23 Wilton, DC. Acrolein, an irreversible active-site-directed inhibitor of deoxyribose 5-phosphate aldolase? *Biochem. J.* 153:495–497 (1976).

24 Gurtoo, HL, AJ Marinello, RF Struck, B Paul, and RP Dahms. Studies on the mechanism of denaturation of cytochrome P-450 by cyclophosphamide and its metabolites. *J. Biol. Chem.* 256:11691–11701 (1981).

25 Patel, JM, JC Wood, and KC Leibman. The biotransformation of allyl alcohol and acrolein in rat liver and lung preparations. *Drug Metab. Dispos.* 8:305–308 (1980).

26 Fjellstedt, TA, RH Allen, BK Duncan, and WB Jakoby. Enzymatic conjugation of epoxides with glutathione. *J. Biol. Chem.* 248:3702–3707 (1973).

27 Hayakawa, T, S Udenfriend, H Yagi, and DM Jerina. Substrates and inhibitors of hepatic glutathione-S-epoxide transferase. *Arch. Biochem. Biophys.* 170:438–451 (1975).

28 Kane, LE, and Y Alarie. Evaluation of sensory irritation from acrolein-formaldehyde mixtures. *Am. Ind. Hyg. Assoc. J.* 39:270–274 (1978).

29 Sedlak, J, and RH Lindsay. Estimation of total, protein-bound, and nonprotein sulfhydryl groups in tissue with Ellman's reagent. *Anal. Biochem.* 25:192–205 (1968).

30 Downie, NM, and RW Heath. *Basic Statistical Methods,* 3rd Ed. New York: Harper and Row, pp. 221–222 (1970).

Chapter 15

Bioactivation and Biotransformation of Xenobiotics in Rat Nasal Tissue

James A. Bond

INTRODUCTION

Biotransformation of xenobiotics, such as polycyclic aromatic hydrocarbons (PAH) found in inhaled environmental pollutants, is generally considered essential for the mutagenic, carcinogenic, and/or toxic effects of these xenobiotics on lung tissue. Biotransformation studies of respiratory tract tissue have focused primarily on lung homogenates (1), cultured lung cells (2), cultured tracheal-bronchial explants (3), and isolated perfused lung preparations (4) to more fully assess the activities of both activating and inactivating lung tissue enzymes responsible for the overall biotransformation of xenobiotics. Only recently, however, have reports appeared in the literature describing nasal tissue metabolism of xenobiotics (5-9), despite its potential role as a first line of defense against inhaled xenobiotics. The importance of studying nasal tissue

This research was supported under U.S. Department of Energy (DOE) Contract No. DE-AC04-76EV01013 and conducted in facilities fully accredited by the American Association for Accreditation of Laboratory Animal Care. The author gratefully acknowledges Drs. B. Smith, A. Dahl, W. Hadley, R. Wolff, R. Henderson, and R. McClellan for their helpful comments and encouragement regarding the work presented in this paper, and the useful discussions with a number of other colleagues at the institute. The author also acknowledges the excellent technical assistance of F. Straus, N. Stephens, A. Federman, R. Shimizu, M. Trujillo, and T. Carmack for their assistance in these studies.

metabolism becomes particularly important when it is recognized that many airborne materials, including environmental pollutants, contain known carcinogens adsorbed onto particles of sizes that deposit in the nasopharyngeal region of the respiratory tract (10, 11).

This report describes the capacity of rat nasal tissue to metabolize PAH and to bioactivate PAH to mutagens. Data are presented on nasal tissue oxidative and nonoxidative enzyme activities, including aryl hydrocarbon hydroxylase (AHH), epoxide hydrolase, UDP-glucuronyltransferase, and glutathione transferase. In addition, the ability of different inducing agents to enhance the nasal tissue enzymes under investigation is described. Results from these studies indicate that rat nasal tissue metabolizes PAH to reactive metabolites that are bacterial mutagens. The data demonstrate that rat nasal tissue may play an important role in the metabolic fate of inhaled xenobiotics.

MATERIALS AND METHODS

Chemicals

[7,10-^{14}C] Benzo[a] pyrene (BaP) (29.7 mCi/mmole) and [7-^{3}H] styrene oxide (90 mCi/mmole) (98 percent pure) were purchased from Amersham Searle Inc., Arlington Heights, IL. 1-Nitro[4,5,9,10-^{14}C] pyrene (NP) (43 mCi/mmole) was custom-synthesized by Amersham Searle, Inc. Both [^{14}C] BaP and [^{14}C] NP were purified by preparative liquid chromatography to a radiochemical purity of $>$99 percent, as determined by high-performance liquid chromatography (HPLC). NP was prepared and purified ($>$99.95 percent) as previously described (12). BaP (98 percent pure) and styrene oxide were obtained from Aldrich Chemical Co., Milwaukee, WI. Umbelliferone, NADPH, NADH, uridine-5′-diphosphoglucuronic acid, glutathione (GSH), phenobarbital (PB), and 3-methylcholanthrene (3-MC) were purchased from Sigma Chemical Co., St. Louis, MO. Aroclor 1254 was purchased from Analabs Inc., North Haven, CT. Tetrachlorodibenzo-*p*-dioxin (TCDD) was a generous gift from Dr. W. Greenlee, Chemical Industry Institute of Toxicology, Research Triangle Park, NC. Methanol (spectro quality) and dimethyl sulfoxide (DMSO) were purchased from Burdick and Jackson Laboratories, Inc., Muskegon, MI. BaP metabolite standards were obtained through the National Cancer Institute Chemical Carcinogen Reference Standard Repository, and NP metabolite standards were a generous gift of Dr. Frederick Beland of the National Center for Toxicological Research, Jefferson, AR. All other chemicals used were of the highest purity commercially available.

Animals

Male F344 rats (18–20 weeks; ~300 g) were used in all studies. Rats (specific pathogen-free) were born and raised in the institute's barrier maintained colony.

At 12-15 weeks of age they were removed from the breeding colony and housed in adult colonies. Rats were housed 2-3 per cage in polycarbonate cages with sterilized hardwood chip bedding and filter tops. Animal rooms were maintained at 20-22°C with a relative humidity of 20-50% and a 12-h light: 12-h dark cycle. Food (Lab-Blox; Allied Mills, Chicago, IL) and water were provided ad libitum, except during the inhalation exposure (see below).

Tissue Preparation

All rats were asphyxiated with CO_2. Rats were exsanguinated by severing the dorsal aorta and the vena cava. Sections of liver and the whole lung were immediately removed and placed in ice-cold 1.15% KCl in 0.1 M sodium phosphate buffer (pH 7.4). The head was split down the midline, and the maxilloturbinates, ethmoturbinates, and nasal epithelial membrane (collectively referred to as nasal tissue) from each rat were picked from the bony structures of the nasal cavity with forceps and immediately placed in ice-cold 0.1 M potassium phosphate buffer (pH 7.4). Liver, lung, and nasal tissue were rinsed in their respective buffers three times and homogenized in buffer using a Tissumizer (Tekmar, Cincinnati, OH). Homogenates were centrifuged at 9000*g* for 20 min at 4°C, and supernatant fractions were collected as previously described (13). For measurements of GSH transferase activity, nasal tissue S-9 was further centrifuged (4°C) for 60 min at 100,000*g*, and the supernatant was collected. Portions of supernatant (S-9 and 100,000*g*) were removed from each sample before freezing at −80°C for determination of protein content by the Lowry method (14).

Salmonella Mutagenesis Assay

Nasal, liver, and lung S-9 tissue were tested for their ability to alter the mutagenicity of BaP and NP in the Ames Salmonella/mammalian microsome assay (15). Tissues were assayed for bioactivation capacity in tester strains TA-98, TA-100, and TA-98NR (nitroreductase-deficient) at four concentrations of BaP (12, 25, 37.5 and 50 μg/plate) and NP (0.25, 0.5, 0.75, and 1.0 μg/plate). The concentrations of promutagens used were previously shown to be below the toxic level for these tester strains. Revertant colonies were counted on an Artek model 880 automatic colony counter interfaced to an Artek-Compuprint programmed to correct counts out of the linear range of the instrument. Results are reported as the slopes ± standard deviation (revertant/μg) of the dose-response curve determined by least-squares linear regression.

Enzyme Assays

Analysis of the rates of formation of NP and BaP metabolites using rat liver, lung, and nasal tissue were determined according to a modified version of a previously published method for BaP (16). Assay mixtures were incubated in the dark by shaking in a Dubnoff incubator at 37°C for 30 min under air. Typical incubation flasks contained (final concentrations) NADPH (800 μM), NADH (1 mM), [^{14}C] BaP (250,000 dpm; 6 μM–nasal tissue, 10 μM–lung, and 20 μM–liver) or [^{14}C] NP (250,000 dpm; 10 μM–lung and nasal tissue, 20 μM–liver), tissue S-9 (1 mg), and sufficient buffer to bring the total reaction volume to 1.0 ml. All samples were run in duplicate, and reactions were started by addition of either BaP or NP. Reaction rates were zero-order with respect to BaP or NP and NADPH, and linear with time and protein concentration.

After incubation of BaP and NP with liver, lung, or nasal tissue, each incubation mixture was extracted twice with ethyl acetate, and organic extracts containing either BaP or NP metabolites from duplicate incubation flasks were pooled. Pooled extracts were evaporated to dryness under gentle nitrogen flow in subdued yellow light. BaP metabolites were separated by HPLC, as previously described (7, 13). NP metabolites were also separated by HPLC, as previously described (17). Fractions (30 sec) of eluate were collected (LKB Instruments, Gaithersburg, MD) directly into mini-liquid scintillation counting vials. Scintillation cocktail was added, and the samples were counted in a Packard model 460C liquid scintillation counter. Quench correction was performed by the automatic external standard method, with counting efficiencies of $>$ 88 percent. Retention times of the radioactive metabolites were compared with authentic BaP or NP metabolites.

Epoxide hydrolase activity in rat nasal tissue S-9, using styrene oxide as substrate, was measured by a modified version (7) of a previously published method (18). Specific activities are expressed as nmole styrene glycol formed per mg protein per min after subtraction of control values.

UDP-glucuronyltransferase activity in rat nasal tissue S-9, using umbelliferone as substrate, was measured by a modified version (7) of a previously published method (19). Quantities of umbelliferone conjugated were expressed as nmole conjugate per mg protein per min after subtraction of background activity.

GSH transferase activity in rat nasal tissue 100,000*g* supernatant, using styrene oxide as substrate, was determined by a modified version (7), of a previously published method (20). Specific activities were expressed as nmole conjugate per mg protein per min after subtraction of values obtained from control incubation.

Treatment of Rats with Inducing Agents

All compounds, except inhaled BaP (see below), were administered i.p. PB was dissolved in 0.9 percent NaCl solution and administered at 80 mg/kg/day for 3 days; rats were killed on day 4. 3-MC was dissolved in corn oil and administered at a dose of 20 mg/kg/day for 2 days; rats were killed on day 3. A single injection of Aroclor 1254 in corn oil (200 mg/kg) was given, and rats were killed on day 5. TCDD in *p*-dioxane was administered as a single dose of 32 μg/kg, and rats were sacrificed 48 h later. Control rats received the appropriate vehicle (1 ml/kg).

To investigate the effects of inhaled BaP on the in vitro metabolism of BaP, rats were exposed to an aerosol concentration of BaP (200 μg/liter of air) in the exposure chamber. Rats were exposed nose-only (21) to BaP aerosols for 30 min for 4 consecutive days. The mass median aerodynamic diameter was 1.7-2.2 μm, with a geometric standard deviation of 1.4-1.9 for the exposures. All rats were sacrificed 24 h after the last exposure, and nasal tissue was immediately removed for assays as described above. Control rats were exposed (nose-only) to air under the same conditions as the BaP-exposed rats.

RESULTS

Enzyme activities of AHH (with either BaP or NP as substrate), epoxide hydrolase, UDP-glucuronyltransferase, and GSH transferase were measured in rat nasal tissue (Table 1). The specific activities for the nonoxidative enzymes were about 10–1000 times greater than those measured for nasal tissue AHH with either BaP or NP as substrate. Rat nasal tissue S-9 metabolized BaP to several oxidized metabolites, including BaP-9,10-diol, BaP-4,5-diol, BaP-7,8-diol, BaP-1,6-quinone, BaP-3,6-quinone, BaP-6,12-quinone, 9-OH-BaP, 3-OH-BaP, and BaP-tetrols (Fig. 1). The major metabolites detected were 3-OH-BaP and BaP-3,6-quinone with rates of about 5-7 pmole/mg protein/min measured for the formation of these metabolites. Rat nasal tissue metabolized NP to oxidized metabolites, including 3-,6- and 8-hydroxynitropyrenes (Fig. 2) with total rates of formation of these metabolites of about 680 pmole/mg protein/min. A comparison of the rates of formation of total BaP and NP metabolites formed by liver, lung, and nasal tissue (Fig. 3) indicates that both BaP and NP are metabolized in liver at rates of about 300-500 pmole/mg protein/min—nearly 5-50 times greater than that measured in lung for each substrate. Formation of

Table 1 Activities of Some Nasal Tissue Enzymes

Enzyme assay	Substrate	Specific activity* (nmole/mg protein/min)
Aryl hydrocarbon hydroxylase	Benzo[a]pyrene	0.02 ± 0.002
	Nitropyrene	0.68 ± 0.03
Epoxide hydrolase	Styrene oxide	6.4 ± 1.3
UDP-glucuronyltransferase	7-Hydroxycoumarin	20.4 ± 1.2
Glutathione transferase	Styrene oxide	24.8 ± 1.0

*Mean ± SE of four separate experiments.

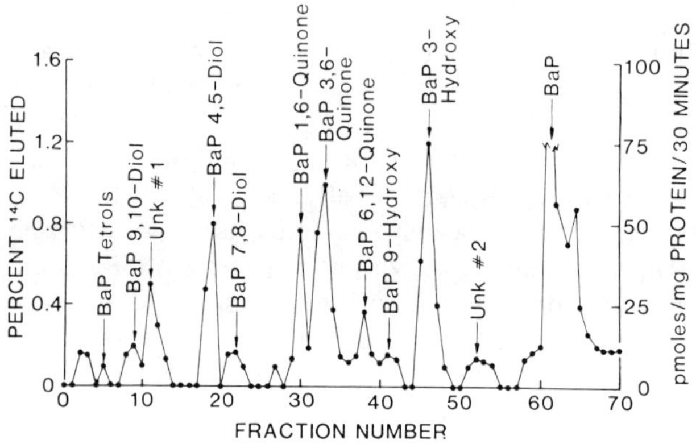

Figure 1 High-performance liquid chromatograph profile of BaP and metabolites formed after incubation for 30 min of nasal tissue S-9 with [^{14}C] BaP. Each point represents a 30-sec collection period. Peak fractions were compared with authentic BaP standards. [*From Bond and Li (13).*]

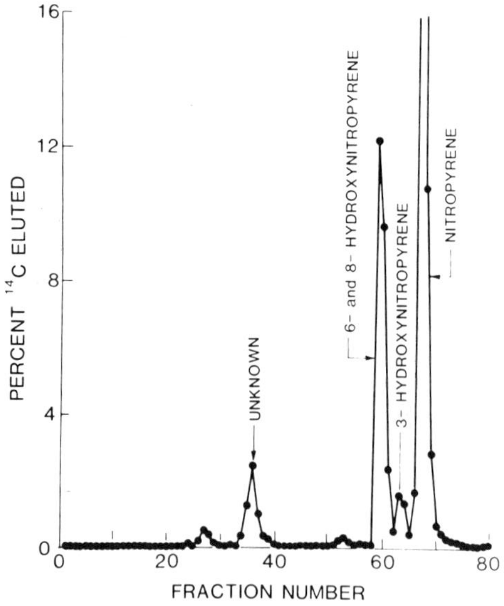

Figure 2 High-performance liquid chromatograph profile of NP and metabolites formed after incubation for 30 min of nasal tissue S-9 with [^{14}C] NP. Each point represents a 30-sec collection period. Peak fractions were compared with authentic NP standards. [*From Bond (17).*]

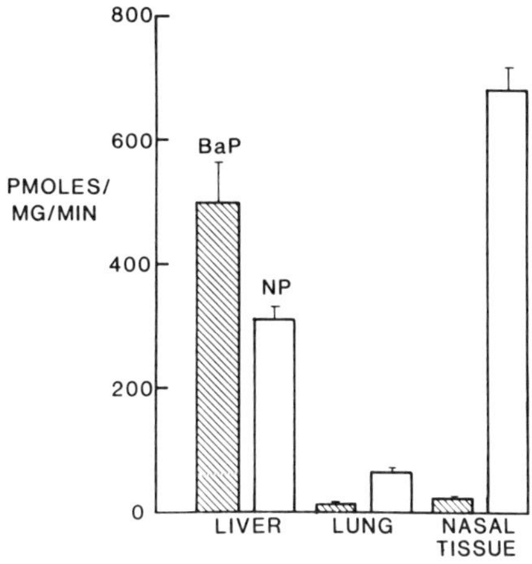

Figure 3 Rates of formation of BaP and NP metabolites in liver, lung, and nasal tissue S-9 of rats. Each bar represents the mean ± SE for 3–5 separate experiments.

NP metabolites in nasal tissue S-9 was about 30 times greater than that measured for BaP in nasal tissue (680 vs. 23 pmole/mg protein/min).

Pretreatment of rats with PB, 3-MC, or Aroclor 1254 resulted in no significant increase in rat nasal tissue AHH activity (BaP as substrate) (Fig. 4). Quantities of BaP metabolites were consistently decreased after pretreatment with these inducing agents, although the changes were not significant ($p > 0.05$).

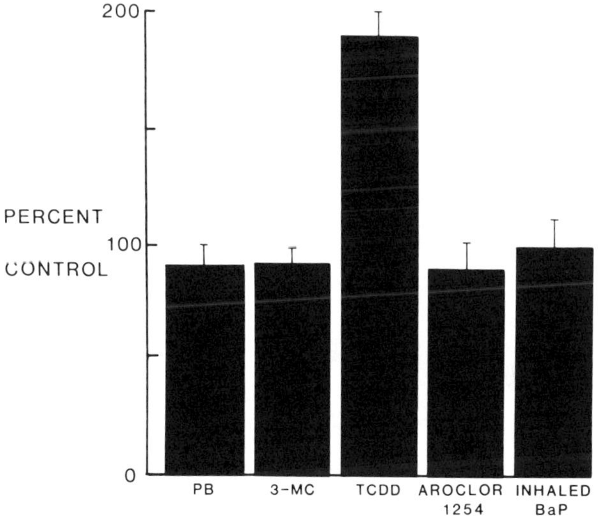

Figure 4 Quantities of BaP metabolites formed in nasal tissue from rats pretreated with phenobarbital (PB), 3-methylcholanthrene (3-MC), 2,3,7,8-tetrachlorodibenzo-*p*-dioxin (TCDD), Aroclor 1254, and BaP aerosol (inhaled BaP). Values are expressed as percent of untreated controls. Each bar represents the mean ± SE of three separate experiments.

Similarly, nasal tissue AHH activity in rats exposed nose-only to BaP aerosols was not significantly changed. Pretreatment of rats with i.p. TCDD, however, resulted in a twofold increase in nasal tissue metabolism of BaP (Fig. 4). TCDD induction of BaP metabolism in nasal tissue S-9 resulted in a slight shift in the quantities of individual BaP metabolites formed in incubation flasks. For example, the formation of BaP-7,8-diol, 9-OH-BaP, and 3-OH-BaP was increased 2.5-3 times (data not shown). Smaller increases in the quantities of the other BaP metabolites were also evident.

Liver, lung, and nasal tissue bioactivated both BaP and NP to mutagens, as detected in the Ames bacterial test system. BaP was weakly mutagenic in strain TA-100 when nasal tissue S-9 was used as the activating system (4 vs. 100 revertants/μg) (Fig. 5). NP has previously been shown to be a direct-acting bacterial mutagen. However, addition of rat liver, lung, and nasal tissue further bioactivated NP to mutagens (about 1.5 times the direct-acting response). NP was consistently more mutagenic than BaP in liver, lung, and nasal tissue. This difference was particularly evident when NP was tested in the presence of nasal tissue S-9. For example, NP was approximately 2-2.5 times more mutagenic than BaP in liver and lung S-9, but more than 100 times more mutagenic than BaP in nasal tissue (4 vs. 500 revertants/μg) (Fig. 5).

When NP was incubated in the presence of liver, lung, or nasal tissue S-9 and nitroreductase-deficient bacteria (TA-98NR), mutagenic responses were significantly decreased, compared to the mutagenic response in the normal tester strain TA-98 (Fig. 6). When liver and nasal tissue S-9 were incubated with NP and TA-98NR, the optimal mutagenic response was decreased about 35 percent. A 75 percent decrease in the mutagenic response was observed when lung tissue S-9 was incubated with NP and TA-98NR.

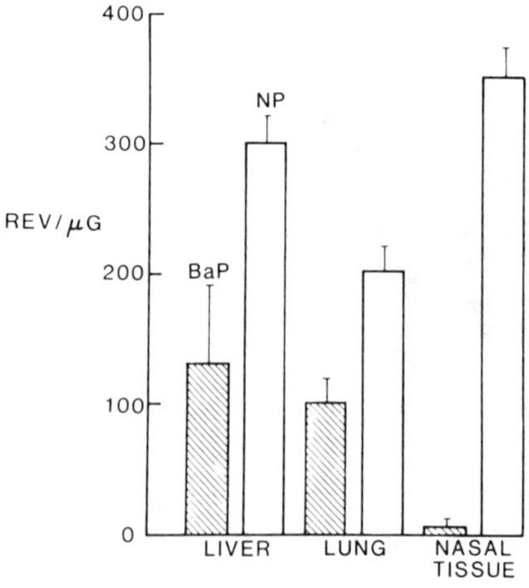

Figure 5 Optimal mutagenic responses of BaP and NP in *Salmonella typhimurium* strain TA-100 using rat nasal tissue, lung, and liver S-9. Values reported represent the mean slope ± SD of the dose-response curve without background revertants subtracted.

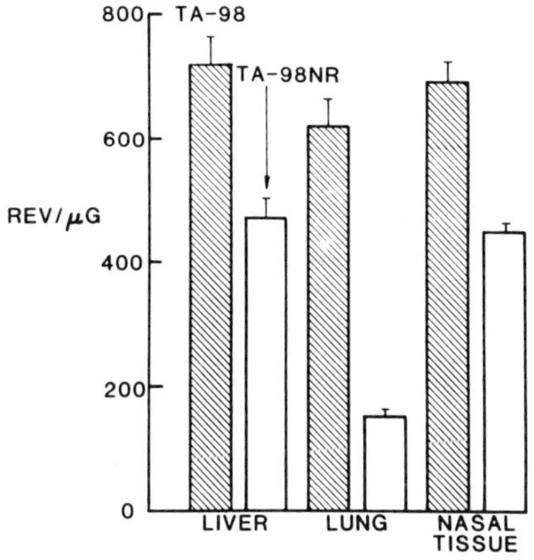

Figure 6 Optimal mutagenic responses of NP in *Salmonella typhimurium* strain TA-98 and TA-98NR using rat nasal tissue, lung, and liver S-9. Values reported represent the mean slope ± SD of the dose-response curve without background revertants subtracted.

DISCUSSION

Nasal tissue is exposed to a variety of atmospheric environmental pollutants, some of which are known carcinogens. The data presented in this report indicate that rat nasal tissue contains enzymes that can biotransform many xenobiotics. Activities of the nonoxidative enzymes measured were 2.5-3 orders of magnitude greater than those measured for the nasal monooxygenase (AHH) with either BaP or NP as substrate. Interestingly, NP appeared to be a better substrate than BaP for the nasal tissue monooxygenases, as evidenced by the observation that NP was metabolized at rates nearly 100 times faster than that measured for BaP.

BaP was metabolized by rat nasal tissue to dihydrodiols, quinones, and phenols at rates approximately twofold greater than that observed for lung microsomes. The in vitro formation of BaP-7,8-diol and BaP-tetrols suggests that rat nasal tissue can produce BaP-7,8-diol-9,10-epoxide, the ultimate carcinogenic metabolite of BaP. Although BaP appears to be actively metabolized by nasal tissue S-9, the results from the mutagenicity studies indicate that BaP is a very weak mutagen for *Salmonella typhimurium* when nasal tissue S-9 is used. The relatively small quantities of BaP-tetrols and the low diol:phenol ratio (2:3) observed in these studies may offer some explanation for the apparent low mutagenicity of BaP.

Nasal tissue metabolized NP at a rate about twice as fast as that seen in rat liver and more than 10 times that observed for rat lung. Nasal tissue metabolism of NP was about 100 times that observed for nasal tissue metabolism of BaP, suggesting that nasal tissue may contain either a single cytochrome P-450 with different affinities to substrates or several different forms of cytochrome P-450. The studies used combined nasal tissues taken from the maxilloturbinates, ethmoturbinates, and nasal epithelial membrane; all may contain different forms of cytochrome P-450. The major metabolites of NP detected were the 6- and 8-hydroxynitropyrenes, with smaller quantities of 3-hydroxynitropyrene. It was recently shown that hydroxynitropyrenes, specifically 3- and 6-hydroxynitropyrene, are mutagenic in the Ames bacterial test system (22). These data, coupled with the observations presented in this report, suggest that ring oxidation may be involved in the mutagenic activity of NP. Presumably, the formation of hydroxynitropyrenes, as catalyzed by nasal tissue S-9, proceeds through epoxide intermediates.

Liver and nasal tissue S-9 increased the mutagenic potency of NP, which in all strains tested was about 50–100 percent greater than that observed in lung tissue S-9. That the mutagenic response to NP in all tissues examined was significantly decreased when tester strain TA-98NR was used suggests that at least a portion of the mutagenic response toward NP in the normal tester strain TA-98 may be the result of bacterial reduction of the nitro group to mutagenic intermediates. It has been suggested that hydroxylaminopyrene, formed by reduction of the nitro group of NP, may be the ultimate mutagenic metabolite of NP. Under conditions of oxygen atmosphere similar to the incubations with bacteria, there was no evidence of the formation of any reduced metabolites of NP (e.g., aminopyrene) in nasal tissue S-9, suggesting that in incubation flasks oxidative metabolism is the predominant metabolic pathway of NP in nasal tissue.

Attempts to increase the metabolism of BaP by pretreating rats with various inducing agents resulted in rat nasal monooxygenases being induced only after pretreatment with TCDD. Further studies, however, are warranted to fully characterize the capacity of various inducing agents to enhance nasal tissue metabolism of xenobiotics.

The data presented here point to the potential importance of nasal tissue metabolism in determining the metabolic fate of inhaled xenobiotics. Several chemicals, including BaP (23), TCDD (24), hexamethylphosphoramide (25), 1,2-dibromo-3-chloropropane (26), 1,4-dioxane (27), and 1,2-dibromoethane (28), induce nasal tumors in experimental animals. Several of these compounds are metabolized by microsomal oxidation. It was recently demonstrated that rat nasal tissue metabolized N′-nitrosonornicotine, a nasal carcinogen, to metabolites that covalently bind to nasal tissue macromolecules (DNA, RNA, and protein) (29, 30). These data support the concept that nasal tissue is capable of bioactivating xenobiotics to reactive intermediates that can interact with nasal tissue macromolecules. The data presented here point to the potential importance of nasal tissue activation of PAH, and possibly other xenobiotics, to reactive intermediates that may be responsible for the formation of nasal tumors. Although no evidence exists that PAHs other than BaP induce nasal tumors, the susceptibility of animals and possibly humans to xenobiotic-induced nasal tumors may be related to the balance of nasal tissue toxification and detoxication enzymes and the role they play in determining the overall metabolic fate of inhaled xenobiotics.

SUMMARY

Respiratory tract biotransformation of many chemicals to inhaled environmental pollutants is generally considered essential for the mutagenic, carcinogenic, and/or toxic response of lung tissue to these chemicals. The metabolic capacity of rat nasal tissue is characterized in this report. Also presented are results that demonstrate that rat nasal tissue can bioactivate polycyclic aromatic hydrocarbons to bacterial mutagens. Oxidative and nonoxidative enzymes, including aryl hydrocarbon hydroxylase (AHH), epoxide hydrolase (EH), uridine 5′-diphosphoglucuronyltransferase (UDPGT), and glutathione transferase, were investigated. Specific enzyme activities (nmole product/mg protein/min) were: (1) AHH, benzo[a]pyrene: 0.02 nitropyrene: 0.68; (2) EH, 6.4; (3) UDPGT, 20.4; and (4) glutathione transferase, 24.8. Rat nasal tissue metabolized benzo[a]pyrene to several oxidized metabolites, including dihydrodiols, quinones, phenols, and tetrols. Nitropyrene, however, was metabolized by rat nasal tissue primarily to phenols. Pretreatment of rats with tetrachlorodibenzo-*p*-dioxin resulted in a twofold increase in nasal tissue metabolism of benzo[a]pyrene. Nasal tissue bioactivated both benzo[a]pyrene and nitropyrene to mutagens, as detected in the Ames bacterial test system. However, nitropyrene was more than 100 times more mutagenic in nasal tissue, compared to the response measured for benzo[a]pyrene (4 vs. 500 revertants/μg). The results indicate that rat nasal tissue contains both oxidative and nonoxidative enzymes capable of metabolizing xenobiotics to mutagens. The data demonstrate that rat nasal tissue may be important in determining the metabolic fate of inhaled xenobiotics.

REFERENCES

1 Watanabe, M, K Bonno, and H Sato. Properties of hydrocarbon (benzo[a]-pyrene) hydroxylase in lung microsomes of mice. *Gann* 69:1–8 (1978).

2 Bond, JA, CE Mitchell, and AP Li. Metabolism and macromolecular covalent binding of benzo[a]pyrene in cultured Fischer-344 rat lung type II epithelial cells. *Biochem. Pharmacol.* 32:3771–3776 (1983).

3 Yang, SK, HV Gelboin, BF Trump, H Autrup, and CC Harris. Metabolic activation of benzo[a]pyrene and binding to DNA in cultured human bronchus. *Cancer Res.* 37:1210–1215 (1977).

4 Ball LM, JL Plummer, BR Smith, and JR Bend. Benzo[a]pyrene oxidation, conjugation, and disposition in the isolated perfused rabbit lung: Role of the glutathione S-transferases. *Med. Biol.* 57:298–305 (1979).

5 Dahl, AR, WM Hadley, FF Hahn, JM Benson, and RO McClellan. Cytochrome P-450–dependent monooxygenases in olfactory epithelium of dogs: Possible role in tumorigenicity. *Science* 216:57–59 (1982).

6 Hadley, WM, AR Dahl, JM Benson, FF Hahn, and RO McClellan. Cytochrome P-450 dependent monooxygenases in nasal epithelial membranes: Effect of phenobarbital and benzo[a]pyrene. *Proc. West. Pharmacol. Soc.* 25:197–199 (1982).
7 Bond, JA. Some biotransformation enzymes responsible for polycyclic aromatic hydrocarbon metabolism in rat nasal turbinates: Effects on enzyme activities of in vitro modifiers and intraperitoneal and inhalation exposure of rats to inducing agents. *Cancer Res.* 43:4805–4811 (1983).
8 Hadley, WM, and AR Dahl. Cytochrome P-450 dependent monooxygenase activity in rat nasal epithelial membranes. *Toxicol. Lett.* 10:417–422 (1982).
9 Brittebo, EG. N-Demethylation of aminopyrene by the nasal mucosa in mice and rats. *Acta Pharmacol. Toxicol.* 51:227–232 (1982).
10 Natusch, DS, and JR Wallace. Urban aerosol toxicity: The influence of particle size. *Science* 186:695–699 (1974).
11 Task Group on Lung Dynamics. Deposition and retention models for internal dosimetry of the human respiratory tract. *Health Phys.* 12:173–207 (1966).
12 Li, AP, and JS Dutcher. Mutagenicity of mono-, di-, tri-nitropyrenes in Chinese hamster ovary cells. *Mutat. Res.* 119:387–392 (1983).
13 Bond, JA, and AP Li. Rat nasal tissue activation of benzo[a]pyrene and 2-aminoanthracene to mutagens in *Salmonella typhimurium*. *Environ. Mutagen.* 5:311–318 (1983).
14 Lowry, OH, NJ Rosebrough, AL Farr, and RJ Randall. Protein measurement with the Folin phenol reagent. *J. Biol. Chem.* 193:265–275 (1951).
15 Ames, BN, J McCann, and E Yamasaki. Methods for detecting carcinogens and mutagens with the *Salmonella*/mammalian microsome mutagenicity test. *Mutat. Res.* 31:347–364 (1975).
16 Bond, JA, CJ Omiecinski, and MR Juchau. Kinetics, activation, and induction of aortic monooxygenases–biotransformation of benzo[a]-pyrene. *Biochem. Pharmacol.* 28:305–311 (1979).
17 Bond, JA. Bioactivation and biotransformation of 1-nitropyrene in liver, lung and nasal tissue of rats. *Mutat. Res.* 124:315–324 (1983).
18 Oesch, F, DM Jerina, and J Daly. A radiometric assay for hepatic epoxide hydrase activity with [7-^{3}H]styrene oxide. *Biochim. Biophys. Acta* 227: 685–691 (1971).
19 Owens, IS. Genetic regulation of UDP-glucuronosyltransferase induction by polycyclic aromatic compounds in mice. *J. Biol. Chem.* 252:2827–2833 (1977).
20 Bond, JA, RM Kocan, EP Benditt, and MR Juchau. Oxidative and non-oxidative metabolism of polycyclic aromatic hydrocarbons in rabbit and chicken aortas and in human fetal smooth-muscle cells. In *Polynuclear Aromatic Hydrocarbons,* edited by PW Jones and P Leber, pp. 489–502. Ann Arbor, MI: Ann Arbor Science (1980).
21 Raabe, OG, JE Bennick, ME Light, CH Hobbs, RL Thomas, and MI Tillery. An improved apparatus for acute inhalation exposure of rodents to radioactive aerosols. *Toxicol. Appl. Pharmacol.* 26:264–273 (1973).

22 El-Bayoumy, K, SS Hecht, and EL Wynder. Identification and mutagenicity of metabolites of 1-nitropyrene formed by a rat liver. *Cancer Res.* 43:3132–3137 (1983).

23 Thyssen, J, J Altoff, G Kimmerle, and U Mohr. Inhalation studies with benzo[a]pyrene in Syrian golden hamsters. *JNCI* 66:575–577 (1981).

24 Kociba, RJ, DG Keyes, JE Beyer, RM Carreon, CE Wade, DA Henber, RP Kalnins, LE Frauson, CN Park, SD Barnard, RA Hummel, and CG Humiston. Results of a two-year chronic toxicity and oncogenicity study of 2,3,7,8-tetrachlorodibenzo-*p*-dioxin in rats. *Toxicol. Appl. Pharmacol.* 46:279–303 (1978).

25 Lee, KP, and HJ Trochimowicz. Induction of nasal tumors in rats exposed to hexamethylphosphoramide by inhalation. *JNCI* 68:157–171 (1982).

26 Reznik, G, H Reznik-Schuller, JM Ward, and SF Stinson. Morphology of nasal-cavity tumors in rats after chronic inhalation of 1,2-dibromo-3-chloropropane. *Br. J. Cancer* 42:772–781 (1980).

27 Kociba, RP, SB McCollister, C Park, and TR Torkelson. 1,4-Dioxane. I. Results of a two-year ingestion study in rats. *Toxicol. Appl. Pharmacol.* 30:275–286 (1974).

28 National Insitutes of Health, U.S. Department of Health and Human Services. Bioassay of 1,2-dibromoethane for possible carcinogenicity (inhalation study). Department of Health and Human Services Publication No. (NIH 80-1766). Washington: Government Printing Office (1980).

29 Brittebo, EB, and H Tjalve. Formation of tissue-bound N′-nitrosonornicotine metabolites by the target tissues of Sprague-Dawley and Fischer rats. *Carcinogenesis* 2:959–963 (1981).

30 Brittebo, EB, A Castomguay, JJ Rafter, B Kowalski, M Ahlman, and I Brandt. Metabolism of xenobiotics and steroid hormones in the nasal mucosa. In *Proceedings of the Seventh CIIT Conference on Toxicology: Toxicology of the Nasal Passages*, edited by CS Barrow, pp. 211–234. Washington: Hemisphere (1985).

Chapter 16

Possible Consequences of Cytochrome P-450-Dependent Monooxygenases in Nasal Tissues

Alan R. Dahl

INTRODUCTION

Nasal cytochrome P-450 occurs in dogs, rats, monkeys, rabbits, mice, Syrian hamsters, guinea pigs, and probably most, if not all, other animal species. In many species, the concentration of cytochrome P-450, averaged over the entire epithelium of the nasal cavity, is second only to that of liver (see Table 1). The concentration in the olfactory mucosa in monkeys, dogs, and rats–the only species in which the intranasal regional distribution has been studied–was much higher than that of the nasal respiratory mucosa (Fig. 1). Indeed, no cytochrome P-450 was found in the nasal respiratory mucosa in monkeys. In dogs, no cytochrome P-450 was detected in the vomeronasal organ, although it

This research was supported by the U.S. Department of Energy under Contract No. DE-AC04-76EV01013 and was conducted in facilities fully accredited by the American Association for Accreditation of Laboratory Animal Care. I thank my colleagues at the Inhalation Toxicology Research Institute for their interest in and support of research in nasal metabolism, and especially Melissa Behr for obtaining vomeronasal tissue from dogs.

Table 1 Concentrations of Cytochrome P-450 in Tissues (nmole P-450/mg microsomal protein)

Organ	Rat	Mouse	Rabbit	Guinea pig	Syrian hamster	Human
Liver	0.22–0.92	0.39–1.10	0.81--1.70	0.43–1.45	1.12	0.26–1.02
Nose	0.11	0.07	0.35	0.09	0.46	—
Kidney	0.05–0.21	0.40	0.14–0.36	0.32	—	0.03
Lung	0.04	—	0.27–0.38	0.07	0.15	—
Intestine	0.01–0.13	0.04	0.07–0.43	0.18	—	—
Skin	0.05	0.02	—	—	—	—

Dashes indicate no data available. [*From Vainio and Hietanen (26).*]

is known to contain high concentrations of smooth endoplasmic reticulum, where cytochrome P-450 usually occurs (1). The vomeronasal organs in other species were not examined for cytochrome P-450 content.

The substrate specificity of nasal cytochrome P-450 is different from that of the liver, so some substrates are more rapidly metabolized by nasal enzymes than by hepatic enzymes with equal amounts of microsomal protein (2-6). In Fig. 2, for example, are compared the rates of oxidation of the potent nasal carcinogen, hexamethylphosphoramide (HMPA), and benzo[a]pyrene (BaP) for dog nasal and liver microsomal enzymes.

Because the nose is the primary entry point for inhaled vapors and particles and is therefore a potential site for extensive metabolism of these materials, it is important to consider the possible consequences of metabolism by nasal cytochrome P-450 and to discuss to what extent the presence of these enzymes might explain observed toxicological phenomena. It is the purpose of this chapter to investigate some of the possible implications from current knowledge of the cytochrome P-450-dependent monooxygenases in nasal tissue.

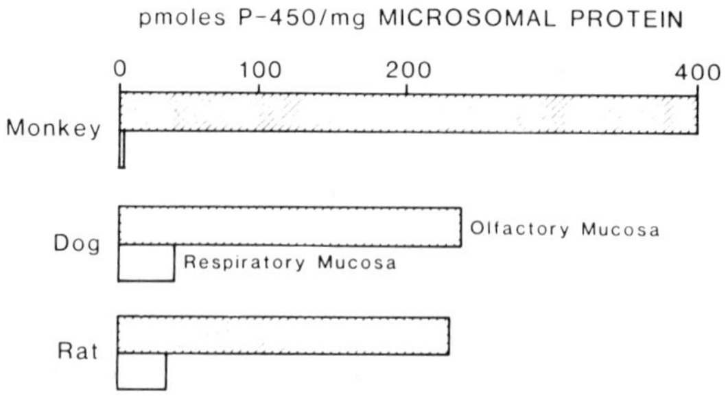

Figure 1 Distribution of nasal P-450 in dogs, rats, and cynomolgus monkeys.

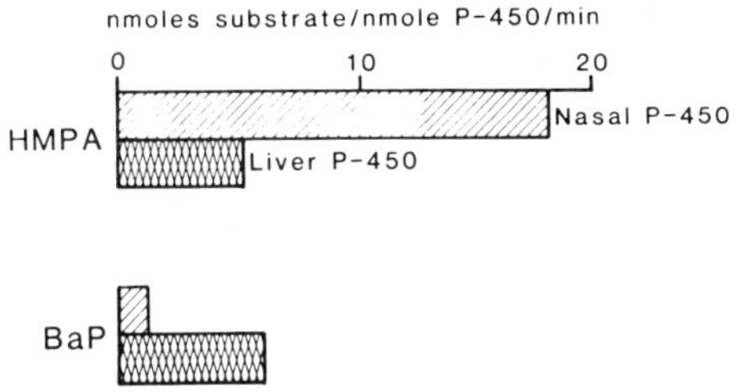

Figure 2 Rates of oxidation of hexamethylphosphoramide (HMPA) and benzo[a]pyrene (BaP) by dog nasal and liver microsomal cytochrome P-450.

MATERIALS AND METHODS

Preparation of Nasal Microsomal Cytochrome P-450

The exposure and dissection of the nasal cavity in preparing nasal microsomes has been described previously (2, 5). Briefly, rabbits and rodents were killed with carbon dioxide, and the skulls were split along the median sagittal line with a scalpel. The halves of the skull were pulled apart, exposing the brain and nasal cavity (Fig. 3). The nasal cavity was then dissected into ethmoturbinates (containing olfactory mucosa) and maxillonasoturbinates (containing respiratory mucosa). The procedure was similar for monkeys and dogs, except that a bone

STRUCTURE OF THE NASAL CAVITY

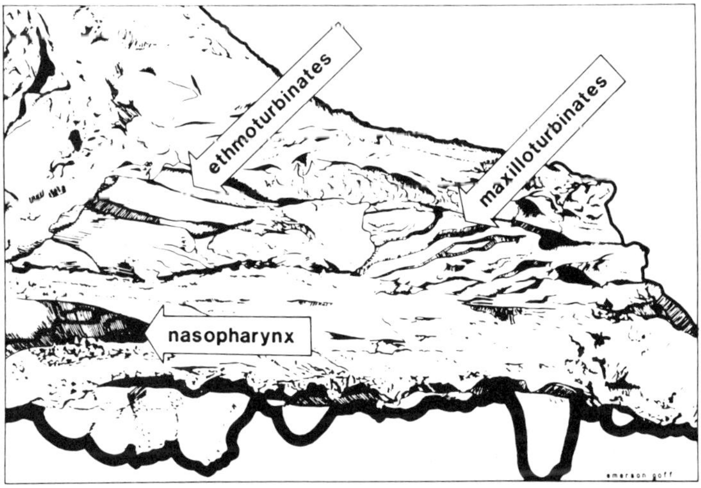

Figure 3 Sagittal median section of the dog nasal cavity.

saw was used to split their heavier skulls. In separate preparations where the dogs' heads were not split, the vomeronasal organs were located by cannulating the incisive ducts and were then exposed by removal of the cartilage shelf ventral to the organs. The stability of nasal microsomal cytochrome P-450 in storage is similar to liver microsomal P-450. Nasal microsomes stored at −75°C in 20% glycerol and Tris buffer pH 7.4 lost less than 10% of their HMPA N-demethylase activity in 2 months.

Enzyme Activity Assays with Nasal Cytochrome P-450

Assays with nasal cytochrome P-450 were like those used for microsomal preparations from other tissues. The following procedures and conditions have been reported: assays with nasal enzymes (2, 4, 5, 7-9); the use of nasal S-9 supernatant in *Salmonella* mutagenicity testing (4, 10); nasal aromatic hydrocarbon hydroxylase activity (AHH) in dogs and rats (2, 4, 9); induction studies with cytochrome P-450 (6, 9); and inhibition of nasal cytochrome P-450 by methylene dioxyphenyl (MDP) compounds (8, 11).

Calculations

The rate of N-nitrosopyrrolidine metabolism to carbon dioxide (Fig. 4) was derived from data from Brittebo et al. (12). The data were originally presented as carbon dioxide produced per gram of tissue. The concentration of cytochrome P-450 in tissue was derived from Hadley and Dahl (5, 7). The data from Brittebo et al. (12) were then converted to rates of carbon dioxide formation per ηmole P-450.

In calculations of the effect of nasal metabolism on the air concentrations of N,N-dimethylaniline reaching the lungs (see Results and Discussion), the following assumptions were made: (1) Only metabolism by nasal respiratory mucosa was considered. This leads to a *conservative* estimate. (2) Ninety percent of the inhaled DMA deposited on the nasal respiratory mucosa. The minute volume was 0.17 liter. (3) Thirteen percent of the total nasal P-450 is in the nasal respiratory mucosa, and the rate of metabolism of DMA was 0.0007 μmole per min (3). (4) Therefore, the maximum air concentration of DMA metabolized by nasal P-450 is 0.0007 μmole DMA/0.15 liter air. This is equivalent to 0.1 ppm. (Note 0.15 liter is 90 percent of the minute volume.)

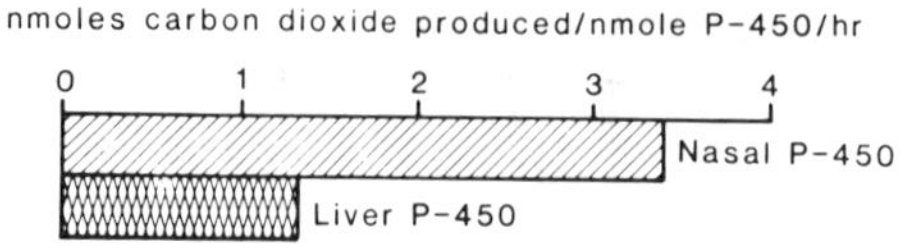

Figure 4 Metabolism of N-nitrosopyrrolidine by rat nasal and liver tissue.

RESULTS AND DISCUSSION

Three implications from the presence of nasal cytochrome P-450 are discussed below: (1) the production of toxic (carcinogenic) metabolites from inhaled compounds; (2) the protection of the lungs from vapors present at low concentrations in the air; and (3) the maintenance of acuity of the sense of smell by the removal of odorants from the olfactory epithelium.

Production of Toxic (Carcinogenic) Metabolites

Five examples that indicate the probable effect of nasal cytochrome P-450 on the toxicity of inhaled compounds are (1) aldehydes released by N- or O-dealkylation; (2) the release of electrophilic metal ions from organometallic compounds; (3) the production of epoxides from aromatic hydrocarbons; (4) the metabolism of methylene dioxyphenyl (MDP) compounds to carbenes that bind to and inhibit nasal cytochrome P-450; and (5) the activation of nitrosamines to carcinogenic alkylating agents.

Figure 5 contains examples of reactions that produce the various toxic metabolites. The first example (reaction A) is HMPA N-demethylation to produce the nasal carcinogen formaldehyde. A variety of other compounds also release formaldehyde in this way (3). Were ethyl groups to replace the methyl groups, acetaldehyde would be produced. Acetaldehyde is also a carcinogen (13). Metabolism by cytochrome P-450 potentially leads to intracellular release of aldehydes. Such aldehydes do not have to penetrate the mucus before causing DNA binding, protein binding, cell death, etc. Perhaps as a consequence, HMPA is a nasal carcinogen at 50 parts per billion (14) whereas carcinogenicity for formaldehyde first occurs at about 6 ppm (15). Many compounds besides HMPA can undergo demethylation to formaldehyde. Included are some commonly inhaled or instilled into the nose (3).

Reaction B in Fig. 5 depicts the release of electrophilic metal ions. The example given is the release of ferrous ion from ferrocene. The metabolism of ferrocene by nasal microsomes has not been directly demonstrated; however, in an experiment in which rats inhaled vapors of iron-59-labeled ferrocene, iron was retained for several weeks in the nose and in the lungs (16). The retention can be explained by metabolism. Ferrocene is metabolized by liver cytochrome P-450 (17) through reaction B in Fig. 5. Iron released intracellularly would rapidly bind protein, DNA, or whatever other nucleophilic biologic macromolecules or small molecules were available. Binding to macromolecules could lead to the observed long-term retention (Fig. 6). Thus, the long-term retention of iron-59 in the lung where P-450 was known to occur was explained. However, to explain the long-term retention in the nose, it was necessary to assume nasal cytochrome P-450. This observation led to the postulation of the presence of nasal cytochrome P-450 (16).

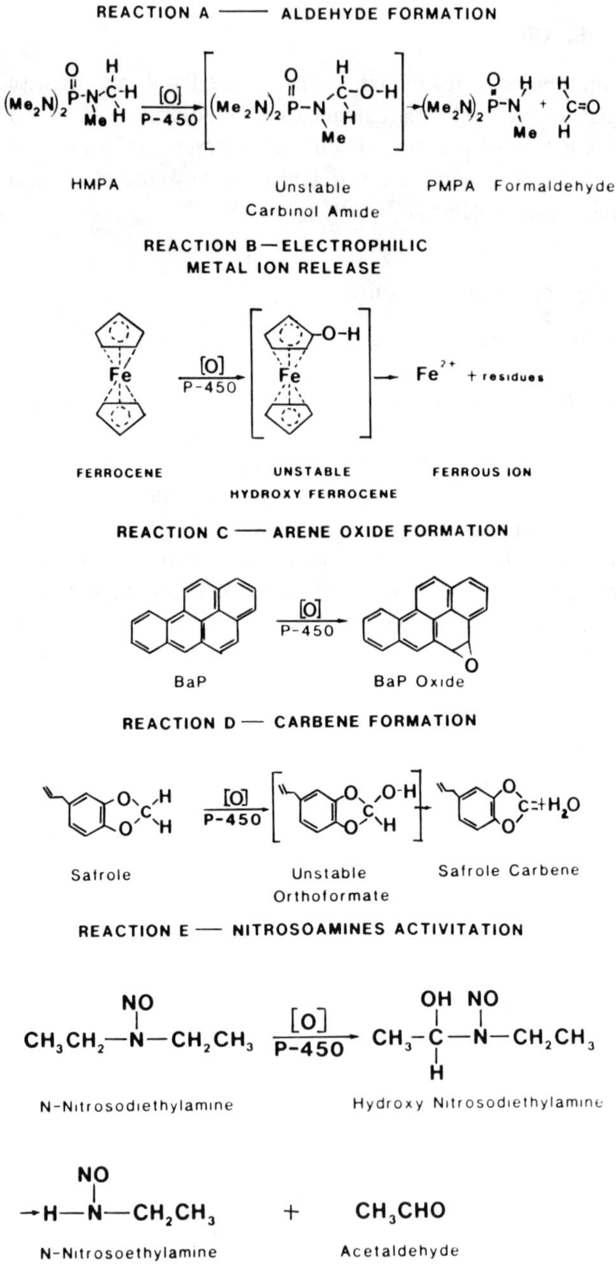

Figure 5 Chemical intermediates and metabolites of some compounds representative of those metabolized by nasal P-450.

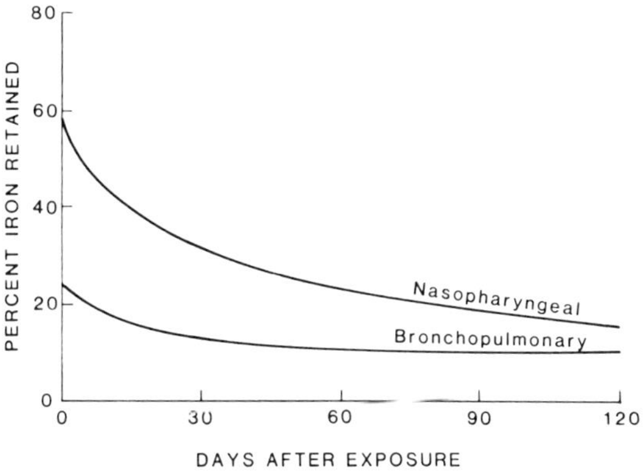

Figure 6 Retention of ^{59}Fe in nasal and pulmonary tissues after inhalation of ferrocene ^{59}Fe vapor.

The intracellular release of iron may have toxicological importance in that iron catalyzes formation of hydroxyl radicals (18). Because unligated metal ions, in general, are strong electrophiles, they potentially can bind to DNA, and are therefore potential mutagens in the cells in which they are released.

Arene oxide formation is illustrated for benzo[a]pyrene (BaP) in Fig. 5, reaction C. Dog and rat nasal microsomes metabolize BaP to arene oxides associated with the carcinogenicity of BaP (2, 9). Nasal cytochrome P-450 may be important in the nasal carcinogenicity of BaP in Syrian hamsters. They have a concentration of nasal cytochrome P-450 (7) four times that of rats. Syrian hamsters are also much more susceptible to nasal cancer after inhalation of BaP aerosol (19, 20). Assuming that BaP AHH activity is proportional to P-450 concentration in these two species, the higher concentration of nasal P-450 in Syrian hamsters may explain their greater susceptibility to nasal cancer from BaP inhalation.

Methylene dioxyphenyl (MDP) compounds are common natural products. They also are synthesized for use in flavorings and as synergists for pyrethrin-based insecticides. Consequently, they are common materials in the air breathed by man. These compounds probably inhibit cytochrome P-450 through binding of the cytochrome P-450 heme iron by a carbene formed by dehydration of an orthoformate (reaction D, Fig. 5) (21-23). They are much more potent inhibitors of rabbit nasal cytochrome P-450 than of liver cytochrome P-450 (11). If inhibition of nasal cytochrome P-450 by MDP compounds occurs in vivo, inhalation of these compounds would lessen the effects, good and ill, of nasal metabolism.

N-nitrosamines, which undergo metabolic activation (for example, reaction E of Fig. 5), are often organ-specific for causing cancers. Several cause cancer in the nasal cavity (24). Little or no data regarding the metabolism of nitrosamines by nasal microsomes is available. However, nasal tissue slices have been used to study the metabolism of nitrosamines (12). Figure 4 illustrates a comparison of the rate of metabolism of N-nitrosopyrrolidine to carbon dioxide by nasal and liver tissue. The data were normalized for P-450 content.

Protection of the Lungs from Vapors

The second role of nasal P-450 is in protection of the lungs. Organic vapors are present in the environment. At sufficiently high concentrations, these compounds saturate the nasal mucus and then pass into the lungs. After saturation of the nasal mucus, the concentration of the vapors reaching the lungs would be the same as that in the inhaled air. Nasal metabolism of inhaled organic vapors can reduce the amount of vapor reaching the lungs. The process can be viewed simply as the conversion of compounds of low solubility, which saturate mucus at low concentrations, to highly soluble metabolites. For example, ethyl acrylate vapor is removed from inhaled air by nasal carboxy-esterases (25). Calculations using N,N-dimethylaniline (DMA) as a representative inhaled compound show that in the rat up to a tenth of a part per million of DMA can be removed from the inhaled air by nasal P-450 metabolism so that the concentration of DMA reaching the lungs is reduced by up to this amount. The toxicological implications of this reduction are not yet clear. However, for example, the susceptibility of monkeys, without P-450 in the nasal respiratory tissue, toward toxic vapors at low concentrations may be different from that of rats, dogs, etc., which do have metabolic capacity in the nasal respiratory tissue.

Maintenance of Acuity of the Sense of Smell

The third implication from the presence of nasal P-450 is its possible role in olfaction. The presence of exceedingly high concentrations of cytochrome P-450 in the olfactory epithelium suggests that metabolism is important in olfaction. Although only 5-20 percent of the inhaled air normally passes over the olfactory mucosa, this tissue contains 80-100 percent of the nasal cytochrome P-450, depending on the animal species. The cytochrome P-450 in the olfactory tissue may be important in the removal of odorants. Without this function, odorants remaining in the mucus covering the sensory organs might produce an unacceptably high background odor, thereby decreasing acuity of the sense of smell. In certain species highly dependent on the sense of smell, the lack of olfactory acuity may have serious debilitating effects.

CONCLUSIONS

In summary, nasal cytochrome P-450 may have three important toxicological implications: (1) the activation of inhaled materials to more toxic forms or to forms which inactivate the cytochrome P-450; (2) the protection of the lungs from inhaled organic vapors; and (3) maintenance of acuity of the sense of smell by removal of odorants.

SUMMARY

Nasal cytochrome P-450 occurs in high concentrations in the olfactory epithelium and in lower concentrations in the nasal respiratory epithelium in most species. The substrate specificity of nasal P-450 is different from that of liver or lung. Nasal cytochrome P-450 may have at least three important toxicological implications: (1) the activation of inhaled materials to more toxic forms or to forms which inactivate the cytochrome P-450; (2) the protection of the lungs from inhaled organic vapors; and (3) maintenance of acuity of the sense of smell by removal of odorants.

REFERENCES

1 Graziadei, PPC. Functional anatomy of the mammalian chemoreceptor system. In *Chemical Signals in Vertebrates,* edited by D Müller-Schwarze, and MM Mozell. New York: Plenum, pp. 435–454 (1977).
2 Dahl, AR, WM Hadley, FF Hahn, JM Benson, and RO McClellan. Cytochrome P-450-dependent monooxygenases in olfactory epithelium of dogs: Possible role in tumorigenicity. *Science* 216:57–59 (1982).
3 Dahl, AR, and WM Hadley. Formaldehyde production promoted by rat nasal cytochrome P-450-dependent monooxygenases with nasal decongestants, essences, solvents, air pollutants, nicotine and cocaine as substrates. *Toxicol. Appl. Pharmacol.* 67:200–205 (1983).
4 Bond, JA. Bioactivation and biotransformation of 1-nitropyrene in liver, lung and nasal tissue of rats. *Mutat. Res.* 124:315–324 (1983).
5 Hadley, WM, and AR Dahl. Cytochrome P-450-dependent monooxygenase activity in rat nasal epithelial membranes. *Toxicol. Lett.* 10:417–422 (1982).
6 Hadley, WM, AR Dahl, JM Benson, FF Hahn, and RO McClellan. Cytochrome P-450-dependent monooxygenases in nasal epithelial membranes: Effect of phenobarbital and benzo(a)pyrene. *Proc. West. Pharmacol. Soc.* 25:197–199 (1982).
7 Hadley, WM, and AR Dahl. Cytochrome P-450-dependent monooxygenase activity in nasal membranes of six species. *Drug Metab. Disposition* 11:275–276 (1983).
8 Dahl, AR. The inhibition of rat nasal cytochrome P-450-dependent monooxygenase by the essence heliotropin (piperonal). *Drug Metab. Disposition* 10:553–554 (1982).
9 Bond, JA. Some biotransformation enzymes responsible for polycyclic aromatic hydrocarbon metabolism in rat nasal turbinates: Effects on enzyme activities of in vitro modifiers and intraperitoneal and inhalation exposure of rats to inducing agents. *Cancer Res.* 43:4805–4811 (1983).

10 Bond, JA, and AP Li. Rat nasal tissue metabolism of benzo(a)pyrene and 2-aminoanthracene to mutagens in *Salmonella typhimurium*. *Environ. Mutagen.* 5:311–318 (1983).
11 Dahl, AR, and DA Brezinski. The inhibition of rabbit nasal and hepatic cytochrome P-450–dependent hexamethylphosphoramide (HMPA) N-demethylase by methylenedioxyphenyl compounds, trivalent oxygenated phosphorus ligands and organic sulfur compounds. *Biochem. Pharm.* 34: 631–636 (1985).
12 Brittebo, E, B Döfberg, and H Tjälve. Extrahepatic sites of metabolism of N-nitrosopyrrolidine in mice and rats. *Xenobiotica* 11:619–625 (1981).
13 Feron, VJ, A Kruysse, and RA Wouterson. Respiratory tract tumours in hamsters exposed to acetaldehyde alone or simultaneously to benzo(a)-pyrene or diethylnitrosamine. *Er. J. Cancer Clin. Oncol.* 18:13–31 (1982).
14 Lee, KP, and HJ Trochimowicz. Induction of nasal tumors in rats exposed to hexamethylphosphoramide by inhalation. *JNCI* 68:157–164 (1982).
15 Kerns, WD, KL Pavkov, DJ Donofrio, EJ Gralla, and JA Swenberg. Carcinogenicity of formaldehyde in rats and mice after long-term inhalation exposure. *Cancer Res.* 43:4382–4392 (1983).
16 Dahl, AR, and TJ Briner. Biological fate of a representative lipophilic metal compound (ferrocene) deposited by inhalation in the respiratory tract of rats. *Toxicol. Appl. Pharmacol.* 56:232–239 (1980).
17 Hanzlik, RP, and WN Soine. Enzymatic hydroxylation of ferrocene. *J. Am. Chem. Soc.* 100:1290–1291 (1978).
18 McCord, JM. Superoxide dismutase and oxygen toxicity. In *Reviews in Biochemical Toxicology,* edited by E Hodgson, JR Bend, and RM Philpot. New York: Elsevier, Vol. I, pp. 109–124 (1979).
19 Laskin, S, M Kuschner, and RT Drew. Studies in pulmonary carcinogenesis. In *Inhalation Carcinogenesis,* AEC Symposium Series No. 18. Oak Ridge: Division of Technical Information. U.S. Atomic Energy Commission, pp. 321–351 (1970).
20 Thyssen, J, J Althoff, G Kimmerle, and U Mohr. Inhalation studies with benzo(a)pyrene in Syrian golden hamsters. *JNCI* 66:575–577 (1981).
21 Dahl, AR, and E Hodgson. The interaction of aliphatic analogs of methylenedioxyphenyl compounds with cytochromes P-450 and P-420. *Chem. Biol. Interact.* 27:163–175 (1979).
22 Mansuy, D, JP Battion, JC Chottard, and V Ullrich. Preparation of a porphyrin iron carbene model for cytochrome P-450 complexes obtained upon metabolic activation of the insecticide synergists of the 1,3-benzodioxole series. *J. Am. Chem. Soc.* 101:3971–3972 (1979).
23 Testa, B, and P Jenner. Inhibitors of cytochrome P-450s and their mechanism of action. *Drug. Metab. Rev.* 12:1–117 (1981).
24 Soderman, JV. *CRC Handbook of Identified Carcinogens and Noncarcinogens: Carcinogenicity-Mutagenicity Database.* Boca Raton, FL: CRC Press (1982).
25 Stott, WT, and MJ McKenna. The comparative absorbtion and excretion of

chemical vapors by the upper, lower, and intact respiratory tract of rats. *Fund. Appl. Toxicol.* 4(4):594-602 (1984).

26 Vainio, H, and E. Hietanen. Role of extrahepatic metabolism. In *Concepts in Drug Metabolism,* edited by P Jenner and B Testa. New York: Dekker, pp. 251-284 (1980).

Chapter 17

Assessment of Genotoxic Effects in Rat Nasal Epithelium

Edilberto Bermúdez

INTRODUCTION

Rats are commonly used as a model for humans. A prerequisite for the assessment of the suitability of the rat model is an understanding of how the target organ functions and responds to stimuli. Various aspects of the structure and function of the nasal organ have been described (1-5), and the capacity of the cells of the nasal cavity to metabolize various chemicals has been examined (6-10). Tumors of the nasal cavity occur in humans at a high incidence in specific occupational groups (11, 12) and are inducible in experimental animals by numerous chemicals (13-18).

Malignant conversion of cells by chemicals is thought to be a multistage process, with an initial interaction between the chemical or its metabolites and the target cell's DNA, leading to permanent genotypic changes. Based on this concept, multiple endpoints have been devised to assess the extent and result of these effects (19, 20). Much of the previous work on the genotoxic effects of chemicals in the respiratory tract has centered on the bronchus and the trachea (21), but little has been done with the nasal tissues.

Interest in this laboratory in the nasal cavity was sparked by the finding that chronic exposure of rats to formaldehyde results in the induction of squamous cell carcinoma in the nose (18). Since DNA damage and DNA repair appear to be important factors in tumor formation, the initial studies concentrated on the development of procedures to assess these events in the nasal epithelium following chemical treatment.

MATERIALS AND METHODS

Animals

The methodology for the experiments discussed here has been described in detail by Bermúdez and Allen (22). Male F-344 rats were purchased from Charles River Breeding Laboratories (Kingston, NY), quarantined for 14 days, and screened for rodent pathogens. Pathogen-free animals were allowed food (NIH 07 open formula diet, Ziegler Bros., Gardners, PA) and water ad libitum, housed in polycarbonate cages, and maintained on a 12-h light/dark cycle with temperature and relative humidity maintained at 21-23°C and 45-55 percent, respectively.

Turbinate Isolation

Nasal turbinates were isolated from the nasal cavity of adult control and treated animals weighing approximately 250 g. Briefly, the animals were decapitated, the heads were skinned, and the skull was split along the medial suture. The nasoturbinates, maxilloturbinates, and ethmoid turbinates were removed (Fig. 1), washed with warm Williams medium E supplemented with 2 mM L-glutamine

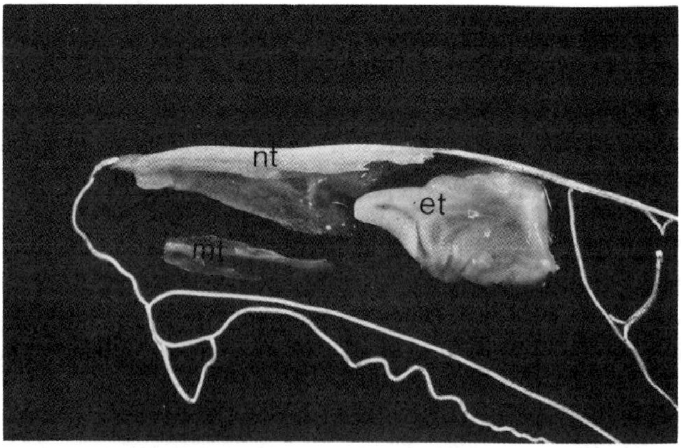

Figure 1 Isolated turbinates. The medial aspect of the nasoturbinate, maxilloturbinate, and ethmoid turbinate is shown. The head is outlined to show the orientation in vivo.

(WEI, Flow Laboratories, McLean, VA), and incubated in the same medium at 37°C in a 95 percent air-5 percent CO_2 incubator. Histologic examination of untreated nasoturbinates and maxilloturbinates indicated that degeneration of the tissue occurred as early as 24 h, particularly in the submucosa. Degenerative changes in the ethmoid turbinates were discernible in the sensory cells of the olfactory epithelium as early as 6 h after being placed in culture, whereas the sustentacular cells appeared unaffected within a 24-h period.

Treatment of Turbinates In Vitro

Isolated turbinates were treated for 3 or 18 h with 1 mM methyl methanesulfonate (MMS, Aldrich Chemical Co., Milwaukee, WI), and the epithelium was examined for the induction of DNA damage and unscheduled DNA synthesis (UDS). Cells from turbinates were treated for 3 h with 0.5, 1, or 5 mM dimethylnitrosamine (DMN, Sigma Chemicals Co., St. Louis, MO), or for 3 and 16 h to 0.5 or 1.0 mM formaldehyde (HCHO, Fisher Scientific, Pittsburgh, PA) and were assayed for DNA damage and UDS. Where the induction of strand breaks was to be determined, the turbinates were washed after the exposure and cell suspensions were prepared for alkaline elution analysis. In the studies of the induction of UDS, the turbinates were treated in medium containing 10 μCi [^{3}H] thymidine/ml ([^{3}H] dThd 40 Ci/mmole, Amersham, Arlington Heights, IL), rinsed with WEI, incubated for 17 h in WEI containing 10 μCi [^{3}H] dThd/ml, and supplemented with 5 percent fetal calf serum (WEC5). Cell suspensions were then prepared and processed through autoradiography.

Treatment of Animals

Male F-344 rats were exposed by inhalation to nominal concentrations of 500 or 1000 ppm DMN for 4 h. Immediately after the exposure the animals were killed and the turbinates were isolated and washed as described above. The turbinates were then incubated for 17 h in the presence of [^{3}H] dThd (10 μCi/ml) and washed, and the cells were isolated for processing through autoradiography.

Cell Isolation

Digest solution was prepared by dissolving 10 mg pronase and 50 units of collagenase (Sigma Chemical Co., St. Louis, MO)/ml Ham's F-12 (Flow Laboratories, McLean, VA) medium buffered to pH 7.10 with 10 mM HEPES (Calbiochem, San Diego, CA) and used to digest the epithelium from the turbinates. The turbinates were placed in 25-ml flasks containing 5 ml of digest solution and shaken at approximately 100 rpm for 20 min in a 37°C water bath. Epithelium digested by this procedure was collected by centrifugation (180*g*, 3 min) and resuspended in medium, and the cell density and viability were determined. Mean cell yields per animal were 0.5, 1.6, and 2.2×10^6 cells for the nasoturbinates, maxilloturbinates, and the ethmoid turbinates, respectively. Cell viabilities, as measured by the exclusion of trypan blue, were 73, 58, and 88 percent for the nasoturbinates, ethmoid turbinates, and maxilloturbinates, respectively. The proportion of the cells traversing S-phase ranged between 0.9 and 1.3 percent. Histologic examination of the remains of digested turbinates revealed that the digestion procedure selectively removed the surface epithelium. Freshly prepared cell suspensions were fixed, pelleted, postfixed with 1 percent OsO_4 in phosphate buffer for 90 min, and embedded in epon/araldite. Thin sections were cut and stained with lead citrate/uranyl acetate and examined by transmission electron microscopy (TEM).

Autoradiography

Fresh suspensions of cells prepared from control and treated turbinates were fixed overnight at 4°C in 10 percent buffered Formalin, washed, and resuspended in 1 ml of 10 percent buffered Formalin. Slides were prepared by placing 3–4 drops of the fixed cell suspension on each slide, air-drying for 24 h, washing the slides twice in distilled water for 4 min, and air-drying for an additional 24 h. The slides were then dipped in NTB2 nuclear track emulsion (Kodak, Rochester, NY) and air-dried, and the emulsion was exposed for 3 weeks at 20°C. The emulsion was developed with Kodak D19 developer, fixed in Kodak fixer, and washed with water. The preparations were stained with methylene blue and scored for the number of grains over the nucleus. Background in the emulsion and cytoplasm was minimal and not adjusted for. The response of the cells was also measured by determining the percent of the treated population that had more grains/nucleus than 90 percent of the control population.

Alkaline Elution

The induction of strand breaks in the DNA of the epithelial cells was assessed using the alkaline elution assay as described by Kohn (23) and modified by Bermúdez et al. (24). Briefly, aliquots of 2×10^5 cells were deposited onto PVC filters (2 μm, BSWP25, Millipore, Bedford, MA), lysed with 0.02 M Na_3EDTA, 2 M NaCl, 0.3 percent Sarkosyl, and eluted for 10 h with 0.02 M H_4EDTA (brought to a pH of 12.2 with 10 percent tetrapropylammonium hydroxide) at a rate of 0.05 ml/min. The formation of DNA crosslinks (DC) was detected by further treating the turbinates with 10 mM MMS for 0.5 h before preparing cell suspensions for alkaline elution. The component of the DC attributable to DNA-protein crosslinks (DPC) was determined by the inclusion of 0.5 mg proteinase K/ml lysing solution during the lysis step. Trans-platinum II (100 μg/ml, Sigma, St. Louis, MO), was used as a positive control for the presence of DPC. The relative amount of DNA remaining on the filters was determined by reacting with 3,5-diaminobenzoic acid hydrochloride (0.3 g/ml, Aldrich, Milwaukee, WI) at 60°C for 1.5 h and measuring the fluorescence of the product with an Aminco SPF-500 spectrofluorometer with the excitation wavelength set at 414 nm and the emission wavelength set at 508 nm. Radiolabeled internal standards were not used. For each treatment and control group at least six filters were prepared, half to be eluted and the other half to serve as a reference for the starting amount of DNA. The final data were expressed as the percent of the control DNA remaining on the control filters.

RESULTS

The olfactory epithelium was more susceptible to degeneration within 6 h of culture than the respiratory epithelium, which showed changes in the submucosa after 24 h in culture. When these tissues were kept in culture for periods of up to 2 weeks, ciliary activity could still be seen in the respiratory epithelium.

Cell isolation procedures, by digestion with a mixture of pronase and collagenase, resulted in the specific removal of the epithelial lining of the turbinates, as assessed by the examination of plastic-embedded sections of digested turbinates (Fig. 2). When the cell suspensions were examined by

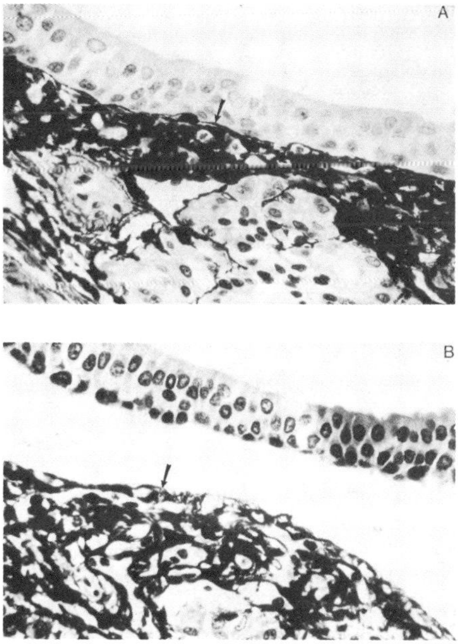

Figure 2 Turbinates before (*A*) and after (*B*) digestion with a mixture of pronase and collagenase. Note the clear separation of the epithelium from the basement membrane (arrow). Jones' silver methenamine, X96.

phase-contrast microscopy, ciliated, goblet, and nonciliated cells were seen. Within the nonciliated group there was a wide range of size, nuclear-to-cytoplasmic ratio, and appearance of the cells. Examination of the cell suspensions by TEM revealed the presence of three distinct cell populations: ciliated, nonciliated, and goblet cells (Fig. 3).

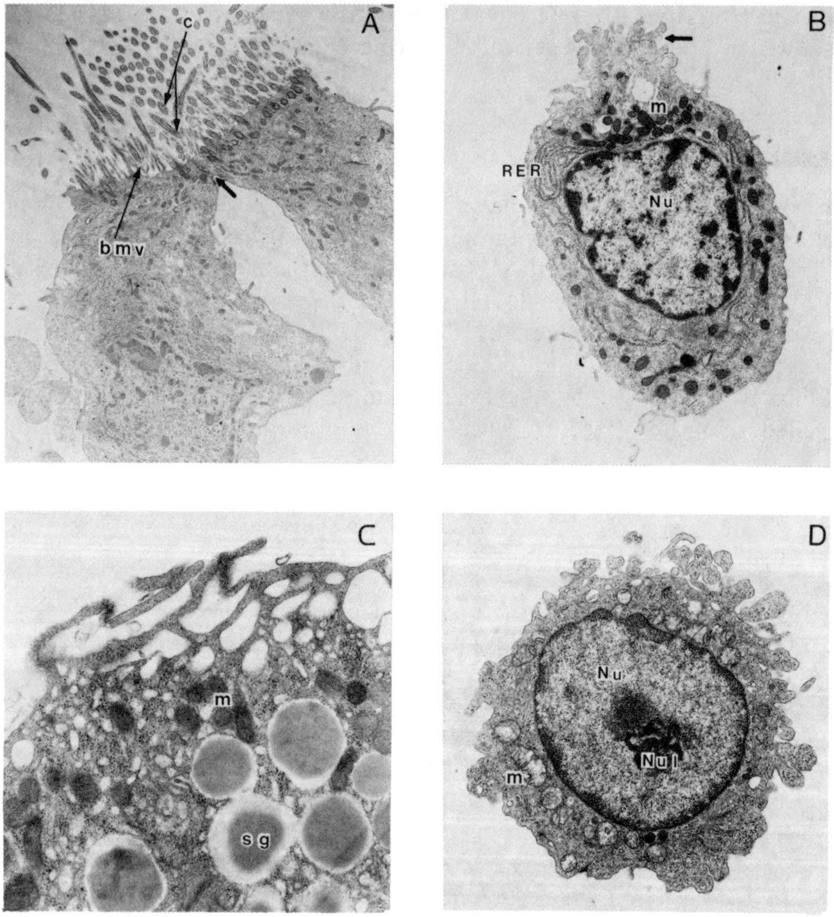

Figure 3 TEM photomicrographs of freshly isolated nasal epithelial cells. (*A*) Ciliated epithelial cells partially joined by a junctional complex (arrow). Cilia (c) and branched microvilli (bmv) are evident. Magnification, X3705. (*B*) Nonciliated epithelial cell with parallel array of rough endoplasmic reticulum (RER), mitochondria (m), nucleus (Nu), and what appears to be remnants of microvilli (arrow). Magnification, X3648. (*C*) High magnification of the cytoplasm of a goblet cell showing the secretory granules (sg) and mitochondria in the cytoplasm. Magnification, X17,700. (*D*) Nonciliated epithelial cell with large nucleus and nucleolus (Nul). This cell has little cytoplasm and contains mitochondria. Magnification, X4560. [*From Bermúdez and Allen (22).*]

Table 1 DNA Damage and Repair Induction in Rat Nasal Respiratory Epithelium Following Exposure In Vitro to Methyl Methanesulfonate (MMS)

	Grains/ nucleus*	Percent responding†	Retention‡ (percent of control)
Control	3.4	10	100
MMS, 1.0 mM	15.0	71	42

*Nasoturbinates and maxilloturbinates were exposed to MMS for 18 h in the presence of [^{3}H]thymidine. The mean grains per nucleus was determined by autoradiography for 600 cells from two separate preparations.

†The percent of the treated population with more grains per nucleus than 90 percent of the control population.

‡Turbinates were exposed to MMS for 3 h, and the DNA of the epithelium was examined for single-strand breaks using the alkaline elution assay. Mean retention for controls was 76 ± 2.0 percent.

Cells from nasoturbinate and maxilloturbinate treated in vitro with 1 mM MMS were examined for the induction of DNA strand breaks and the induction of UDS. Strand breaks were detected in the cells of the respiratory epithelium, and UDS was observed in the majority of the cells (Table 1).

Exposure of rats to 500 or 1000 ppm DMN by inhalation resulted in the induction of DNA damage and UDS in the cells of the epithelium from each of the three turbinates. A decrease in the percent of the population responding was observed with an increase in nominal concentration (Fig. 4). DMN was also used to treat the turbinates in vitro for 3 h. Statistically significant increases in the induction of DNA damage were observed in the DNA from the cells of the nasoturbinate treated with 0.5, 1, or 5 mM concentrations of DMN. Consistent with these findings, the induction of UDS was observed at the same concentrations in approximately 50 percent of the population (Fig. 5). In contrast to the respiratory epithelium of the nasoturbinate, the respiratory epithelium of the maxilloturbinate had significant induction of strand breaks and UDS only after treatment with 5 mM DMN (Fig. 6). Increases in the induction of DNA strand breaks and UDS in the ethmoid turbinate were observed following treatment with 1 and 5 mM DMN; however, there was no statistically significant increase in the percent of the population responding (Fig. 7).

Nasoturbinates were treated with 0.5 and 1 mM concentrations of HCHO or 100 μg/ml trans-platinum II for 3 h, and the cells of the epithelium were assayed for the presence of DPC. All treatments resulted in the formation of DC in the cells of the respiratory epithelium. Treatment with proteinase K

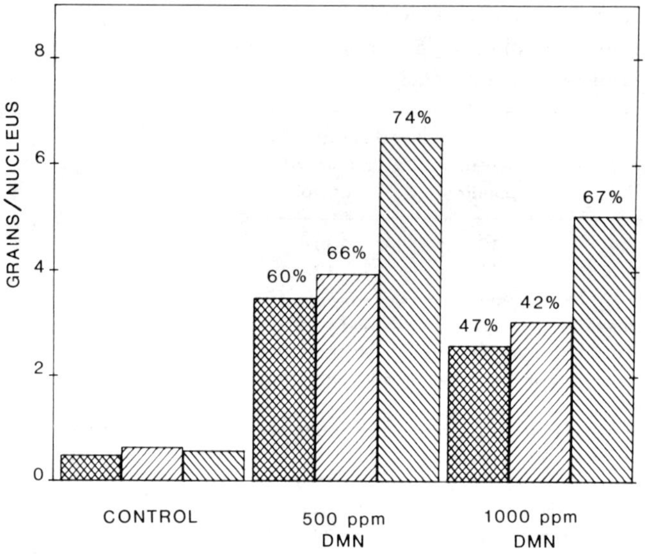

Figure 4 The induction of unscheduled DNA synthesis (UDS) in nasal turbinates following in vivo administration of dimethylnitrosamine (DMN) by inhalation. Male F-344 rats were exposed to nominal concentrations of 500 and 1000 ppm DMN for 4 h. Immediately after exposure, the turbinates were isolated, washed, and incubated for 17 h in the presence of [^{3}H]thymidine. Incubation was followed by digestion of the epithelium, fixation of the cells, and the performance of autoradiography. The induction of UDS was assessed by determining the number of grains/nucleus in cells from the naso- (left columns), maxillo- (center), and ethmoid turbinates (right). The percent of the population responding, defined as the portion of the treated population having more grains per nucleus than 90 percent of the control population, was also determined and is shown at the top of each bar.

revealed that most of the observed crosslinking for both compounds was due to DPC and that single-strand breaks were apparently also present (Table 2). Treatment of turbinates with HCHO resulted only in a slight increase in UDS in the cells exposed to 0.5 mM HCHO, but no difference from control was observed when 1.0 mM HCHO was employed (Table 3). No significant difference was seen between control and treated cells in ciliary activity or the ability to exclude trypan blue.

DISCUSSION

There has been a lack of techniques to assess the genotoxicity of chemicals in nasal epithelium despite the fact that the general population is exposed to many chemicals where the primary site of contact is the upper airways. The present studies were designed to develop the means to assess genotoxicity in the nasal cavity of the rat using the induction of DNA damage and repair as endpoints.

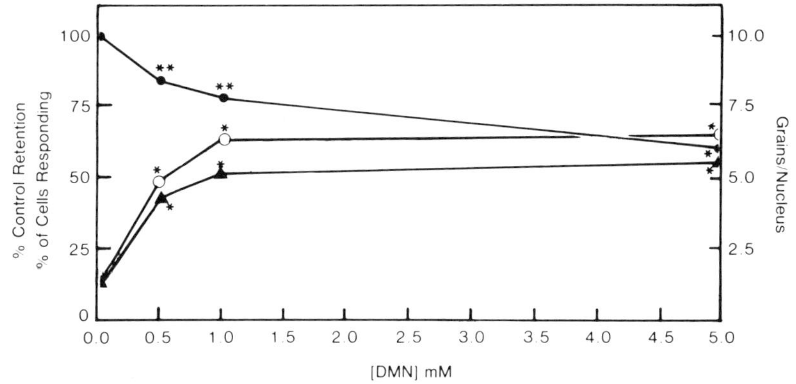

Figure 5 The induction of DNA damage and unscheduled DNA synthesis (UDS) in rat nasal epithelium, by dimethylnitrosamine (DMN) in vitro, isolated from the nasoturbinate. Whole, isolated nasoturbinates were incubated with DMN alone or with DMN in the presence of [^{3}H]thymidine for 3 h. The induction of DNA damage in the cells from treated turbinates was assessed using the alkaline elution assay (solid circles). For the induction of UDS, the turbinates were incubated after treatment for an additional 17 h in the presence of [^{3}H]-thymidine. The tissue was then digested, and autoradiography was performed on fixed preparations of the cells. The data are presented as the mean grains per nucleus (open circles) and the percent of the cells responding (triangles, the percent of the treated cells with more grains per nucleus than 90 percent of the control population) of 200 cells from each of three preparations per data point. Statistical significance: $*p < 0.05$; $**0.10 > p > 0.05$.

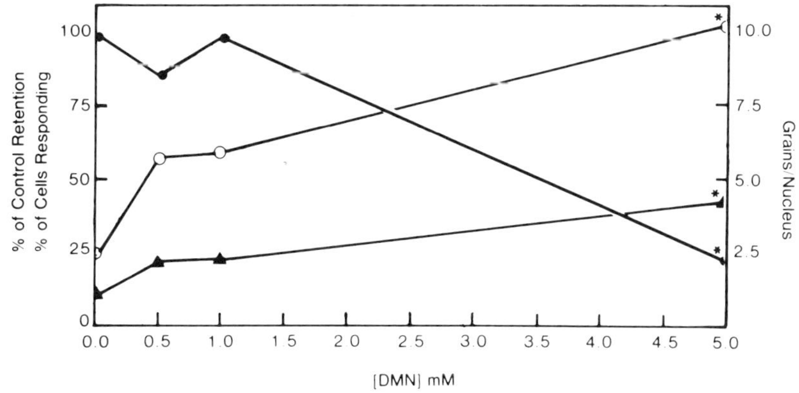

Figure 6 The induction of DNA damage and unscheduled DNA synthesis (UDS) in rat nasal epithelium, isolated from maxilloturbinates, by dimethylnitrosamine (DMN), in vitro (for experimental detail and symbols see the legend to Fig. 4).

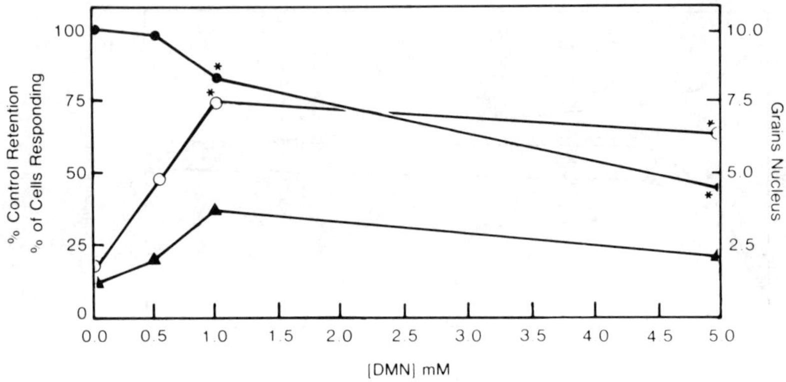

Figure 7 The induction of DNA damage and unscheduled DNA synthesis (UDS) in rat nasal epithelium, isolated from ethmoid turbinates, by dimethylnitrosamine (DMN), in vitro (for experimental detail and symbols see the legend for Fig. 4).

Nasal turbinates were isolated as a means of sampling the major epithelial types encountered in the nasal cavity: respiratory and olfactory epithelium. The nasoturbinate and maxilloturbinate are lined with respiratory epithelium and lie well within the airway, whereas the ethmoid turbinate is lined mainly with olfactory epithelium and is not directly in the airway (2). Incubation of these tissues in culture medium indicated that changes in the tissue occurred in the sensory cells of the olfactory epithelium within 6 h of isolation, but that changes

Table 2 Induction of DNA Damage in Nasoturbinates Treated In Vitro with Formaldehyde (HCHO)*

	Retention as percent of MMS†-treated control			
	(−)Proteinase K‡	(*n*)§	(+)Proteinase K	(*n*)
MMS	100‖	(5)	100	(3)
0.5 mM HCHO/MMS	389	(3)	78	(3)
1.0 mM HCHO/MMS	552	(4)	188	(3)
Trans-platinum II#/MMS	169	(3)	54	(2)

*Isolated nasoturbinates were treated with formaldehyde in serumless medium for 3 h.

†Turbinates were treated with 10 mM methyl methanesulfonate for 30 min after the formaldehyde was washed off.

‡0.5 mg/ml of lysing solution.

§n = Number of preparations.

‖Mean retention for controls was 11 ± 5 percent and 9 ± 4 percent for (−) and (+) proteinase K, respectively.

#Isolated turbinates were treated with 100 μg/ml trans-platinum II in serumless medium for 3 h.

Table 3 Unscheduled DNA Synthesis in Rat Nasal Turbinates Treated In Vitro with Formaldehyde (HCHO)*

	Grains/nucleus†			
	Nasoturbinate	Maxilloturbinate	Ethmoturbinate	n‡
Control	0.41 (0.37)§	0.46 (0.12)	0.57 (0.01)	2
0.5 mM HCHO	1.02 (0.37)	1.05 (0.67)	1.58 (0.19)	3
1.0 mM HCHO	0.42 (0.02)	0.35 (0.12)	0.99 (0.33)	3

*Isolated turbinates were treated with formaldehyde for 16 h in the presence of [^{3}H]thymidine followed by a 3-h incubation in medium alone.

†Mean of 300 cells per preparation.

‡n = Number of preparations.

§Standard deviation.

in the sustentacular cells of the olfactory epithelium and the cells of the respiratory epithelium were not discernible within a 24-h period in culture. These results were similar to those described for the culture of the rat nasal septum (25) and punctuated the necessity of carrying out the in vitro procedures as soon as possible after the isolation of the tissues.

To limit the study of the effects of chemical treatment to the surface epithelium, a digestion procedure was devised which selectively removed the cells above the basement membrane and resulted in the production of single-cell suspensions. Examination of the suspensions by electron microscopy revealed the presence of three distinct populations: ciliated, nonciliated, and goblet cells. Ultrastructural studies of intact rat nasal tissues have shown that at least six distinct morphological cell types can be found in the respiratory epithelium and three in the olfactory (3). The loss of shape, orientation, and surface characteristics with digestion precludes the application of the same criteria used for identification of intact cells to isolated cell populations. Although it is unlikely that the digestion of the epithelium results in the selective loss of a particular cell type, until definitive identification can be made of all the cells present in the cell suspensions, the presence of all cell types can only be assumed.

The susceptibility of respiratory epithelium to DNA damage by the direct-acting mutagen MMS and the ability of these cells to repair the damage were assessed. Incubation with 1 mM MMS resulted in DNA strand breaks and the induction of UDS. This indicates that these cells have the ability to excise and repair methylated base adducts. The repair of some methylated base damage is thought to be mediated by a methyl transferase enzyme rather than by an excision mechanism (26, 27), and the presence of this enzyme in the nasal epithelium (J. Swenberg, personal communication) indicates that these cells can repair this type of damage.

DMN can induce tumors in the nasal cavity of the rat whether it is administered by inhalation (28) or i.p. injection (29), suggesting that DMN or its metabolites are preferentially localized in the nasal cavity. Localization of other nitrosamines has been demonstrated in the hamster (30) and rat (31) in vivo and in rat nasal septum in vitro (25). Consistent with these studies the exposure of rats to nominal concentrations of 500 or 1000 ppm results in the induction of UDS in the cells isolated from the nasoturbinates, maxilloturbinates, and ethmoid turbinates (Fig. 4). This is an interesting finding in that it may indicate the existence of a mechanism to rid the animal of these types of compounds. The supposition that the nasal cavity may be a site of detoxification is also supported by the substantial capacity of these cells to metabolize various chemicals (6-10).

In vitro exposure of the nasal turbinates to DMN resulted in the induction of DNA strand breaks and UDS in the cells of the respiratory and olfactory epithelium (Figs. 5-7). These results are consistent with the metabolism of DMN by the cells of respiratory and olfactory epithelium, or the cells of the submucosa, and the capacity of the cells of the rat nasal septum to metabolize tobacco-specific nitrosamines (25). The determination of which specific cell type(s) are capable of metabolizing DMN must await techniques to separate the various cell types found in these tissues. Differences in the response observed with the cells from the three turbinates were apparent following treatment, in vitro, with DMN. The cells isolated from the maxilloturbinates had a pattern of response distinct from those of the nasoturbinates and ethmoid turbinates (Figs. 5-7). A difference in response between the maxilloturbinates and the ethmoid turbinates is not surprising considering that the cells making up these tissues are very distinct in morphology and function. The nasoturbinates and maxilloturbinates, however, are both lined by respiratory epithelium, the difference being only in distribution of the various cell types (4). It may be that the cells found on the maxilloturbinates uptake, metabolize, and/or excrete DMN in a manner different from the cells in other areas. DMN induced virtually the same response in the cells of the nasoturbinates and the ethmoid turbinates. Considering the difference in cell types being examined, it is interesting that no substantial dissimilarities were observed. The lack of a significant increase in the percent of the cells responding in the cells of the ethmoid turbinates, however, indicates that the observed response may arise from the respiratory epithelium found on the anterior edge of this turbinate.

Treatment of nasoturbinates with HCHO resulted in the generation of DNA-protein crosslinks and DNA strand breaks. These results are in agreement with the induction of similar lesions by HCHO in *E. coli* (32), yeast (33, 34), and human bronchial epithelium (35). Formaldehyde also induced a small but significant UDS response in the cells of the respiratory epithelium at the lower concentration tested (Table 3), consistent with the observation that these lesions are repairable by the excision repair mechanism (34-37). Higher concentrations of HCHO appeared to suppress the UDS response with a concomitant increase in the occurrence of DNA lesions (Table 3), suggestive of a toxic response. The occurrence of general toxicity, however, is negated by the lack of effect on ciliary activity and the exclusion of trypan blue. Grafstrom et al. (35) have suggested that HCHO may inhibit the ligase enzyme necessary for the closure of repair gaps, but this would not appear to be the case here, as an increase in the proportion of single-strand breaks with dose was not observed and incorporation of radiolabel would have resulted in apparent increases in UDS. However, the possibility of specific inhibition of the repair mechanism at some other step cannot be ruled out. Another explanation may be that DPCs are repaired by a mechanism other than the excision repair mechanism. Further work in this area is under way to clarify the mechanism of action of HCHO.

SUMMARY

Methods to isolate and maintain in culture the nasal turbinates of rats were developed to examine the cells of the nasal epithelium for chemically induced genotoxic effects. Two endpoints were selected as measures of genotoxicity: alkaline elution analysis for the detection of strand breakage, and the induction of unscheduled DNA synthesis. Strand breakage and the induction of unscheduled DNA synthesis resulted when the cells of the epithelium were exposed in vitro to 1 mM methyl methanesulfonate or 0.5-, 1.0-, or 5.0-mM concentrations of dimethylnitrosamine. DNA damage and unscheduled DNA synthesis were also observed in the epithelium from rats exposed to nominal concentrations of 500 or 1000 ppm dimethylnitrosamine by inhalation. Treatment with 0.5- or 1-mM concentrations of formaldehyde resulted in the detection of two distinct lesions in the cells of the nasoturbinates: single-strand breaks and DNA-protein crosslinks. The amount of crosslinking increased with concentration. Little induction of UDS by 0.5 mM formaldehyde was observed, and an increase in the concentration to 1 mM resulted in the absence of any UDS, although ciliary action and viability of the cells were unaffected. The ability to determine the induction of DNA damage and repair in the nasal epithelium provides a valuable opportunity to examine the effects of various airborne chemicals at the primary site of exposure.

REFERENCES

1 Proctor, DF, and I Andersen. The mucociliary system. In *The Nose, Upper Airway Physiology and the Atmospheric Environment*, edited by DF Proctor, and I Andersen. Amsterdam: Elsevier, pp. 245–278 (1982).

2 Proctor, DF, and JFC Chang. Comparative anatomy and physiology of the nasal cavity. In *Nasal Tumors in Animals and Man*, Vol. I: *Anatomy, Physiology, and Epidemiology*, edited by G Reznik and SF Stinson. Boca Raton, FL: CRC Press, pp. 1–33 (1983).

3 Monteiro-Riviere, NA, and JA Popp. Ultrastructural characterization of the nasal respiratory epithelium in the rat. *Am. J. Anat.* 169:31–43 (1984).
4 Popp, JA, and JT Martin. Surface topography and distribution of cell types in the rat nasal respiratory epithelium: Scanning electron microscopic observations. *Am. J. Anat.*, 169:425–436 (1984).
5 Morgan, KT, XZ Jiang, DL Patterson, and EA Gross. The nasal mucociliary apparatus: Correlation of structure and function in the rat. *Am. Rev. Respir. Dis.* 130:275–281 (1984).
6 Bond, JA. Bioactivation and biotransformation of 1-nitropyrene in liver, lung, and nasal tissue of rats. *Mutat. Res.* 124:315–324 (1983).
7 Bond, JA. Some biotransformation enzymes responsible for polycyclic aromatic hydrocarbon metabolism in rat nasal turbinates: Effects on enzyme activities of in vitro modifiers and intraperitoneal and inhalation exposure of rats to inducing agents. *Cancer Res.* 43:4805–4811 (1983).
8 Bond, JA, and AP Li. Rat nasal tissue activation of benzo(a)pyrene and 2-aminoanthracene to mutagens in *Salmonella typhimurium. Environ. Mutagen.* 5:311–318 (1983).
9 Hadley, WM, AR Dahl, JM Benson, FF Hahn, and RO McClellan. Cytochrome P-450 dependent monooxygenases in nasal epithelial membranes: Effect of phenobarbital and benzo(a)pyrene. *Proc. West. Pharmacol. Soc.* 25:197–199 (1982).
10 Hadley, WM, and AR Dahl. Cytochrome P-450 dependent monooxygenase activity in rat nasal epithelial membranes. *Toxicol. Lett.* 10:417–422 (1982).
11 Buiatti, E, M Geddes, F Carnevale, and E Merier. Nasal cavity and paranasal sinus tumors in woodworkers and shoemakers in Italy compared to other countries. In *Nasal Tumors in Animals and Man*, Vol. I: *Anatomy, Physiology and Epidemiology*, edited by G Reznik and SF Stinson. Boca Raton, FL: CRC Press, pp. 111–149 (1983).
12 Doll, R, JD Matthews, and LG Morgan. Cancer of the lung and nasal sinuses in nickel workers: A reassessment of the period of risk. *Br. J. Ind. Med.* 34: 102–105 (1977).
13 Kociba, RJ, SB McCollister, C Park, and TR Torkelson. 1,4-Dioxane. I. Results of a two-year ingestion study in rats. *Toxicol. Appl. Pharmacol.* 30: 275–286 (1974).
14 Lee, KP, and HJ Trochimowicz. Induction of nasal tumors in rats exposed to hexamethylphosphoramide by inhalation. *JNCI* 68:157–171 (1982).
15 Reznik, G, H Reznik-Schuller, JM Ward, and SF Stinson. Morphology of nasal-cavity tumors in rats after chronic inhalation of 1,2-dibromo-3-chloropropane. *Br. J. Cancer* 42:772–781 (1980).
16 Reznik-Schuller, HM. Cancer induced in the respiratory tract of rodents by N-nitroso compounds. In *Comparative Respiratory Tract Carcinogenesis*, Vol. II: *Experimental Respiratory Tract Carcinogenesis*, edited by HM Reznik-Schuller. Boca Raton, FL: CRC Press, pp. 109–134 (1983).
17 Takano, T, T Shirai, T Ogiso, H Tsuda, S Baba, and N Ito. Sequential changes in tumor development induced by 1,4-dinitrosopiperazine in the nasal cavity of F344 rats. *Cancer Res.* 42:4236–4240 (1982).

18 Swenberg, JA, WD Kerns, RI Mitchell, EJ Gralla, and KL Pavkov. Induction of squamous cell carcinomas of the rat nasal cavity by inhalation exposure to formaldehyde vapor. *Cancer Res.* 40:3398–3402 (1980).

19 Hollstein, MJ, MJ McCann, FA Angelosano, and WW Nichols. Short term tests for carcinogens and mutagens. *Mutat. Res.* 65:133–226 (1979).

20 Hsie, AW, JP O'Neill, and VK McElheny (eds). *Mammalian Cell Mutagenesis: The maturation of Test Systems, Banbury Reports 2.* Cold Spring Harbor NY: Cold Spring Harbor Laboratory, 504 pp. (1979).

21 Tice, R, DL Costa, and KM Schaich (eds). *Genotoxic Effects of Airborne Agents.* New York: Plenum, 658 pp. (1982).

22 Bermúdez, E, and PF Allen. The assessment of DNA damage and repair in rat nasal epithelial cells. *Carcinogenesis,* 15:1453–1458 (1984).

23 Kohn, KW. DNA as a target in cancer chemotherapy: Measurement of macromolecular damage produced in mammalian cells by anticancer agents and carcinogens. *Methods Cancer Res.* 16:291–345 (1979).

24 Bermúdez, E, JC Mirsalis, and HC Eales. Detection of DNA damage in primary cultures of rat hepatocytes following in vivo and in vitro exposure to genotoxic agents. *Environ. Mutagen.* 4:667–679 (1982).

25 Brittebo, EB, A Castonguay, K Furuya, and SS Hecht. Metabolism of tobacco-specific nitrosamines by cultured rat nasal mucosa. *Cancer Res.* 43: 4343–4348 (1983).

26 Mehta, JR, DB Ludlum, A Renard, and WG Verly. Repair of O^6-ethylguanine in DNA by a chromatin fraction from rat liver: Transfer of the ethyl group to an acceptor protein. *Proc. Natl. Acad. Sci. USA* 78:6766–6770 (1981).

27 Olsson, M, and T Lindahl. Repair of alkylated DNA in *Escherichia coli. J. Biol. Chem.* 255:10569–10571 (1980).

28 Druckery, H, R Preussmann, S Ivankovic, and D Schmall. Organotrope Carcinogene Wirkung bei 65 verschiedenen N-Nitroso-Verbindungen and BD Ratten. *Z. Krebsforch.* 69:103 (1967).

29 Noronha, RFX, and CM Goodall. Nasal tumours in starved rats injected once with dimethylnitrosamine. *N.Z. Med. J.* 75:374 (1972).

30 Reznik-Schuller, HM. Labeling in the cells of the nasal cavity of hamsters treated with tritiated N-nitrosodiethylamine. *Cancer Lett.* 16:109–114 (1982).

31 Loefberg, B, EB Brittebo, and H Tjaelve. Localization and binding of N'-nitrosonornicotine metabolites in the nasal region and in some other tissues of Sprague-Dawley rats. *Cancer Res.* 42:2877–2883 (1982).

32 Wilkins, RJ, and HD MacLeod. Formaldehyde induced DNA-protein crosslinks in *Escherichia coli. Mutat. Res.* 38:2621–2627 (1976).

33 Magana-Schwencke, N, B Ekert, and E Moustacchi. Biochemical analysis of damage induced in yeast by formaldehyde. I. Induction of single-strand breaks in DNA and their repair. *Mutat. Res.* 50:181–193 (1978).

34 Magana-Schwencke, N, B Ekert, and E Moustacchi. Biochemical analysis of damage induced in yeast by formaldehyde. II. Induction of cross-links between DNA and protein. *Mutat. Res.* 51:11–19 (1978).

35 Grafstrom, RC, Fornace, AJ Jr., H Autrup, JF Lechner, and CC Harris.

Formaldehyde damage to DNA and inhibition of DNA repair in human bronchial cells. *Science* 220:216–218 (1983).

36 Fornace, AJ Jr. Detection of DNA single-strand breaks produced during the repair of damage by DNA-protein cross-linking agents. *Cancer Res.* 42:145–149 (1982).

37 Ross, WE, and N Shipley. Relationship between DNA damage and survival in formaldehyde-treated mouse cells. *Mutat. Res.* 79:277–283 (1980).

Chapter 18

Localization and Quantitation of Cell Proliferation Following Exposure to Nasal Irritants

James A. Swenberg, Elizabeth A. Gross, and Holly W. Randall

INTRODUCTION

Cell proliferation is a critical response following exposure of epithelial surfaces to irritants, for it is through cell proliferation that broken epithelial barriers are healed and thickened to help prevent subsequent insult. An intact epithelium is considered the body's first line of defense against infection. It is therefore not surprising that homeostatic mechanisms that initiate cell proliferation begin shortly after an insult occurs. Little information has been reported on the proliferative response of nasal epithelium following exposure to single or multiple insults by respiratory irritants. This chapter will focus on alterations in cell proliferation following acute exposures to nasal irritants. As the number of exposures increases from days to weeks or months, the magnitude of the increase in cell proliferation decreases, such that only exposure to concentrations resulting in continued cell killing maintains increased numbers of replicating cells.

The authors wish to acknowledge Dr. C. S. Barrow and his staff for providing the inhalation exposures for these investigations and for providing the data on acrylic acid.

Understanding what factors affect cell proliferation is important in chronic studies for several reasons. Cell replication is believed to be required to "fix" promutagenic DNA lesions into heritable alterations of the genetic code (1). These mutations are generally thought to represent the initiation step in carcinogenesis. Cell replication also provides a mechanism for tumor promotion through selective amplification of initiated cells. Moreover, current theories of multistage carcinogenesis require sequential mutational events in such expanded cell populations for progression to malignancy (2-6). Thus, in order to evaluate thoroughly the toxic potential of nasal irritants, it will be necessary to understand the complex interrelationships between cell proliferation and exposure concentration, exposure duration, and length of study.

The nasal epithelium markedly differs in composition between the respiratory and olfactory regions. In both regions, it is the basal cells that retain the capacity for regeneration. More differentiated cells such as ciliated or olfactory sensory cells have little or no ability to replicate. Thus, if they are killed by toxic exposures, they will only be replaced if the basal cells can differentiate. The lack of such differentiation in the case of olfactory sensory cells leads to their replacement by basal cells or respiratory metaplasia.

MATERIALS AND METHODS

Male F-344 rats or B6C3F1 mice were exposed by inhalation to 0.5-15 ppm formaldehyde gas for 3-12 h per day for 1-10 days. These animals, including unexposed controls, were pulse-labeled with [^{3}H]thymidine (2 μCi/g, 6.7 Ci/mmole, New England Nuclear) by intraperitoneal injection 2 or 18 h after their last exposure to formaldehyde. The animals were killed 2 h later and the mandible, tongue, skin, and excess muscle over the head were removed. The nasal passages were flushed and fixed with Helly's fixative, rinsed in water, decalcified in formic acid, and rinsed. Two to four levels of nasal passage were embedded in glycol methacrylate (GMA) and 1-2 μm sections were cut, dipped in Kodak NTB-2 emulsion, exposed at $-20°$C for 12 weeks, developed using Kodak D-19 developer, stained with hematoxylin and eosin, coverslipped, and evaluated. Cells having five or more grains over the nucleus were considered labeled. Approximately 4000 and 1500 cells were counted per section of rat and mouse nose, respectively.

RESULTS

The respiratory epithelium of nasal passages of unexposed control rats and mice has little cell replication, as only 0.1-0.5 percent of the cells were labeled with [^{3}H]thymidine. Nearly all labeled cells were basal in location. The labeling index was higher in the anterior and ventral squamous-lined portion of the nasal passages, where 1-3 percent of the cells had silver grains over the nucleus. The olfactory epithelium of mice contained 0.1–0.5 percent labeled cells, and that of rats had 1.0–1.5 percent. In both cases, the labeled cells were basally located.

Effects of Formaldehyde on Cell Proliferation

Previous investigations had demonstrated that acute cytotoxicity was induced in the nasal passages of rats after a single 6-h exposure to 15 ppm formaldehyde (7). Multiple exposures to formaldehyde produced concentration related cellular changes ranging from mild rhinitis and epithelial hyperplasia to severe ulceration. These lesions were of greater severity in rats than in mice. Early studies on the time course of restorative cell proliferation and hyperplasia had demonstrated the highest number of labeled cells after 3–5 days of formaldehyde exposure. Thus, a 3-day exposure was used for the initial concentration-response study in rats and mice (8). In this study the animals were injected with [^{3}H]thymidine 2 h after the third day of exposure (6 h/day), and the middle portion of the respiratory mucosa was examined. Figure 1 shows that rats were more sensitive than mice, because rats exposed to 6 or 15 ppm formaldehyde exhibited 10- to 20-fold increases in their labeling index, whereas only mice exposed to 15 ppm showed a similar response. No increase was noted for lower concentrations of formaldehyde. It was important, however, to investigate whether or not the [^{3}H]thymidine pulse administered 2 h after the last exposure was the most sensitive time period for detecting exposure related cell proliferation, since it was well known that *de novo* DNA synthesis could be inhibited by exposure to carcinogens (9). To investigate the time of labeling versus time since last exposure, rats were exposed to 6 ppm formaldehyde for 3 days and injected with [^{3}H]thymidine either 2 or 18 h after the third day of exposure. The number of labeled cells increased nearly twofold

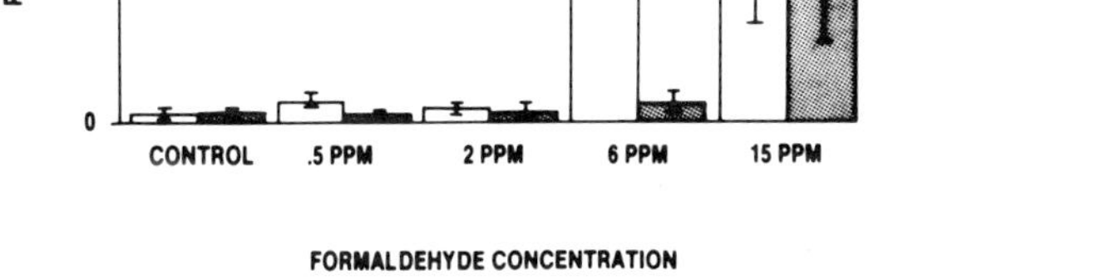

Figure 1 Effect of formaldehyde exposure on cell proliferation in level 2 of the nasal passages. All animals were exposed for 6 h/day for 3 days. [^{3}H] Thymidine was administered 2 h after the third exposure. Data shown are means ± standard error.

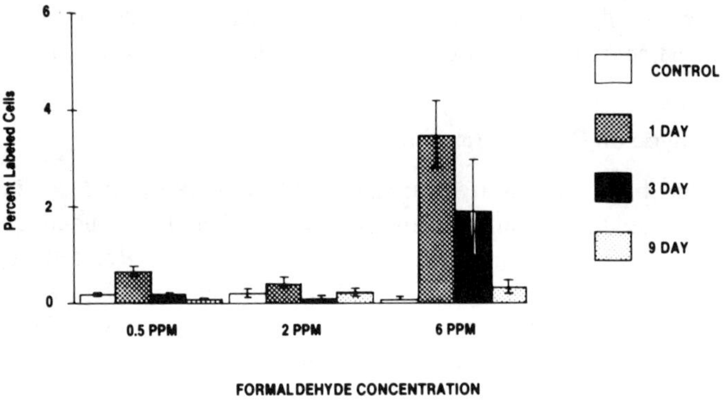

Figure 2 Effect of formaldehyde exposure on cell proliferation in level 2 of the rat nasal passages. All animals were exposed for 6 h/day. [^{3}H]Thymidine was administered 18 h after the last exposure. Data shown are means ± standard error.

with the 18-h postexposure period compared to the 2-h period (8). Studies by Chang et al. (10) demonstrated that as little as a single 6-h exposure to 15 ppm formaldehyde resulted in a tenfold increase in ,cell proliferation in both rats and mice when the [^{3}H]thymidine pulse was administered 18 h after the exposure. Silver grains were confined to basal cells. The labeling index increased to more than 20 times that of the controls in rats and mice exposed to 15 ppm formaldehyde for 5 days.

Since the earlier concentration-response study had not used the optimal time for [^{3}H]thymidine labeling, the concentration response over time was repeated using the 18-h postexposure period before the pulse. A transient increase in cell proliferation was seen in rats exposed to 0.5 or 2 ppm formaldehyde for just 1 day (Fig. 2). This increase disappeared after 3 and 9 days of exposure. Rats exposed to 6 ppm formaldehyde had a massive increase in labeling index after one 6-h exposure, had a lesser response after three exposures, and nearly returned to control rates after nine exposures.

Effect of Formaldehyde Concentration versus Cumulative Exposure

A review of pathology slides from two 6-month exposure studies on formaldehyde revealed striking differences between rats exposed to 15 ppm, 6 h/day, 5 days/week (450 ppm-h/week) (11) and 3 ppm, 22 h/day, 7 days/week (462 ppm-h/week) (12), with animals in the latter study showing much less toxicity. A study was designed to determine whether concentration or cumulative exposure was the dominant factor in cell proliferation. An 18-h postexposure period before the [^{3}H]thymidine pulse was used to compare cell proliferation in groups of rats and mice exposed to the same daily dose (ppm-h), but to different concentrations and durations of exposure (CxT; concentrations times time), i.e., 12 ppm X 3 h, 6 ppm X 6 h, and 3 ppm X 12 h.

In the most anterior section of the nasal passage, where mucociliary clearance is minimal (13), cell replication in both rats and mice was increased following 3 days of exposure to all CxT products (Fig. 3*a*). In the mice the increase was between 5- and 10-fold and in the rats it was slightly higher, but not significantly different for the different exposure groups. Thus, in the absence of effective mucociliary clearance, cytotoxicity and increased cell turnover were dependent on cumulative exposure (CxT product). This is in marked contrast to level 2, where mucociliary clearance is prominent. At this level in both rats and mice cell proliferation was strictly concentration dependent (Fig. 3*b*).

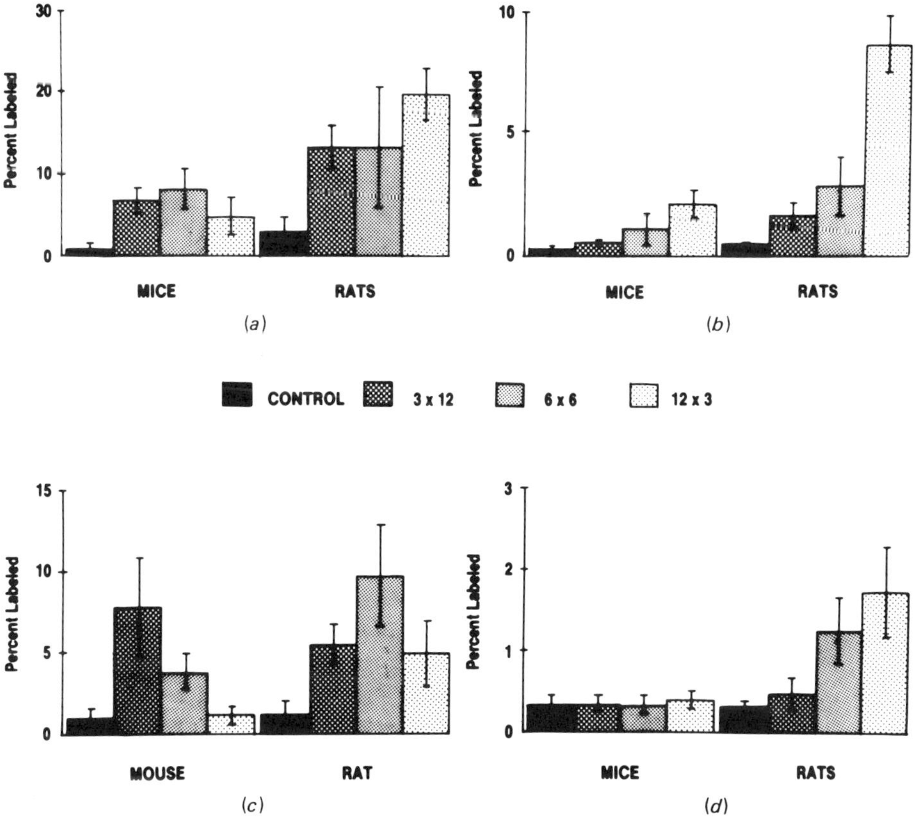

Figure 3 Effect of formaldehyde exposure on cell proliferation of the respiratory mucosa of rats and mice. Figures 3*a* and 3*b* are data following 3 days of exposure; 3*c* and 3*d* are for 9 days of exposure. Figures 3*a* and 3*c* are from level 1 (most anterior); 3*b* and 3*d* are from level 2. [^{3}H] Thymidine was administered 18 h after the last exposure.

Data from rats and mice exposed under the same conditions for 9 days are more complex. In both rats and mice the level of cell proliferation is reduced from that of animals exposed for 3 days (Figs. 3*c* and *d*). This is true at both levels in the nose and at all CxT products except for the mice exposed to 3 ppm for 12 h. This may be explained by differences in minute volumes for mice exposed to 3 ppm vs. 6 or 12 ppm (8). Mice exposed to 3 ppm for 12 h were predicted to receive over 50 percent more formaldehyde each day versus rats from this CxT group or rats and mice at the other two CxT groups. This difference in exposure may help to explain the greater response in mice at the 3-ppm X 12-h exposure. Cytotoxicity was similar to or greater in the 3-ppm mice than in the 6- and 12-ppm groups, whereas cell turnover was greatly increased in level 1 of the 3-ppm mice, but not the 12-ppm animals (Fig. 3*c*). A decrease in cell turnover and no cytotoxicity was demonstrable in level 2 of all groups. This decrease in labeling index noted after 9 days of exposure reflects the establishment of a hyperplastic response, since the epithelial thickness had also increased. The differences in labeling index in the 9-day exposed versus control animals of both species were minimal and, in section 2 of the 9-day rats, reflects a concentration dependence for increased cell loss and regeneration (Fig. 3*d*). Other factors such as higher linear velocity of the airstream through the nose of rats and/or the presence of better mucociliary flow and cellular repair mechanisms in mice may also play a role in the species and concentration differences observed in these studies. This apparent site difference, in view of similar "dose" predictions, requires further study.

From the above studies it is clear that cell proliferation is dependent on concentration, dose, and time. Species differences in upper respiratory tract reflexes exert considerable influence on the response to formaldehyde exposure. Concentration is the major contributor to the extent of toxicity and cell turnover in respiratory epithelium in rats, where a similar respiratory minute volume is breathed over formaldehyde exposures of 3–15 ppm. The concentration effect is less clear in the mouse because different doses occur even though CxT products of exposure are the same. The greatest response to formaldehyde exposure occurs in the most anterior respiratory epithelium, the region of the nasal passages having the least protection by mucociliary clearance. At low concentrations such as 0.5 and 2 ppm, only a slight transitory increase in cell proliferation is seen, and it disappears after 3 or 9 days of exposure. This is in contrast to the response at higher concentrations (Fig. 4). The response was maximal after a 1-day exposure, but remained elevated after 3 days of exposure to 6 ppm formaldehyde. The maximum increase in cell proliferation for rats exposed to 12–15 ppm formaldehyde occurred after 5 days, but increased proliferation was still evident after 9 days of exposure. Thus, the extent and duration of increased cell proliferation correlate well with earlier findings on cytotoxicity and impaired mucociliary clearance (7, 8, 14, 15).

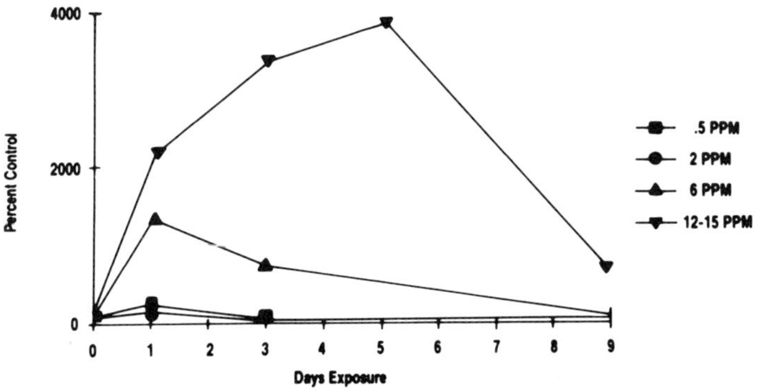

Figure 4 Compilation of all rat cell turnover data using the 18-h [^{3}H]thymidine pulse. Exposures were 0.5, 2, and 6 ppm formaldehyde 6 h/day and the combined data from 12 ppm 3 h/day and 15 ppm 6 h/day.

Effects of Acrylic Acid on Olfactory Cell Proliferation

Much less is known about the effects of nasal irritants on olfactory cell proliferation. As mentioned earlier, the proliferating cells are basal in location, and unexposed rats have a higher labeling index than mice. As discussed in the chapter by Barrow et al. (16) in this volume, mice exposed to 75 ppm acrylic acid were predicted to receive 88 percent more acrylic acid per cm^2 of nasal epithelium than rats. Indeed, mice had more severe pathology than rats and had a greater loss of olfactory cells. Both rats and mice showed increased cell proliferation when they were pulsed with [^{3}H]thymidine 18 h after five 6-h/day exposures to 75 ppm acrylic acid (Fig. 5); however, the increase was 17 times greater than control in mice, but only four times greater in rats. Furthermore,

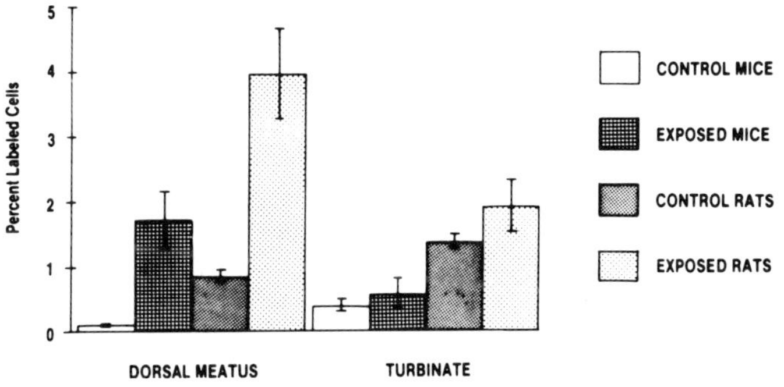

Figure 5 Effect of 5 days of exposure to 75 ppm acrylic acid on cell turnover in the olfactory mucosa of rats and mice.

the region most severely affected was the olfactory epithelium lining the dorsal meatus. Only a slight increase was detectable in olfactory epithelium lining the turbinates.

DISCUSSION

Cell proliferation is a normal homeostatic mechanism that maintains the integrity of the epithelium lining the nasal passages. Under normal conditions, this requires replacement of only a small percentage of cells each day. However, toxic insult can damage and kill large numbers of cells, which must be rapidly replaced. In the case of continued toxic insult, compensatory hyperplasia results in thickening of the epithelium, eventually leading to squamous hyperplasia or metaplasia. In addition to these morphologic changes, cells develop enhanced biochemical pathways for detoxification. When specially differentiated cells are killed, they may not be replaced, leading to a new type of epithelial lining–i.e., respiratory metaplasia of the dorsal meatus.

Increased cell proliferation may also play a major role in nonlinear dose responses for nasal carcinogenesis, since increased cell proliferation can increase both initiating and promoting events. It is therefore important that the dose-response relationship for increases in cell proliferation due to toxicity be factored into quantitative risk assessment. Cell proliferation is likely to be of much greater importance under conditions of high exposure. The use of cumulative dose as an index of exposure may grossly overestimate the risk in cases of prolonged low-level exposure, but may underestimate the risk of brief high-level exposure. It is therefore prudent to incorporate what is known about the biological processes of each exposure situation into the risk assessment process.

SUMMARY

Cell proliferation is an important homeostatic mechanism responsible for the repair and replacement of cells lost from aging as well as from toxic insults. This chapter summarizes what is known about cell proliferation in the nasal passages of rats and mice and how exposure to formaldehyde or acrylic acid alters the amount of replication. Briefly, it demonstrates that exposure concentration, exposure duration, and length of study influence the proliferative response. Increases in cell proliferation may play a major role in nonlinear dose responses for nasal carcinogens and should therefore be factored into the quantitative risk assessment process.

REFERENCES

1 Farber, E. Chemical carcinogenesis. A biologic perspective. *Am. J. Pathol.* 106:271–296 (1982).

2 Hennings, H, R Shores, ML Wenk, EF Spangler, R Tarone, and SH Yuspa. Malignant conversion of mouse skin tumors is increased by tumor initiators and unaffected by tumor promoters. *Nature (Lond.)* 304:67–69 (1983).

3 Moolgavkar, SH, and AG Knudson Jr. Mutation and cancer: A model for human carcinogenesis. *JNCI* 66:1037–1052 (1981).

4 Potter, VR. Initiation and promotion in cancer formation: The importance of studies on intercellular communication. *Yale J. Biol. Med.* 53:367–384 (1980).

5 Potter, VR. Commentary: A new protocol and its rationale for the study of initiation and promotion of carcinogenesis in rat liver. *Carcinogenesis* 2:1375–1379 (1981).

6 Potter, VR. Use of two sequential applications of initiators in the production of hepatomas in the rat: An examination of the Solt-Farber protocol. *Cancer Res.* 44:2733–2736 (1984).

7 Swenberg, JA, EA Gross, J Martin, and JA Popp. Mechanisms of formaldehyde toxicity. In *Formaldehyde Toxicity,* edited by JE Gibson. New York: Hemisphere, pp. 132–147 (1983).

8 Swenberg, JA, EA Gross, HW Randall, and CS Barrow. The effect of formaldehyde exposure on cytotoxicity and cell proliferation. In *Formaldehyde: Toxicology, Epidemiology and Mechanisms,* edited by JJ Clary, JE Gibson, and RS Waritz. New York: Marcel Dekker, pp. 225–236 (1983).

9 Painter, RB. DNA synthesis inhibition in mammalian cells as a test for mutagenic carcinogens. In *Short-term Tests for Chemical Carcinogens,* edited by HF Stich and RHC San. New York: Springer-Verlag, pp. 59–64 (1981).

10 Chang, JCF, EA Gross, JA Swenberg, and CS Barrow. Nasal cavity deposition, histopathology, and cell proliferation after single or repeated formaldehyde exposures in B6C3F1 mice and F-344 rats. *Toxicol. Appl. Pharmacol.* 68:161–176 (1983).

11 Kerns, WD, DJ Donofrio, and KL Pavkov. The chronic effects of formaldehyde inhalation in rats and mice. A preliminary report. In *Formaldehyde Toxicity,* edited by JE Gibson. New York: Hemisphere, pp. 111–131 (1983).

12 Rusch, GM, HF Bolte, and WE Rinehart. A 26-week inhalation toxicity study with formaldehyde in the monkey, rat and hamster. In *Formaldehyde Toxicity,* edited by JE Gibson. New York: Hemisphere, pp. 98–110 (1983).

13 Morgan, KT, XZ Jiang, DL Patterson, and EA Gross. The nasal mucociliary apparatus: Correlation of structure and function in the rat. *Am. Rev. Resp. Dis.* 130:275–281 (1984).

14 Morgan, KT, DL Patterson, and EA Gross. Formaldehyde and the nasal mucociliary apparatus. In *Formaldehyde: Toxicology, Epidemiology and Mechanisms,* edited by JJ Clary, JE Gibson, HS Waritz. New York: Marcel Dekker, pp. 193–208 (1983).

15 Morgan, KT, DL Patterson, and EA Gross. Responses of the nasal mucociliary apparatus to airborne irritants. In *Toxicology of the Nasal Passages,* edited by C Barrow. New York: Hemisphere (1985).

16 Barrow, CS, LA Buckley, RA James, WH Steinhagen, and JCF Chang. Sensory irritation: Studies on correlation to pathology, structure-activity, tolerance development and prediction of species differences to nasal injury. In *Toxicology of the Nasal Passages,* edited by CS Barrow. New York: Hemisphere (1985).

Panel Discussion

Moderator—Dr. Alarie

Moderator: Dr. Acheson, in your wood dust study, what proportion of nasal cancer occurred in workers who were exposed prior to World War II?

Dr. Acheson: There have been about 500 cases of adenocarcinoma of the nasal mucosa reported in furniture workers in the world literature. I would judge that perhaps 450 of those started their exposure before World War II. But only a small proportion completed their exposure before World War II. You have to remember that the mean induction time of this tumor is about 40 years.

Moderator: What are the criteria for classifying a malignant tumor arising from the olfactory epithelium, as a neuroepithelioma or as an esthesioneuroepithelioma?

Dr. Feron: The problem is, do we consider the olfactory epithelium complete in that the basal cells, sustentacular cells, and sensory cells represent neuroepithelium? If this is so, I agree with others that all tumors arising from the olfactory epithelium should be called neuroepitheliomas. This could be modified if there is differentiation–e.g., sustentacular differentiation. When there is no differentiation they could perhaps be called undifferentiated neuroepitheliomas and so on. The other question is: Do adenocarcinomas of the olfactory epithelium really exist? To complicate the situation even more, we have glands of Bowman. Are these part of neuroepithelium or do they come from another type of tissue? I am really hoping that the ultrastructural people in the audience or in the panel would give us some more information about this.

Dr. Swenberg: I think that if tumors are arising from Bowman's glands they are appropriately called adenocarcinomas. I think that we are probably going to have to wait for some data with monoclonal antibodies to identify whether or not these stem cells truly have markers for neuroectodermal tissues. These are becoming available. It is very interesting that the same stem cell can give rise to the sensory cells and the sustentacular cells, which would support your position. But I think that when you look at the toxic insult and you see these polyhedral cells or basal cell hyperplasias, they don't look much like neuroepithelial cells, and nobody really knows.

Dr. Acheson: I am not a pathologist, and I would hesitate to attempt an answer to a question about the classification of tumors, but it seems to me it would be a pity if this conference broke up without mention being made of the most interesting of the epidemiological findings in relation to formaldehyde. I think that now seven studies in four different professional groups involved with the preparation of human tissues provide evidence of an increased incidence of gliomas. All of these groups use formaldehyde as well as other compounds. Although this is very far from proof, there is sufficient concern from these studies to justify further work. Of course one of the possibilities is that there is bias in that professional groups get better medical care than the population at large. But in some of the studies, attempts have been made to correct for this, and this has not extinguished the apparent relative risk.

Moderator: Would someone discuss the reversibility of various pathological changes seen in the nasal cavity and the significance of this issue in risk estimation?

Dr. Swenberg: In the CIIT bioassay you will recall that we stopped the exposures at 24 months and then continued some of those animals out to 30 months. In these animals we found that dysplasia and squamous metaplasia were reversible with the exception of the latter in the 15-ppm-treated animals. We assume that what has happened is that the stem cells that have the potential to differentiate into ciliated epithelium and nonciliated cells have lost this and are only able to be squamous cells. It appears these are probably reversible unless you get to such a severe amount of damage that only one kind of cell population remains. However, these are not precancerous lesions and may not have a great deal to do with risk estimation.

Moderator: Is it likely that the olfactory epithelium will proliferate or regenerate in excess following necrosis or "virtually near complete loss" of the epithelium?

Dr. Young: I would like to comment on this question as well as the previous one. First, the respiratory metaplasia that we see in olfactory epithelium, at least in our experience, is a relatively innocuous lesion other than losing sense of smell in that area. However, it appears to be irreversible once that area has lost its ability to regenerate the olfactory portion. In some studies we have stopped exposure at 6 months, held the animals for as long as 27 months, and you could not tell the difference between the animals the day exposure stopped and 27 months later. As to whether or not it can proliferate in excess, I think that the basal cell hyperplasia that is seen in the rats appears to be excessive sometimes. However, in my experience the epithelium never appeared to exceed what the normal height of the epithelium would have been, nor did it look like any early proliferative focal lesion.

Dr. Morgan: I think we have a lot to learn about the olfactory epithelium. In the last 7 or 8 months I have been asked to examine a number of slides. It's interesting to note that sometimes these lesions look very proliferative. I think what is lacking is information and experience on our part concerning the range of changes you get in olfactory epithelium.

Moderator: When experimental animals (rats, mice, etc.) are used to extrapolate effects to humans should the total surface area of the nasal epithelium be used, or should only the surface area where the lesion appears, be used? I recall that Dr. Jiang presented summaries of pathology in the nose for approximately 11 different chemicals. Dr. Jiang, which areas of the nose do you see as the most significant ones to use for this calculation, or which areas are the most often involved with these irritants?

Dr. Jiang: We find that most lesions are at the front of the nose, which is mainly respiratory epithelium. Another location often affected is the tip of the naso-turbinate and maxilloturbinate.

Dr. Popp: The point is that the calculations that have been made have been very useful to address the issue of dose to the nasal epithelium. However, Dr. Jiang's data clearly show that there is never any lesion that is uniformly distributed over a specific cell type. Therefore, I think we have to remember that these are estimates that are helpful, but we need to be careful about using these as absolute numbers.

Dr. Barrow: Yes, I agree with Dr. Popp, and as I said yesterday, the surface area information really has to be taken in concert with other kinds of information such as mucus effects, metabolism, etc. I believe it has proved to be very useful in terms of seeing differences in what could be called the "amount delivered" to the nasal epithelium surface area. However, I can't see any scientific justification right now for using squamous versus respiratory versus olfactory and just using that particular portion of the epithelium in doing these calculations. I feel more comfortable doing it on a total surface area basis at this time.

Dr. Feron: To further complicate this situation, I think it also depends on the level of toxicity. For instance, at high concentrations of acetaldehyde, effects are seen in the olfactory epithelium and the respiratory epithelium but at lower levels only the olfactory epithelium is affected. So this is another aspect which needs to be taken into consideration.

Dr. Swenberg: I personally don't think we have any justification at this time to make comparisons beyond the rat and mouse. Although anatomical features of their noses are very close, when we go to a primate or to a human it is very different. I made that point yesterday. We recently conducted a 1-year inhalation study of chlorine by inhalation. At 2.5 ppm the only effects found were slight lacrimation and very focal areas of nonkeratinizing metaplasia in the nasal cavity. In rodents, particularly female rats, the picture is quite different. So I don't think we have any business at this time extrapolating very far using this dose calculation.

Moderator: Dr. Andersen, what is your view in terms of airflow patterns and surface area information regarding extrapolation to man?

Dr. Andersen: There is certainly less than 150 cm^2 (which is the total surface area of the nasal epithelium in man) exposed to the main part of the airstream, probably 50 percent or something of that magnitude. I think from our point of view we would probably opt to use a lesser area than the total area in the human nose.

Dr. Morgan: It seems quite likely that airflow patterns are causing delivery to different sites in the nose. For example, in our studies with dye, which simulates airflow patterns, a very good approximation of turbulence can be seen. I think this accounts for lesions on the lateral nasoturbinates and back on the septum. Additionally, reactivity, water solubility, the functioning of the mucociliary apparatus, and blood supply undoubtedly play important roles. So it is an extremely complicated issue, and it seems to me that the surface area calculations are the best thing we've got for now.

Moderator: Dr. Dahl, what is the best animal model to use from a cytochrome P-450 standpoint in terms of the nasal mucosa?

Dr. Dahl: I guess it depends on whether you want results or you want to mimic the human situation. If I were going to do an exposure with a compound that I knew had to be activated by cytochrome P-450 before it was a carcinogen, I would use the Syrian hamster. If I wanted to make the best argument for this being relevant to human exposure, I'd use the monkey.

Moderator: Dr. Brittebo, in which cell type do you think nitrosamines are metabolized?

Dr. Brittebo: As I mentioned during my lecture, we have been working with ^{14}C-labeled compounds but we have poor resolution of ^{14}C so it is not clear what cell type it could be. Considering ultrastructural studies, there has been work showing that there is smooth endoplasmic reticulum in sustentacular cells. I don't know if smooth endoplasmic reticulum exists in the Bowman's glands. Cells that have a lot of smooth endoplasmic reticulum should, in general, have a lot of metabolic activity.

Dr. Feron: I know from a recent study performed by Dr. Reznik-Schüller that in hamsters diethylnitrosamine was present only in the glands of Bowman in the olfactory region and, if I remember well, in the mucus glands in the respiratory epithelium. But the tumors occur from the supporting cells in the olfactory epithelium. She speculated that the diethylnitrosamine needs to be metabolized by the glands of Bowman, and then, in one way or the other, active metabolites diffuse to other surrounding cells.

Moderator: Are there other enzyme inducers of cytochrome P-450 and monooxygenase beside TCDD and also glutathione-S-transferase in the nose?

Dr. Bond: We looked at phenobarbital, methylcholanthrene, and Aroclor. We found they didn't induce, but I think we need to keep in mind that the regimen used was based on hepatic induction. Perhaps a different type of regimen may give nasal induction. The only one we were successful with was TCDD, but you have to remember that it is approximately 10,000-30,000 times more potent than something like methylcholanthrene. It may be that higher doses are needed for induction by those compounds, or perhaps longer periods of time are necessary. Diesel exhaust exposure for 1 month also caused induction, and that was very exciting because for the first time we found an environmental type of compound that was able to induce. Unfortunately, there is probably no way we can identify the individual constituent, if one even exists, in diesel exhaust.

There are also other types of inducers that one could use. I just selected a few that have been classical agents, but I think that there will eventually be other ones that we simply have not looked at.

Dr. Heck: I would like to add on that point that the induction of cytochrome P-450 enzymes in the nasal tissue may be more a function of whether the inducing agent gets to the tissue than whether the particular enzymes are more or less acceptable to that agent. The fact that phenobarbital and two or three other compounds didn't succeed in inducing but TCDD did seems to me to go along with Dr. Brittebo's findings that TCDD does go to the nasal tissue. We don't know whether these other compounds do, however. Another point I might add is that we have been doing studies on glutathione depletion in the nasal tissue. We have tried three different agents that are very good depleters of glutathione in the liver. With diethylmaleate we saw practically no effect on the nose. Buthionine sulfoximine had practically no effect on the nose, but phorone, another depleting agent, depleted glutathione on the nose virtually completely to $\approx$ 10 percent of the control value.

Moderator: Why is the mouse less sensitive in inhalation studies? I am not sure that this is a correct statement, however.

Dr. Barrow: That is obviously not the case with acrylic acid. In that instance the mouse tends to be more sensitive than the rat, which is just the opposite of formaldehyde.

Dr. Young: As far as I am concerned, there is no generalization that can be made from the standpoint that rats are more or less sensitive than mice or vice versa.

Moderator: I would agree with that. I don't think that you can make a general statement that one species is always less or more sensitive than another. What is the most appropriate animal with which to study nasal toxicology? Although I don't think we are going to resolve that particular question today, perhaps we can make some headway. Let's begin by first discussing this in terms of biochemistry.

Dr. Dahl: The cynomolgus monkey did not have any cytochrome P-450 that was measurable by our techniques in the respiratory tissues. In olfactory tissues, they do have as much on a per-milligram microsomal protein basis as dogs and some rodents. Assuming man and monkey are similar in that primary biotransforming activities in the respiratory tissues are minimal, then you might be biasing the results if you use a rodent, which does have the ability to biotransform compounds.

Moderator: It has been clear over the course of this conference that the rat has been used extensively. Can anyone comment on this?

Dr. Dahl: We used rats first because they were there. We used dogs second because it is easy to dissect out various portions of the epithelium for separate studies. We have also used a number of other species. However, on balance the rat is a very convenient species.

Dr. Heck: We use rats first and foremost because it is the only species that we are able to get enough tissue out of to perform our experiments. Other people have been successful in studying enzymatic reactions in mice, and perhaps in 2 or 3 years we may know more about monkeys.

Dr. Stott: As with most things, I find that we wind up working with the rodents to try to explain toxic effects in that species and then we look to the human. We are first trying to explain bioassay data obtained in rodents, not necessarily coming at it from the standpoint of going to humans first but rather from the standpoint of how to explain the effect in rodents first.

Moderator: From the physiological point of view, in terms of measuring sensory irritation, we used mice quite frankly because they were there and they were cheap, easy to handle, and, as it turns out, probably the best species to use anyway. They are very sensitive to sensory irritants. You don't get a mixed respiratory pattern, for example, as in guinea pigs, which also bronchoconstrict quite easily. Rabbits are very sensitive, have good reproducibility, and are slightly more sensitive than mice. Of course they are also more expensive, more difficult to handle, etc. Dogs are probably the most sensitive species I have worked with to study sensory irritation. They are extremely sensitive to sensory irritants. But once again, they are very expensive and difficult to handle, and as the concentration is raised, you get a tremendous amount of salivation and bronchoconstriction. Rats, in general, are much less sensitive than mice perhaps by a factor of 10 although there are some exceptions. Monkeys, as I mentioned before, are very insensitive to sensory irritants.

Dr. Swenberg: To me the interesting question is, using Cl_2 as an example, why is the monkey less sensitive than smaller laboratory animals (e.g., the rat) when it breathes the same concentration? Perhaps that is a fruitful area for future research. Maybe its differences lie in mucociliary clearance or detoxification, but the key question in my opinion is which is more like man—the rat or the monkey? That is probably what we should be studying.

Index

Numbers in italics denote figures; numbers followed by "t" denote tables.